PROCEDURES IN COSMETIC DERMATOLOGY

LASERS, LIGHTS, and ENERGY DEVICES

FIFTH EDITION

Edited by

Elizabeth L. Tanzi, MD, FAAD
Director, Capital Laser & Skin Care
Chevy Chase, MD, United States
Associate Clinical Professor of Dermatology
George Washington University School of Medicine
Washington, DC

Jeffrey S. Dover, MD, FRCPC
Director, SkinCare Physicians,
Chestnut Hill, MA, United States
Associate Clinical Professor of Dermatology,
Yale University School of Medicine,
Providence, RI, United States
Adjunct Associate Professor of Dermatology,
Brown Medical School, Providence, RI, United States

Video Editor

Leah K. Spring, DO, FAAD
Head of Procedural Dermatology,
Mohs Micrographic Surgery,
Cosmetic Dermatologic Surgery
Naval Medical Center Portsmouth,
Portsmouth, VA, United States
Commander, United States Navy

Series Editors

**Jeffrey S. Dover, MD, FRCPC and
Murad Alam, MD, MSCI**

ELSEVIER

Elsevier
1600 John F. Kennedy Blvd.
Ste 1800
Philadelphia, PA 19103-2899

PROCEDURES IN COSMETIC DERMATOLOGY: LASERS, LIGHTS, AND ENERGY DEVICES, FIFTH EDITION

ISBN: 978-0-323-82905-2

Notice

Practitioners and researchers must always rely on their own experience and knowledge in evaluating and using any information, methods, compounds, or experiments described herein. Because of rapid advances in the medical sciences, in particular, independent verification of diagnoses and drug dosages should be made. To the fullest extent of the law, no responsibility is assumed by Elsevier, authors, editors, or contributors for any injury and/or damage to persons or property as a matter of products liability, negligence or otherwise, or from any use or operation of any methods, products, instructions, or ideas contained in the material herein.

Previous Editions 2013, 2009, and 2005.

Content Strategist: Charlotta Kryhl
Content Development Specialist: Akanksha Marwah
Content Development Manager: Somodatta Roy Choudhury
Publishing Services Manager: Shereen Jameel
Project Manager: Haritha Dharmarajan
Design Direction: Patrick Ferguson

Printed in India

Last digit is the print number: 9 8 7 6 5 4 3 2

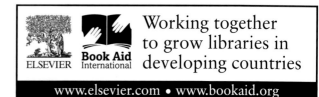

Working together to grow libraries in developing countries

www.elsevier.com • www.bookaid.org

LASERS, LIGHTS, and ENERGY DEVICES

PROCEDURES IN COSMETIC DERMATOLOGY

*To my parents, Joe and Lyn, who taught me through example the power of an
unpretentious yet unwavering work ethic.
To my wonderful husband, Big Pete, whose love, support and attitude inspire
me to always take on the next challenge.
To my children, Peter and Katie, who remind me every day what is truly important in life.
Oh, how I love those smiles!*

Elizabeth L. Tanzi, MD, FAAD

*To the women in my life: my grandmothers, Bertha and Lillian; my mother, Nina; my daughters,
Sophie and Isabel; and especially to my wife, Tania.
For their never-ending encouragement, patience, support, love, and friendship.
To my father, Mark—a great teacher and role model; to my mentor, Kenneth A. Arndt for his generosity,
kindness, sense of humor, joie de vivre, and above all else curiosity and enthusiasm.*

Jeffrey S. Dover, MD, FRCPC

*Elsevier's dedicated editorial staff has made possible the continuing success of this ambitious project.
The team led by Charlotta Kryhl and the production staff have refined the concept for this
new edition while maintaining the series' reputation for quality and cutting-edge relevance.
In this, they have been ably supported by the graphics shop, which has created the signature high-quality
illustrations and layouts that are the backbone of each book. We are also deeply grateful to the volume editors,
who have generously found time in their schedules, cheerfully accepted our guidelines, and recruited
the most knowledgeable chapter authors. And we especially thank the chapter contributors, without
whose work there would be no books at all. Finally, I would also like to convey my debt to my teachers,
Kenneth Arndt, Jeffrey Dover, Michael Kaminer, Leonard Goldberg, and David Bickers,
and my parents, Rahat and Rehana Alam.*

Murad Alam, MD, MSCI

LIST OF CONTRIBUTORS

The editor(s) acknowledge and offer grateful thanks for the input of all previous editions' contributors, without whom this new edition would not have been possible.

Murad Alam, MD, MSCI
Associate Professor of Dermatology,
   Otolaryngology, and Surgery; Chief,
   Section of Cutaneous and Aesthetic Surgery,
   Northwestern University, Chicago, IL,
   United States

Macrene Alexiades, MD, PhD
Associate Clinical Professor, Yale University
   School of Medicine
   Adjunct Clinical Professor,
   Syngros Hospital, University of Athens
   Founder and Director, Dermatology and Laser
   Surgery Center of New York
   CEO, Founder, Dr. Macrene Skin Results
   New York, NY, United States

Rawaa Almukhtar, MD, MPH
ASDS Cosmetic and Laser Fellow Dermatology
   Cosmetic and Laser Dermatology,
   San Diego, CA, United States

Lisa Arkin, MD
Director of Pediatric Dermatology; Associate Professor
   of Dermatology and Pediatrics, University of
   Wisconsin School of Medicine,
   Madison, WI, United States

Bradley S. Bloom, MD
Clinical Assistant Professor, Ronald O. Perelman
   Department of Dermatology at NYU
   Grossman School of Medicine
   New York, NY, United States

Erica G. Baugh, BA
Dermatology Resident, University of California
   Irvine, CA, United States

Lauren Meshkov Bonati, MD
Mountain Dermatology Specialists Edwards, CO,
   United States

Jeremy Brauer, MD
Clinical Associate Professor, Ronald O.
   Perelman Department of Dermatology,
   NYU School of Medicine, New York
   Founder and Director, Spectrum Skin and Laser,
   New York, United States

Emily Wood, MD
Westlake Dermatology, Austin, TX, United States

Anne Chapas, MD
Dermatology, Union Square Laser Dermatology,
   New York, NY, United States

Joel L. Cohen, MD
Director, AboutSkin Dermatology and DermSurgery
   Director, AboutSkin Research
   Associate Clinical Professor, University of California
   Irvine Department of Dermatology
   Greenwood Village, Colorado, CO, United States

Kelly O'Connor, BS, MD
South Shore Skin Center
   Plymouth, MA, United States

Shraddha Desai, MD, FAAD
Adjunct Clinical Professor, Dermatology Loyola
   University, Maywood, IL, United States
   Director of Dermatologic Cosmetic
   & Laser Surgery Duly Health and Care
   Naperville, IL, United States
   Instructor, Department of Otolaryngology,
   Division of Dermatology, Rush University Chicago,
   IL United States

Karen J. Dover, MD
Physician, CEO & President, Dr. Karen J. Dover, Laser
   and Cosmetic Medicine and Surgery
   Dover Medicine Professional Corporation
   Ottawa, ON, Canada

Jeffrey S. Dover, MD, FRCPC
Director, SkinCare Physicians, Chestnut Hill, MA,
    United States
Associate Clinical Professor of Dermatology,
    Yale University School of Medicine
    Adjunct Associate Professor of Dermatology, Brown
    Medical School, Providence, RI, United States

David J. Goldberg, MD, JD
Skin Laser & Surgery Specialists
    Director, Cosmetic Dermatology and
    Clinical Research
    Schweiger Dermatology Group
    Clinical Professor of Dermatology
    Former Director of Mohs Surgery and
    Laser Research
    Icahn School of Medicine
    Adjunct Professor of Law
    Fordham Law School
    New York, NY, United States

Mitchel Goldman, MD
Volunteer Clinical Professor, Dermatology University
    of California, San Diego, CA, United States
    Medical Director, Cosmetic Laser Dermatology,
    San Diego, CA, United States
    Medical Director, West Dermatology, CA,
    United States

Courtney Gwinn, MD
Physician, Dermatology, Advanced Dermatology
    and Skin Surgery, Spokane WA and Coeur d'Alene,
    ID, United States

Kerry Heitmiller, MD, FAAD
Allura Skin & Laser Center, San Mateo,
    California, CA, United States

Omar A. Ibrahimi, MD, PhD
Medical Director, Connecticut Skin Institute, Stamford,
    CT, United States

Omer Ibrahim, MD
Associate and director of research Chicago Cosmetic
    Surgery and Dermatology
    Chicago, IL, USA

Jacob J. Inda, MD
Associate Consultant, Department of Dermatology,
    Mayo Clinic Health System, La Crosse, WI,
    United States

Michael S. Kaminer, MD
Associate Clinical Professor of Dermatology,
    Yale University School of Medicine
    New Haven, CT, United States
    Adjunct Assistant Professor of Medicine
    (Dermatology), Dartmouth Medical School,
    Hanover, NH, United States
    Adjunct Assistant Professor of Dermatology,
    Brown Medical School
    Managing Partner, SkinCare Physicians,
    Chestnut Hill, MA, United States

Kristen M. Kelly, MD
Chair Department of Dermatology,
    Professor, Dermatology and Surgery, University of
    California, Irvine, CA, United States

Shilpi Khetarpal, MD
Assistant Professor of Dermatology,
    Cleveland Clinic Foundation, Cleveland,
    OH, United States

Suzanne L. Kilmer, MD
Director, Laser and Skin Surgery Center of Northern
    California, Sacramento, CA, United States
    Clinical Professor, Department of Dermatology
    University of CA, Davis School of Medicine
    Sacramento, CA, United States

Steven Krueger, MD
Resident Physician, Department of Dermatology
    University of Massachusetts Medical School
    Worcester, MA, United States

Kachiu Lee, MD, MPH
Cosmetic Dermatologist and Laser Specialist, Main
    Line Center for Laser Surgery,
    Ardmore, PA, United States
    Assistant Professor, Department of Dermatology,
    Temple University Philadelphia, PA United States

Jennifer MacGregor, MD
Dermatologist, Union Square Laser Dermatology,
    Columbia University Medical Center, New York,
    NY, United States Assistant Professor, Department
    of Dermatology, Temple University
    Philadelphia, PA United States

Farah Moustafa, MD, FAAD
Director of Laser & Cosmetic Center, Assistant
    Professor, Tufts Medical Center, Boston,
    MA, United States

Deborah Paul, MD
Mohs Surgery Fellow, Mayo Clinic
    Rochester, MN, United States

John D. Peters, MD, FAAD
Lieutenant Commander, Medical Corps,
    United States Navy
Chairman, Department of Dermatology,
    Naval Medical Center Portsmouth
Asst. Professor of Dermatology, Uniformed Services
    University of Health Sciences

Saleh Rachidi, MD, PhD
Skin Laser and Surgery Specialists, New York, NY,
    United States

Thomas E. Rohrer, MD
Director of Dermatologic Surgery, SkinCare Physicians,
    Chestnut Hill, MA, United States

Mona Sadeghpour, MD
Co-Founder, SkinMed Institute,
    Denver, Colorado, CO, United States

Leah Spring, DO, FAAD
Head of Procedural Dermatology, Mohs Micrographic
    Surgery, Cosmetic Dermatologic Surgery
    Naval Medical Center Portsmouth, Portsmouth, VA,
    United States
    Commander, United States Navy

Marcus G. Tan, MD, FRCPC
Division of Dermatology, University of Ottawa and The
    Ottawa Hospital, Ottawa, ON, Canada

Elizabeth L. Tanzi, MD, FAAD
Director, Capital Laser & Skin Care,
    Chevy Chase, MD, United States
Associate Clinical Professor of Dermatology,
    George Washington University School of Medicine,
    Washington, DC, Unites States

Jennifer M. Tran, MD
Dermatology Resident, University of Wisconsin School
    of Medicine and Public Health, Madison, WI,
    United States

Mara Weinstein Velez, MD
Assistant Professor, Dermatology Department,
    University of Rochester,
    Rochester, NY, United States
Director, Cosmetic and Laser Dermatology
    University of Rochester Medical Center
    Rochester, NY, United States

Jacqueline Watchmaker, MD
Physician, Dermatology, SouthWest Skin Specialists,
    Scottsdale, AZ, United States

Much has changed since the first edition of this series. Noninvasive and minimally invasive cosmetic procedures, as pioneered by dermatologists, have become increasingly adopted by physicians and well-accepted by patients.

Cosmetic dermatologic surgery procedures have been refined and improved. Interventions have become more effective and also safer and more tolerable with increasing benefit:risk ratios. Combination cosmetic regimens that include multiple procedure types have been shown to achieve results comparable to those with more invasive procedures. And new devices and technologies continue to be introduced.

And how best to keep up with these advances and to ensure your offerings are state of the art and at the cutting edge? The newest edition of the *Procedures in Cosmetic Dermatology* series keeps you there, and for those starting out in the field these texts quickly introduce you and bring you to the state of the art. Each book in this series is designed to quickly impart basic skills as well as advanced concepts in an easy-to-understand manner.

We focus not on theory but on how to. Our expert book editors and chapter authors will guide you through the learning process efficiently, so you can soon get back to treating patients.

The authors are leading dermatologists in the field. Dermatologists' role in cosmetic medicine has continued to expand. Research has revealed that primary care physicians and the general public view dermatologists as the experts in less invasive cosmetic procedures. A nationwide advanced fellowship program in cosmetic dermatologic surgery has been initiated to train the next generation of dermatologists to the highest standards.

What has not changed is physicians' need for clear, concise, and current direction on procedure techniques.

Physicians need to be proficient in the latest methods for enhancing appearance and concealing the visible signs of aging.

To that end, we hope that you, our reader, find the books enjoyable and educational.

We thank our many contributors and wish you well on your journey of discovery.

Jeffrey S. Dover, MD, FRCPC, and
Murad Alam, MD, MSCI

SERIES PREFACE FOR THE FIRST EDITION

Although dermatologists have been procedurally inclined since the beginning of the specialty, particularly rapid change has occurred in the past quarter century. The advent of frozen section technique and the golden age of Mohs skin cancer surgery have led to the formal incorporation of surgery within the dermatology curriculum. More recently, technological breakthroughs in minimally invasive procedural dermatology have offered an aging population new options for improving the appearance of damaged skin.

Procedures for rejuvenating the skin and adjacent regions are actively sought by our patients. Significantly, dermatologists have pioneered devices, technologies, and medications, which have continued to evolve at a startling pace. Numerous major advances, including virtually all cutaneous lasers and light-source-based procedures, botulinum exotoxin, soft tissue augmentation, dilute anesthesia liposuction, leg vein treatments, chemical peels, and hair transplants, have been invented or developed and enhanced by dermatologists. Dermatologists understand procedures, and we have special insight into the structure, function, and working of skin. Cosmetic dermatologists have made rejuvenation accessible to risk-averse patients by emphasizing safety and reducing operative trauma. No specialty is better positioned than dermatology to lead the field of cutaneous surgery while meeting patient needs.

As dermatology grows as a specialty, an ever-increasing proportion of dermatologists will become proficient in the delivery of different procedures. Not all dermatologists will perform all procedures, and some will perform very few, but even the less procedurally directed among us must be well versed in the details to be able to guide and educate our patients. Whether you are a skilled dermatologic surgeon interested in further expanding your surgical repertoire, a complete surgical novice wishing to learn a few simple procedures, or somewhere in between, this book and this series are for you.

The volume you are holding is one of a series entitled *Procedures in Cosmetic Dermatology*. The purpose of each book is to serve as a practical primer on a major topic area in procedural dermatology. If you want to make sure you find the right book for your needs, you may wish to know what this book is and what it is not. It is not a comprehensive text grounded in theoretical underpinnings. It is not exhaustively referenced.

It is not designed to be a completely unbiased review of the world's literature on the subject. At the same time, it is not an overview of cosmetic procedures that describes these in generalities without providing enough specific information to actually permit someone to perform the procedures. Importantly, it is not so heavy that it can serve as a doorstop or a shelf filler. What this book and this series offer is a step-by-step, practical guide to performing cutaneous surgical procedures. Each volume in the series has been edited by a known authority in that subfield. Each editor has recruited other equally practical-minded, technically skilled, hands-on clinicians to write the constituent chapters. Most chapters have two authors to ensure that different approaches and a broad range of opinions are incorporated. On the other hand, the two authors and the editors also collectively provide a consistency of tone. A uniform template has been used within each chapter so that the reader will be easily able to navigate all the books in the series. Within every chapter, the authors succinctly tell it like they do it. The emphasis is on therapeutic technique; treatment methods are discussed with an eye to appropriate indications, adverse events, and unusual cases. Finally, this book is short and can be read in its entirety on a long plane ride. We believe that brevity paradoxically results in greater information transfer because cover-to-cover mastery is practicable.

We hope you enjoy this book and the rest of the books in the series and that you benefit from the many hours of clinical wisdom that have been distilled to produce it. Please keep it nearby, where you can reach for it when you need it.

Jeffrey S. Dover, MD, FRCPC, and
Murad Alam, MD, MSCI

PREFACE

The remarkable advances in the field of laser, light, and device-based dermatologic treatments continue at a speed that can make it difficult for even the most diligent dermatologic surgeon to stay abreast of the most important developments. The *Procedures in Cosmetic Dermatology* series was created to deliver practical information in a succinct fashion by experts in the field. This fifth edition of *Lasers, Lights, and Energy Devices* captures the numerous developments in our field since the last edition. Written by key opinion leaders in the field of cutaneous laser surgery, chapters have been thoroughly revised and added to include the latest breakthroughs in both technology and technique for each topic.

Several chapters have been expanded to capture new treatments that were not available during the writing of the last edition. There is expanded coverage of pigment-specific lasers and tattoos and treatment with intense pulsed-light sources. New chapters include radiofrequency microneedling, photodynamic therapy, muscle-toning and contouring, and the treatment of acne with laser and energy-based devices. However, in keeping with previous editions, the book begins with an excellent overview of the fundamentals and basic science of cutaneous laser, light, and device-based treatments. The chapters devoted to ablative laser resurfacing and the laser treatment of ethnic skin have been updated with the most current information. A review of complications and legal considerations of cutaneous laser and device-based treatments concludes the book.

In keeping with the philosophy of the entire *Procedures in Cosmetic Dermatology* series, the book is written to provide comprehensive, yet practical information on a variety of topics. The chapters highlight proper patient selection, treatment considerations, practical pearls, and expert tips and outline potential side effects and complications. Written for the benefit of the novice and experienced cutaneous laser surgeon alike, the authors include basic and advanced techniques discussed in a concise and straightforward manner. With the addition of clinical photographs, graphic illustrations, practice pearls, tables, clinical cases, tables, clinical cases, and key points, the reader will gain valuable insight beyond the written text. The newly expanded digital component of the book complements the text and provides the viewer with a deeper understanding of technique and insight into the thought process of experts in the field. We are confident that the fifth edition of *Lasers, Lights, and Energy Devices* will provide the reader with an outstanding and timely overview of the use of lasers, light sources, and other energy-based devices within the rapidly evolving field of cosmetic dermatology.

Elizabeth L. Tanzi, MD, FAAD and
Jeffrey S. Dover, MD, FRCPC

CONTENTS

1. **Understanding Lasers, Light Sources, and Other Energy-Based Technology,** 1
   Kelly O'Connor and Jeffrey S. Dover

2. **Laser Treatment of Vascular Lesions,** 11
   Kristen M. Kelly, Lisa Arkin, Erica G. Baugh, and Jennifer M. Tran

3. **Laser Treatment of Pigmented Lesions and Tattoos,** 25
   Kerry Heitmiller, Thomas E. Rohrer, and Mona Sadeghpour

4. **Laser Hair Removal,** 54
   Omar A. Ibrahimi, Suzanne L. Kilmer, and Farah Moustafa

5. **Treatment of Skin With Intense Pulsed Light Sources,** 72
   Jeremy Brauer, Karen J. Dover, Jacqueline Watchmaker, and Courtney Gwinn

6. **Nonablative Fractional Laser Skin Rejuvenation,** 85
   Jacqueline Watchmaker, Jeffrey S. Dover, Bradley S. Bloom, and Leah Spring

7. **Nonsurgical Skin Tightening,** 104
   Michael S. Kaminer, Courtney Gwinn, and Karen J. Dover

8. **Photodynamic Therapy,** 127
   Macrene Alexiades

9. **Ablative Laser Skin Resurfacing,** 137
   Jacob J. Inda and Joel L. Cohen

10. **Nonsurgical Body Contouring of Fat,** 152
    Lauren Meshkov Bonati and Omer Ibrahim

11. **Muscle Toning and Contouring,** 167
    Leah Spring and John Peters

12. **Radiofrequency Microneedling,** 176
    Marcus G. Tan, Anne Chapas, Jennifer MacGregor, and Shilpi Khetarpal

13. **Laser Treatment of Ethnic Skin,** 192
    Kachiu Lee, Shraddha Desai, Mara Weinstein Velez, and Deborah Paul

14. **Treatment of Acne With Light and Energy-Based Devices,** 206
    Mitchel P. Goldman, Emily Wood, Rawaa Almukhtar, and Steven Krueger

15. **Complications and Legal Considerations of Laser, Light, and Energy-Based Treatments,** 221
    Saleh Rachidi and David J. Goldberg

Index 229

VIDEO CONTENTS

2.1 **Laser Treatment of Rosacea**
Kristen Kelly, MD

2.2 **Corneal Eye Shield Placement Prior to Port Wine Birthmark Treatment**
Kristen Kelly, MD

3.1 **Treatment of Pigmented Lesions and Tattoos**
Thomas Rohrer, MD

4.1 **Laser Hair Removal in a Skin Type II Patient**
Farah Moustafa, MD

5.1 **Intense Pulsed Light Treatment Demonstration**
Jacqueline Watchmaker, MD

6.1 **Treatment of the Neck and Chest With NAFL**
Jacqueline Watchmaker, MD

7.1 **Demonstration of Thermage**
Courtney Gwinn, MD

7.2 **Nonsurgical Skin Tightening With High-Intensity Focused Ultrasound**
Elizabeth Tanzi, MD

8.1 **Blue Light PDT for Actinic Keratoses, Part 1: Preoperative Assessment**
Macrene Alexiades, MD, PHD

8.2 **Blue Light PDT for Actinic Keratoses, Part 2: Acetone Prep & ALA Application**
Macrene Alexiades, MD, PHD

8.3 **Blue Light PDT for Actinic Keratoses, Part 3: Blue Light Application**
Macrene Alexiades, MD, PHD

8.4 **Blue Light PDT for Actinic Keratoses, Part 4: Posttreatment Recommendations**
Macrene Alexiades, MD, PHD

8.5 **Red Light PDT With Ameluz, Part 1: Preoperative Assessment & Preparation**
Macrene Alexiades, MD, PHD

8.6 **Red Light PDT With Ameluz, Part 2: Treatment**
Macrene Alexiades, MD, PHD

8.7 **Red Light PDT With Ameluz, Part 3: Treatment**
Macrene Alexiades, MD, PHD

8.8 **Red Light PDT With Ameluz, Part 4: Posttreatment Recommendations**
Macrene Alexiades, MD, PHD

8.9 **Blue Light PDT With ALA, Part 1: Preoperative Assessment & Preparation**
Macrene Alexiades, MD, PHD

8.10 **Blue Light PDT With ALA, Part 2: Application of ALA**
Macrene Alexiades, MD, PHD

8.11 **Blue Light PDT With ALA, Part 3: Post-Application of ALA**
Macrene Alexiades, MD, PHD

8.12 **Blue Light PDT With ALA, Part 4: Treatment**
Macrene Alexiades, MD, PHD

8.13 **Blue Light PDT With ALA, Part 5: Post-Illumination**
Macrene Alexiades, MD, PHD

9.1 **Laser Skin Resurfacing**
Thomas Rohrer, MD

10.1 **Informational Video on TruSculpt ID (Copyrights Retained by Cutera)**

10.2 **Informational Video on SculpSure (Copyrights Retained by Cynosure)**

10.3 **Demonstration of Application of Coolsculpting Handpiece to Lower Abdomen (Copyrights Retained by ZELTIQUE Aesthetics)**

10.4 **Demonstration of Application of Coolsculpting Handpiece to Submentum (Copyrights Retained by ZELTIQUE Aesthetics)**

11.1 **Muscular Contractions During Treatment With Neuromuscular Electrical Stimulation (TruSculpt Flex)**
Leah Spring, DO

12.1 Treatment of Acne Scars With Radiofrequency Microneedling
Jennifer MacGregor, MD

13.1 1927-nm Diode Laser for Facial Rejuvenation in Skin Type IV Asian Female
Kachiu Lee, MD

13.2 Port Wine Stain Treated With the 595 Pulsed-Dye Laser
Deborah Paul, MD and Mara Weinstein, MD

13.3 1470/2940-nm Hybrid for Acne Scarring in Skin Type V
Deborah Paul, MD and Mara Weinstein, MD

13.4 1064-nm Nd:YAG in Skin Type IV Asian Female Treated for Axillary Hair Removal
Kachiu Lee, MD

13.5 Laser Hair Removal Using the Long Pulsed 1064-nm Nd:YAG With Contact Cooling
Deborah Paul, MD and Mara Weinstein, MD

13.6 Picosecond Laser for Melasma in Skin Type V
Deborah Paul, MD and Mara Weinstein, MD

13.7 Fractional Plasma Radiofrequency for Photoaging—Glide Tip in Skin Type IV
Shraddha Desai, MD

13.8 Fractional Plasma Radiofrequency for Photoaging—Focus Tip in Skin Type IV
Shraddha Desai, MD

14.1 Demonstration of Photodynamic Therapy Treatment
Emily Wood, MD

Understanding Lasers, Light Sources, and Other Energy-Based Technology

Kelly O'Connor and Jeffrey S. Dover

SUMMARY AND KEY FEATURES

- Laser is an acronym that stands for Light Amplification by Stimulated Emission of Radiation.
- Laser light is a concentrated beam of electromagnetic radiation that travels at a single wavelength.
- The therapeutic value of a laser rests on the principle that specific compounds in the skin (chromophores) absorb laser light more readily at specific wavelengths. This process is known as selective photothermolysis.
- The user can manipulate laser parameters, such as fluency, pulse duration, and spot size, to optimize destruction of the target chromophore.
- Understanding the properties of laser light will help guide laser selection, determine clinical endpoints, and avoid adverse reactions.

CHARACTERISTICS OF LIGHT

Light is a form of energy that is made up of photons. Photons are particles that travel in space as electromagnetic waves. Photons will eventually come into contact with atoms, which exist in nature in their lowest state of energy, the "ground state." When atoms absorb photons, they are propelled into higher energy states because their orbiting electrons are displaced further from the nucleus. When photons stop hitting atoms, the atoms instantaneously fall back toward their ground states, and in so doing, release energy in the form of photons. The process of energy transfer from energized atoms back to their resting states via the emission of photons is called electromagnetic radiation. It was originally described by Albert Einstein in "The Quantum Theory of Radiation."

ELECTROMAGNETIC SPECTRUM

The photons that are released as electromagnetic radiation move at a specific wavelength and frequency based on properties of the emitting atom. The electromagnetic spectrum is the range of frequencies at which photons travel in nature (Fig. 1.1). It encompasses low-frequency radio waves, visible light, ultraviolet radiation, and high-frequency gamma rays.

Light, composed of a stream of photons, travels at a constant velocity "the speed of light" in a vacuum. The speed of light is a product of wavelength and frequency ($c = \lambda \times f$). Since the speed of light is constant, the energy of the photon is proportional to its frequency and inversely proportional to its wavelength. Therefore, high energy photons have higher frequencies and lower wavelengths. Lasers take advantage of the different properties of photon frequencies and wavelengths to treat a wide variety of dermatologic diseases.

LASERS

Laser is an acronym that stands for *Light Amplification by Stimulated Emission of Radiation*. A laser is

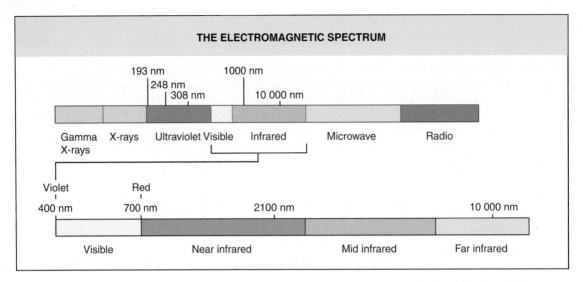

Fig. 1.1 The electromagnetic spectrum. The electromagnetic spectrum is the collection of wavelengths at which photons travel in space. (From Sakamoto FH, Avram MM, Anderson RR. Lasers and other energy-based technologies—principles and skin interactions. In: Bolognia JL, Schaffer JV, Cerroni L, eds. *Dermatology*. 4th ed. Philadelphia: Elsevier; 2018.)

comprised of an energy source and an optical resonator. The energy source, which may be an electrical current, flashlamp, or a second laser, functions to excite atoms within the optical resonator into high energy states. The optical resonator contains a medium (gas, liquid, solid, or crystal) that provides the source of atoms (Fig. 1.2). The medium determines the wavelength of the photons that are emitted as electromagnetic radiation. Lasers often take the names of the specific medium they contain: Neodymium-doped: Yttrium Aluminium Garnet (Nd:YAG), Ruby, carbon dioxide (CO_2), etc.

The medium is enclosed in a tube between two parallel mirrors, one that is completely reflective and one that is semi-transparent. The energy source fires photons at the atoms in the medium which displaces their electrons further from the nuclei and brings them to higher energy levels. Atoms then emit photons of a specific wavelength when the atoms fall back into their ground states. If an emitted photon collides with an atom already in the excited state, another photon of the same wavelength will be emitted. This chain reaction leads to photons of the same wavelength bouncing off the walls and reflective mirror in the optical resonator until they are in parallel with the semi-transparent mirror. The semi-transparent mirror acts as a filter to emit only photons of a specific wavelength that are traveling

in the same phase and direction. The exiting stream of photons is known as the laser beam.

Properties of Laser Light

Laser light is unique because it is monochromatic, which means that the stream of photons is composed of a single wavelength of light. This differs from other light sources, such as sunlight, light bulbs, and intense pulsed light, which emit photons with many different wavelengths. Monochromaticity carries great therapeutic importance because it allows for laser light to target specific compounds in the skin.

Laser light is also coherent and collimated (Fig. 1.3). Coherence is the state in which photons travel together in both time and space, while collimation is the state in which photons travel in parallel to one another. Coherent and collimated light is able to travel longer distances without significant divergence or loss of intensity. In this manner, lasers are able to treat spot sizes that are near-equivalent to the wavelength of light.

INTENSE PULSED LIGHT (IPL)

Lasers are unique in that they are monochromatic. Intense pulsed light (IPL) devices are not lasers—they are light sources that produce electromagnetic

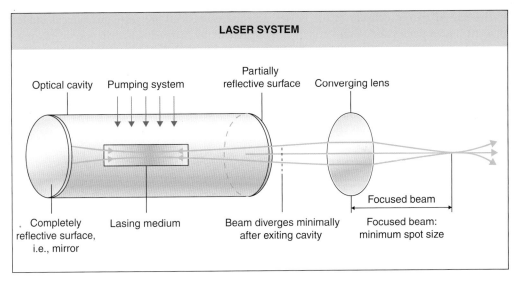

Fig. 1.2 Anatomy of an optical resonator. The energy source (pumping system) stimulates the laser medium to emit photons. The mirrors at either end of the cavity reflect traveling photons until they are in alignment with the filter of the partially reflective surface. The exiting photons then meet on a converging lens, which focuses the beam to a specific spot size. (From Sakamoto FH, Avram MM, Anderson RR. Lasers and other energy-based technologies—principles and skin interactions. In: Bolognia JL, Schaffer JV, Cerroni L, eds. *Dermatology*. 4th ed. Philadelphia: Elsevier; 2018.)

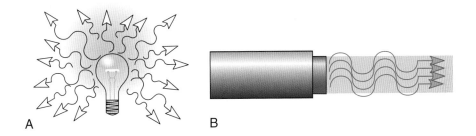

Fig. 1.3 Properties of laser light. (A) A conventional light bulb emits light that is made up of multiple wavelengths, travels in different phases of time and space, and moves in multiple directions. (B) A laser emits light that is monochromatic, coherent, and collimated. (From Flint PW, Haughey BH, Lund VJ, et al. Laser surgery: basic principles and safety considerations. In *Cummings Otolaryngology Head and Neck Surgery*. 6th ed. Philadelphia: Saunders; 2015.)

radiation that spans a range of wavelengths, approximately 500–1200 nanometers (nm). Different filters are inserted into the IPL device to allow for a more specific range of wavelengths. A specific filter permits light of that wavelength and longer wavelengths to pass through. For example, a 560 nm filter permits light with wavelengths 560 nm and above to exit the device.

RADIOMETRY: MEASURE OF ELECTROMAGNETIC RADIATION

Fluence is the measurement of laser energy delivered to an area of skin, expressed in Joules per centimeter squared (J/cm^2). The time over which the energy is delivered is known as the pulse duration, expressed in seconds. The rate of energy delivery is the power, expressed in watts (Joules per second [J/s]).

BEAM TYPE

Laser light can be delivered in a continuous or pulsed fashion. A continuous beam has no to minimal variation in power output over the pulse duration. The beam may be intermittently blocked by shutters that shield the light from exiting the device. The major drawback to continuous beams is that they are limited by the amount of power they can produce over time.

As opposed to a shuttered continuous beam, a pulsed beam is a discrete and intermittent output of laser light. Pulsed beams are able to generate higher power outputs than continuous beams by limiting the time period over which the light is generated and emitted. Greater peak powers can generate more targeted destruction and improved clinical outcomes.

Q-switched lasers are an extreme form of pulsed beams. They can produce even higher peak powers by allowing energy to build up in the laser cavity before being discharged at very short pulse durations in the nanosecond domain. The build-up of energy in the laser cavity is achieved by the use of an attenuator, a device inside the optical resonator that prevents the discharge of energy without changing the waveform of that energy. Most commonly, the attenuator is either an acousto-optic or electro-optic device. The former uses sound waves to deflect the light beams away from the mirrors in the cavity, while the latter applies a voltage to a non-linear crystal (separate from the laser medium) to block transmission of the light beam through the exit. When the attenuator is turned off the high energy laser beam is quickly released from the device cavity. This may be likened to shaking up a bottle of carbonated water— energy is built up inside the bottle because there is no way for it to exit the bottle. Once the top is unscrewed, the water (energy) rushes out of the bottle much faster, and with more power, than it would have if the top were unscrewed without shaking it beforehand. The "Q" in Q-switching denotes the *quality* factor of the optical resonator and is defined by the rate of energy discharged over the rate of energy lost.

Further advances in laser technology have resulted in lasers with pulse durations in the long picosecond domain, between 300 and 750 ps. These lasers have peak powers exceeding those of Q-switched lasers, and

the tissue effects are more mechanical and less thermal potentially increasing benefit and decreasing unwanted thermal tissue effects.

LASER-TISSUE INTERACTIONS

When laser light hits tissue one of four things can occur: absorption, reflection, transmission, and scatter (Fig. 1.4). Absorption occurs when the stream of photons interacts with certain components of the skin, and there is a transfer of energy from the photons to those components. The components of the skin that absorb light energy are known as chromophores.

Reflection is the redirection of light when it strikes the skin at an angle. Even when a laser is positioned to strike perpendicular to the skin, up to 5% of the light is reflected due to microscopic curvatures of elements within the stratum corneum. Reflection is the main reason why safety googles, blocking the corresponding wavelength of laser light, are needed for eye protection.

Scatter is the deviation of light as it interacts with microscopic elements of the skin. These elements may include very small particles, such as cellular organelles and membranes, or larger ones, such as hair follicles and sweat glands. The amount of scatter is dependent of the light's wavelength and the spot size of the beam. More scatter occurs at shorter wavelengths and smaller spot sizes, respectively.

Transmission is the continuation of laser light that is not absorbed in the tissue. Transmission is dependent on both wavelength and spot size: it occurs more readily at longer wavelengths and larger spot sizes (6). It is worthwhile to note that the relationship between the penetration depth of laser light and the wavelength of the light are inverted at wavelengths greater than 1100 nm. Penetration actually decreases at wavelengths greater than 1100 nm because the laser light starts being absorbed by water molecules, which are present in all levels of the skin.

TYPES OF TISSUE DESTRUCTION

When laser light is absorbed by particles in the skin several different types of energy transfer and reactions can occur, including photochemical, photoacoustic, and photothermal reactions. A photochemical reaction induces a physiologic response in the absorbing chromophore. For example, laser light induces mitochondria

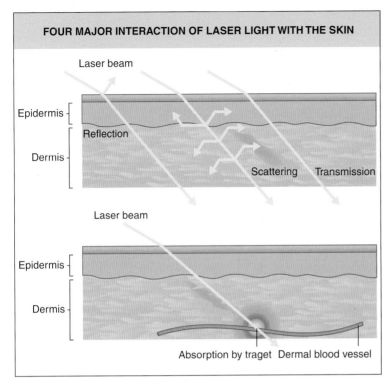

FOUR MAJOR INTERACTION OF LASER LIGHT WITH THE SKIN

Laser beam

Epidermis

Reflection

Dermis

Scattering   Transmission

Laser beam

Epidermis

Dermis

Absorption by traget   Dermal blood vessel

Fig. 1.4 The four main laser-tissue inter-actions. Laser light may be reflected, scattered, transmitted, or absorbed in the tissue. Absorption is responsible for the clinical efficacy of lasers. (From Sakamoto FH, Avram MM, Anderson RR. Lasers and other energy-based technologies—principles and skin interactions. In: Bolognia JL, Schaffer JV, Cerroni L, eds. *Dermatology*. 4th ed. Philadelphia: Elsevier; 2018.)

inside cells on the scalp to start cellular respiration, which can lead to the regrowth of hair follicles. A photo-acoustic reaction occurs when the impact of high energy laser light photons on treated tissue is strong enough to create reverberating acoustic waves. The repetitive compressions and rarefactions of the acoustic waves within the tissue create shearing forces that enable destruction and dispersion of pigment particles in melanocytic lesions or tattoos. This type of reaction is most consequential with nano- or picosecond lasers because their short pulse durations create peak powers that are high enough to elicit this type of response.

Most lasers rely on the effects of a photothermal reaction. In this reaction, the transfer of energy from laser light to a chromophore occurs in the form of heat- the bombardment of photons generates molecular vibrations which heat the molecules that absorb them. The goal of the laser is to heat chromophores to temperatures that cause the desired amount of destruction. Temperatures below 50 degrees Celsius cause local vasodilation and initiate the inflammatory cascade. Temperatures between 50°C and 100°C cause protein denaturation and tissue coagulation, both of which may

be irreversible. Temperatures exceeding 100°C cause vaporization of the water in tissue—the steam that is generated can cause tissue cavitation and expansion, which lead to formation of "vacuoles" within the epidermis and dermis. This destruction can both break up pigment or hemoglobin and establish a remodeling environment through new collagen formation in the skin.

SELECTIVE PHOTOTHERMOLYSIS

The theory of selective photothermolysis was described by Anderson and Parrish in 1983. The theory states that laser wavelength and pulse duration can be manipulated to target specific chromophores in the skin, while avoiding unnecessary destruction of surrounding tissue. A chromophore is any light absorbing compound that is found in the skin—including melanin, hemoglobin, tattoo ink, deposited drug, fat, and water. Each chromophore has a unique absorptive spectrum, which means that it will absorb certain wavelengths of light more readily than other wavelengths (Fig. 1.5) (Table 1.1).

Fig. 1.5 Absorption spectra of common chromophores. Chromophores absorb laser light more readily at certain wavelengths. *Er,* Erbium; *KTP,* potassium titanyl phosphate; *Nd,* neodymium-doped; *PDL,* pulsed dye laser; *YAG,* yttrium aluminum garnet; *YSGG,* yttrium scandium gallium garnet. (From Sakamoto FH, Avram MM, Anderson RR. Lasers and other energy-based technologies—principles and skin interactions. In: Bolognia JL, Schaffer JV, Cerroni L, eds. *Dermatology.* 4th ed. Philadelphia: Elsevier; 2018.)

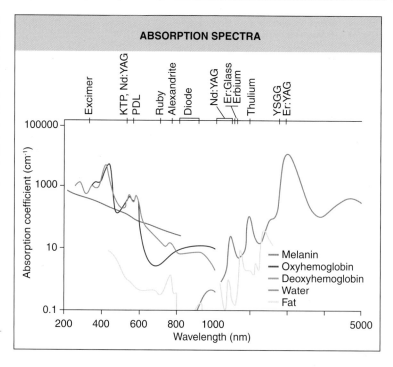

TABLE 1.1	Commonly Used Lasers in Dermatology and Their Target Chromophores	
Type of Laser	**Wavelength (nm)**	**Major Target Chromophore(s)**
Carbon dioxide (CO_2)	10,600	Water
Erbium-doped yttrium aluminum garnet (Er:YAG)	2940	Water
Thulium fiber	1927	Water
Diode	1720	Water, fat, sebum
Erbium glass	1550	Water, fat, sebum
Erbium glass	1540	Water, fat, sebum
Neodymium-doped yttrium aluminum garnet (Nd:YAG)	1440	Water, fat
Neodymium-doped yttrium aluminum garnet (Nd:YAG)	1064	Melanin, hemoglobin
Diode	1060	Fat
Diode	810	Melanin in hair follicle
Alexandrite	755	Melanin in hair follicle
Ruby	694	Melanin
Pulsed dye	585, 595	Hemoglobin, melanin
Potassium titanyl phosphate, lithium triborate	532	Hemoglobin, melanin
Argon	488, 514	Hemoglobin, melanin
Excimer (xenon chloride)	308	Epidermal melanin

Pulse duration is crucial in selective photothermolysis due to its relationship with the thermal relaxation time (TRT) of the targeted chromophore. A chromophore's TRT is time needed for a laser-treated chromophore to cool to half of its peak temperature. It is derived from the equation,

$$TRT = d^2 / 16\,\alpha$$

where d is the target diameter and α is the tissue diffusivity. Since the TRT is greatly influenced by the size of the chromophore, longer pulse durations are required to heat up and break down larger chromophores (Table 1.2). If the pulse duration exceeds a chromophore's TRT, the excess heat will spill over into the surrounding tissue. This can result in unwanted tissue damage and adverse side effects. On the other hand, underheating chromophores will keep in them intact, resulting in no clinically observed changes. Picosecond lasers have emerged as the standard treatment for tattoo removal because the pulse duration is shorter than the TRT of tattoo pigment, and the peak power is high enough to break-up pigment particles.

Another key variable in selective photothermolysis is the depth of the chromophore—light must be able to reach the targeted chromophore before it is scattered, reflected, or absorbed by other molecules in more superficial skin (Fig. 1.6). The most appropriate wavelength must be selected not only for the absorptive properties of the target chromophore, but also the ones of untargeted chromophores. For example, if one is using a laser to remove tattoo ink, then selection of the wavelength should strongly absorb the color of the tattoo pigment, while only weakly absorbing the patient's normal melanin pigment.

TABLE 1.2   Target Chromophore and Optimal Treatment Pulse Duration

Target Chromophore	Chromophore Diameter	Pulse Duration
Hair follicle	0.02–0.2 mm	10–50 ms
Melanocyte	7 μm	ms, ns
Melanosome	1–1.5 μm	ns, ps
Tattoo pigment	100 nm	ns, ps

ABLATIVE AND NON-ABLATIVE LASERS

Ablative layers create damage to the epidermis and superficial dermis resulting in the removal, or ablation, of tissue, while non-ablative lasers leave the epidermis fully intact. Ablative lasers achieve this level of damage by vaporizing water, which is found in all layers of the skin. Erbium-doped:Yttrium Aluminum Garnet (Er:YAG; 2940 nm) and CO_2 (10,600 nm) are examples of ablative lasers because their wavelengths are strongly absorbed by water molecules. Non-ablative lasers have wavelengths that do not strongly absorb water molecules; instead, their wavelengths target chromophores that are found in more discrete locations in the skin (melanin, hemoglobin, tattoo pigment, etc.).

The CO_2 laser became very popular after it was first discovered by Kumar Patel in 1964—it was used extensively in the treatment of photodamage and skin laxity. The destruction of ablative lasers induces a change in the treated tissue's cytokine milieu that promotes the deposition of new collagen and elastin in the superficial dermis. The new collagen fibers are arranged in a tighter and more bundled fashion, as seen in younger and non-photodamaged skin. Furthermore, high energy pulsed CO_2 laser treatments result in heat-induced tightening of the existing collagen fibers found in loose and folded skin of facial wrinkles. The downsides of achieving this level of destruction are more patient discomfort, prolonged recovery times, and a relatively high incidence of side effects. These factors gave way to the rise of fractionation, as well as other non-ablative methods.

FRACTIONATION

The concept of fractionation with an ablative laser was described by Manstein et al. in 2004. In fractionation, only thin columns of laser light come in contact with the skin. This creates grid-like pattern in the treatment area, where only a small percentage of the skin is damaged. The unaffected tissue provides the injured tissue with growth factors and for rebuilding and remodeling, decreasing the wound healing time and resulting in fewer side effects when compared to fully ablative lasers.

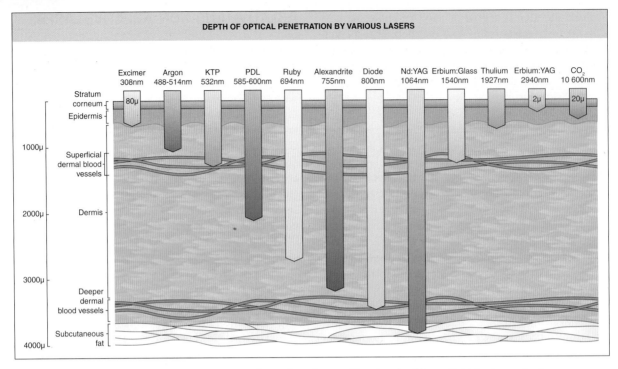

Fig. 1.6 Depth of optical penetration by various lasers. The depth of laser light is dependent on its wavelength. *KTP*, Potassium titanyl phosphate; *Nd*, neodymium-doped; *PDL*, pulsed dye laser; *YAG*, yttrium aluminum garnet. (From Sakamoto FH, Avram MM, Anderson RR. Lasers and other energy-based technologies—principles and skin interactions. In: Bolognia JL, Schaffer JV, Cerroni L, eds. *Dermatology*. 4th ed. Philadelphia: Elsevier; 2018.)

CLINICAL ENDPOINTS

Tissue reactions that occur immediately or shortly after laser treatments can be used to judge efficacy, as well as side effects. Clinical endpoints depend on the target chromophore, laser wavelength, pulse width, fluence, and patient's skin type. In general, the lowest fluence that generates the expected clinical endpoint should be used to limit unwanted and unnecessary tissue effects.

The clinical endpoints of vascular lesions vary based of the type of lesion. Immediate purpura is the goal when treating port wine stains, while immediate vessel disappearance or vessel coagulation is the goal with telangiectasias. For pigmented lesions, the type of laser dictates the endpoints: Q-switch and picosecond lasers result in immediate whitening, while long pulsed lasers or IPLs cause darkening after several minutes.

Fractionated and non-fractionated non-ablative lasers also have specific clinical endpoints, although it can be more difficult to assess treatment efficacy and excessive tissue damage. Fractionated non-ablative lasers tend to produce grids of subtle skin whitening and erythema. Fractionated ablative lasers produce grids of ablated tiny defects with a rim of whitening followed by mild focal hemorrhage from some of the ablated columns.

ADVERSE EFFECTS

Short- and long-term side effects from laser therapy include crusting, erythema, edema, pain, dyspigmentation, burns, infections, and scarring. Formulaic approaches to laser settings may be well intentioned, but they may lead to side effects due to failure of cooling measures inappropriate pulse stacking, loss of laser calibration, or variations in skin pigmentation. While clinical endpoints should be used as guidelines when they are known, each individual patient should be closely monitored during and after laser treatment.

COOLING

The rate of photon absorption by the target chromophore is important because overheating result in undesired destruction of the surrounding tissue. As soon the target chromophore absorbs photons it begins conduction heating, dispersing heat to cooler (untreated) components of the skin. To maximize thermal damage to the target chromophore and minimize damage to surrounding tissue, the temperature of the tissue must be kept below the degree that would evoke thermal injury. This problem is encountered when dermal chromophores are targeted for destruction, but the epidermis is sought to be preserved.

One of the most employed methods to decrease the risk of overheating is to cool the epidermis. This can occur before (pre), during (parallel), and/or after (post) laser treatment. Cooling may be applied by direct solid contact (i.e., ice or a cold sapphire window), automated cryogen spray, or blown cold air (Fig. 1.7). A specific method and its accompanying parameters should be chosen based on the depth of the targeted chromophore and the known temperature increase of the epidermis from each specific laser. Deeper target chromophores require longer applications of cooling. In addition to preventing side effects, cooling allows for higher energy settings to be used to destroy targeted chromophores and decreases the amount of pain associated with treatment.

CONCLUSIONS

The diversity of laser mediums and plethora of treatment settings make lasers an ideal platform to treat a wide variety of dermatologic conditions. Knowledge of wavelength, fluence or energy, and pulse duration can lead to targeted and efficacious treatments. The remainder of this book will give you a deeper appreciation for the wonderful world of lasers, lights, and energy devices in dermatology and esthetic medicine.

FURTHER READING

Anderson RR, Parish JA. Selective photothermolysis: precise microsurgery by selective absorption of pulsed radiation. *Science*. 1983;220(4596):524–527.

Anderson RR, Parrish JA. Microvasculature can be selectively damaged using dye lasers: a basic theory and experimental evidence in human skin. *Lasers Surg Med*. 1981;1(3):263–276.

Anderson RR, Parrish JA. The optics of human skin. *J Invest Dermatol*. 1981;77(1):13–19.

Anvari B, Milner TE, Tanenbaum BS, Kimel S, Svaasand LO, Nelson JS. Selective cooling of biological tissues: application for thermally mediated therapeutic procedures. *Phys Med Biol*. 1995;40(2):241–252.

Choi B, Welch AJ. Analysis of thermal relaxation during laser irradiation of tissue. *Lasers Surg Med*. 2001;29(4):351–359.

Deng Y, Chu D. Coherence properties of different light sources and their effect on the image sharpness and speckle of holographic displays. *Sci Rep*. 2017;7:5893. https://doi.org/10.1038/s41598-017-06215-x.

Einstein A. Zur Quantentheorie der Strahlung (On the Quantum Theory of Radiation). *Phys Zeitschrift*. 1917;18:121–128.

Fitzpatrick RE, Goldman MP, Satur NM, Tope WD. Pulsed carbon dioxide laser resurfacing of photoaged facial skin. *Arch Dermatol*. 1996;132(4):395–402.

Franck P, Henderson PW, Rothaus KO. Basics of lasers: history, physics, and clinical applications. *Clin Plast Surg*. 2016;43(3):505–513.

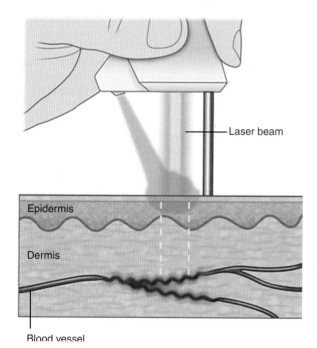

Laser beam

Epidermis

Dermis

Blood vessel

Fig. 1.7 Automated cryogen spray. An automated cryogen spray is often used with a pulsed dye laser (PDL) to prevent epidermal injury. (From Chun Yin Chan J and Hin Lee Chan H. Laser and light treatment of acquired and congenital vascular lesions. In: June KR, ed. *Surgery of the Skin*. Philadelphia: Elsevier; 2015.)

Goldman L, Wilson RG, Hornby P, Meyer RG. Radiation from Q-switched ruby laser: effect of repeated impacts of power output of 10 megawatts on a tattoo of man. *J Invest Dermatol.* 1965;44:69–71.

Gupta AK, Foley KA. A Critical Assessment of the evidence for low-level laser therapy in the treatment of hair loss. *Dermatol Surg.* 2017;43(2):188–197.

Herd RM, Alora MB, Smoller B, Arndt KA, Dover JS. A clinical and histologic prospective controlled comparative study of the picosecond titanium:sapphire (795 nm) laser versus the Q-switched alexandrite (752 nm) laser for removing tattoo pigment. *J Am Acad Dermatol.* 1999;40(4):603–606.

Herd RM, Dover JS, Arndt KA. Basic laser principles. *Dermatol Clin.* 1997;15(3):355–372.

Høgsberg T, Loeschner K, Löf D, Serup J. Tattoo inks in general usage contain nanoparticles. *Br J Dermatol.* 2011;165(6):1210–1218.

Kaplan I. The CO_2 surgical laser. *Photomed Laser Surg.* 2010;28(6):847–848.

Koechner W, Bass M. *Chapter 9: Q-Switching. Solid-State Lasers.* Springer; 2003:279–307.

Longo C, Galimberti M, De Pace B, Pellacani G, Bencini PL. Laser skin rejuvenation: epidermal changes and collagen remodeling evaluated by in vivo confocal microscopy. *Lasers Med Sci.* 2013;28(3):769–776.

Manstein D, Herron GS, Sink RK, et al. Fractional photothermolysis: a new concept for cutaneous remodeling using microscopic patterns of thermal injury. *Lasers Surg Med.* 2004;34(5):426–438.

Nahm WK, Tsoukas MM, Falanga V, Carson PA, Sami N, Touma DJ. Preliminary study of fine changes in the duration of dynamic cooling during 755-nm laser hair removal on pain and epidermal damage in patients with skin types III-V. *Lasers Surg Med.* 2002;31(4):247–251.

Nanni CA, Alster TS. Complications of carbon dioxide laser resurfacing. An evaluation of 500 patients. *Dermatol Surg.* 1998;24(3):315–320.

Nelson JS, Majaron B, Kelly KM. Active skin cooling in conjunction with laser dermatologic surgery. *Semin Cutan Med Surg.* 2000;19(4):253–266.

Orringer JS, Sachs DL, Shao Y, et al. Direct quantitative comparison of molecular responses in photodamaged human skin to fractionated and fully ablative carbon dioxide laser resurfacing. *Dermatol Surg.* 2012;38:1668–1677.

Polla LL, Margolis RJ, Dover JS, et al. Melanosomes are a primary target of Q-switched ruby laser irradiation in guinea pig skin. *J Invest Dermatol.* 1987;89(3):281–286.

Preissig J, Hamilton K, Markus R. Current Laser Resurfacing Technologies: A review that delves beneath the surface. *Semin Plast Surg.* 2012;26(3):109–116.

Ross V, Naseef G, Lin G, et al. Comparison of responses of tattoos to picosecond and nanosecond Q-switched neodymium:YAG lasers. *Arch Dermatol.* 1998;134(2):167–171.

Saedi N, Metelitsa A, Petrell K, Arndt KA, Dover JS. Treatment of tattoos with a picosecond alexandrite laser: a prospective trial. *Arch Dermatol.* 2012;148(12):1360–1363.

Thong HY, Jee SH, Sun CC, Boissy RE. The patterns of melanosome distribution in keratinocytes of human skin as one determining factor in skin colour. *Br J Dermatol.* 2003;149(3):498–505.

Tsai MT, Yang CH, Shen SC, Lee YJ, Chang FY, Feng CS. Monitoring of wound healing process of human skin after fractional laser treatments with optical coherence tomography. *Biomed Opt Express.* 2013;4(11):2362–2375.

Varghese B, Bonito V, Jurna M, Palero J, Verhagen MH. Influence of absorption induced thermal initiation pathway on irradiance threshold for laser induced breakdown. *Biomed Opt Express.* 2015;6(4):1234–1240.

Waldorf HA, Alster TS, McMillan K, Kauvar AN, Geronemus RG, Nelson JS. Effect of dynamic cooling on 585-nm pulsed dye laser treatment of port-wine stain birthmarks. *Dermatol Surg.* 1997;23:657–662.

Waldorf HA, Kauvar AN, Geronemus RG. Skin resurfacing of fine to deep rhytids using a char-free carbon dioxide laser in 47 patients. *Dermatol Surg.* 1995;21:940–946.

Wanner M, Sakamoto FH, Avram MM, et al. Immediate skin responses to laser and light treatments: therapeutic endpoints: how to obtain efficacy. *J Am Acad Dermatol.* 2016;74(5):821–833.

Zandi S, Lui H. Long-term removal of unwanted hair using light. *Dermatol Clin.* 2013;31(1):179–191.

Zenzie HH, Altshuler GB, Smirnov MZ, Anderson RR. Evaluation of cooling methods for laser dermatology. *Lasers Surg Med.* 2000;26(2):130–144.

2

Laser Treatment of Vascular Lesions

Kristen M. Kelly, Lisa Arkin, Erica G. Baugh, and Jennifer M. Tran

SUMMARY AND KEY FEATURES

- Vascular lesions are among the most common indications for laser treatment.
- Treatment relies on the theory of selective photothermolysis and aims to confine thermal injury to targeted vessels.
- Pulsed dye laser (PDL) is the treatment of choice for port-wine birthmarks (PWBs), but multiple vascular targeting devices can be used. Early treatment is thought to enhance response. Resistant or hypertrophic lesions can be treated with an alexandrite laser.
- β-blockers are standard of care for treatment of infantile hemangiomas.

- Combined treatment with β-blockers and PDL can be considered for infantile hemangiomas, particularly those which are ulcerated or in cosmetically sensitive areas. Low energies should be used for proliferative lesions treated with PDL. Involuted lesions with residual telangiectasias and/or textural change can be treated with PDL and fractional lasers.
- Erythema and telangiectasias associated with rosacea may be treated with vascular targeting light sources, including PDL or intense pulsed light.

INTRODUCTION AND HISTORY

The treatment of vascular lesions was among the first applications of lasers in dermatology. Laser surgery has since become the treatment of choice for many vascular lesions, including port-wine birthmarks (PWBs), rosacea, and poikiloderma. Laser can also be used for infantile hemangiomas (IH).

Vascular-specific lasers have evolved considerably. The 1960s saw the emergence of ruby and argon lasers, which improved the color of PWBs and IH, but relatively nonspecific heating of the skin resulted in scarring. In 1983, the theory of selective photothermolysis proposed a way to confine thermal injury to the target of interest while minimizing damage to surrounding tissue.

Three components are necessary for selective photothermolysis: a laser wavelength with preferential absorption

of the target chromophore, appropriate pulse duration matched to the target size, and a fluence that both treats the target and minimizes nonspecific thermal injury. Thermal relaxation time is roughly defined as time needed for the heated target to cool approximately halfway to its initial temperature. The ideal pulse duration is shorter than or equal to the thermal relaxation time of the target. A pulse duration that is too short may not be effective, whereas one that is too long may cause heat to dissipate to surrounding structures and cause unwanted thermal injury. The target chromophore for vascular lesions is oxyhemoglobin which has greatest absorption peaks at 418, 542, and 577 nm (Fig. 2.1). Laser light is absorbed by oxyhemoglobin and converted to heat, which is transferred to the vessel wall causing coagulation and vessel closure. Other hemoglobin species can also be targeted. For example, venous lesions may benefit from wavelengths that

11

target deoxyhemoglobin. The alexandrite laser at 755 nm is close to a deoxyhemoglobin absorption peak and has been used for refractory or hypertrophic PWBs, venocapillary malformations, and venous lakes. Methemoglobin absorption (which forms after 585 or 595 nm treatment at or above 5 J/cm²) has been recognized as another potential target chromophore.

The pulsed dye laser (PDL) became available in 1986 and was initially developed at 577 nm to target oxyhemoglobin's yellow absorption peak. It was later realized that selective photothermolysis could be achieved with wavelengths near absorption peaks, if preferential absorption still occurred. PDLs shifted to 585 nm, allowing for a depth of penetration of approximately 1.16 mm; 595 nm PDLs later became available to achieve greater depth of penetration. PDLs also evolved to incorporate longer pulse durations. Early PDLs had a fixed pulse duration of 0.45 ms, whereas currently available PDLs have pulse durations from 0.45 to 40 ms. Longer pulse durations can minimize posttreatment purpura.

Epidermal cooling was introduced in the 1990s to protect the epidermis, minimizing pigmentary changes and scarring. Cooling also permits use of higher fluences and provides greater treatment efficacy while minimizing discomfort. Modern cooling methods include cryogen spray, contact, and forced cold air.

Because PDL reaches a depth of only 1–2 mm, other lasers can be used to treat vascular lesions with greater depth. For example, the 755 nm alexandrite laser and 1064 nm neodymium:yttrium-aluminum-garnet (Nd:YAG) laser penetrate up to 50%–75% deeper into the skin. Given that the absolute absorption of hemoglobin is lower at these wavelengths, higher fluences are required and risk of injury is greater.

Intense pulsed light (IPL) devices emit polychromatic noncoherent broadband light from 420 to 1400 nm with varying pulse durations. Filters are implemented to remove unwanted wavelengths.

Other potential vascular targeting lasers include potassium titanyl phosphate (KTP) (532 nm), other near-infrared, long-pulsed lasers such as diode (including 800–810 nm, 940 nm), and dual wavelength lasers such as PDL and Nd:YAG (595 nm and 1064 nm).

VASCULAR ANOMALIES CLASSIFICATION

The International Society for the Study of Vascular Anomalies (ISSVA) publishes a widely accepted standard for classification of vascular anomalies that was updated in 2018. Lesions are broadly grouped as either vascular tumors characterized by a proliferation of blood vessels, or vascular malformations characterized by vessels with abnormal structure. IH, a type of vascular tumor, and PWB, a type of vascular malformation are common vascular anomalies that present to the dermatologist (Table 2.1).

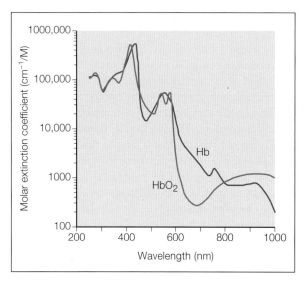

Fig. 2.1 Optical absorption of hemoglobin. (Source: Dr. Scott Prahl. http://omlc.ogi.edu/spectra/hemoglobin.)

TABLE 2.1 Comparison of Infantile Hemoglobin and Port-Wine Birthmark

	Infantile Hemangioma	Port-Wine Birthmark
Onset	• First few weeks of life • Precursor may be present at birth	• Present at birth
Course	• Proliferative period in first months of life, followed by slow involution	• Does not regress • May become hypertrophic, more violaceous with age • May develop vascular blebs
Tissue marker	• GLUT1 positive	• GLUT1 negative

GLUT1, Glucose transporter 1.

Of note, certain rare lesions seem to defy precise classification under these terms and have been listed in a provisional category. The classification also provides a list of known causal genes related to each vascular anomaly, which is an exciting area of evolving research.

PORT-WINE BIRTHMARKS

Overview

PWBs are vascular malformations that are composed of ectatic capillaries and postcapillary venules in the superficial vascular plexus. PWB vessels vary in size from 7 to 300 μm, with older patients, particularly those naive to laser treatment, tending to demonstrate larger vessels. In most cases, PWBs are congenital, although acquired cases are reported. PWBs occur in approximately 0.3%–0.5% of newborns. They often involve cosmetically sensitive areas including the head and neck but may appear anywhere on the body. Over time, some PWBs darken in color with acquisition of secondary changes including soft tissue overgrowth and development of vascular nodules (Fig. 2.2). In untreated patients, the mean age of hypertrophy has been reported as 37 years, and by the fifth decade approximately 65% of lesions are hypertrophic or nodular. Over time, significant soft tissue overgrowth, if it occurs, can lead to functional impairment in areas such as the lip or eyelid. Vascular nodules or blebs may develop. Some are pyogenic granulomas, which are proliferative and associated with second genetic hits, but others defy classification and may bleed with minimal trauma. Early treatment of PWBs can improve outcomes and is restorative in nature, minimizing disfigurement and psychosocial morbidity.

The natural history of PWB is explained by the recent discovery of mosaic mutations in highly conserved genes including *GNAQ, GNA11, PIK3CA,* and others that control cell-cycle proliferation and survival. Their mosaic origin accounts for low familial recurrence risk. Gain-of-function mutations in PWBs activate oncogenic pathways that result in synchronous, tightly regulated cellular proliferation and growth. These genes are known to be critical regulators of fetal vascular development, and very low allele frequency is required for alterations in embryonic vasculature.

Genotype-phenotype correlations exist but are not yet well characterized due to varied phenotype expression. Contributing factors to varied phenotype expression are hypothesized to include low variant allele frequency, anatomical location, age, prior treatment,

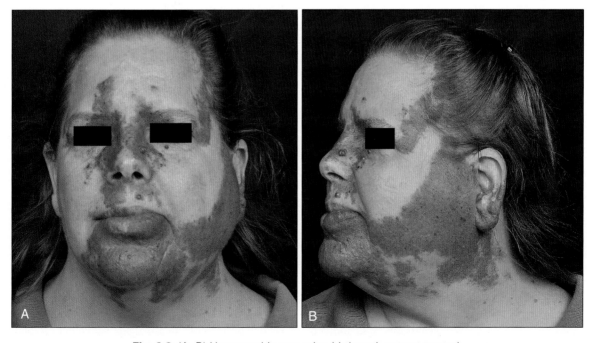

Fig. 2.2 (A, B) Hypertrophic port-wine birthmark not yet treated.

and ancestry. In general, *GNAQ* mutations yield PWBs which are often red and moderately demarcated. PWBs resulting from *PIK3CA* hotspot mutations are generally deep red, sharply demarcated, and often associated with overgrowth, particularly leg length discrepancy. Lighter pink and blotchy or reticulated lesions are often associated with *GNA11* mutations.

PWBs can be isolated or associated with various genetic syndromes. Sturge-Weber syndrome involves a facial PWB with associated eye and/or cerebral nervous system involvement, including glaucoma, seizures, and developmental delay. Numerous studies have indicated that facial PWBs follow embryologic vascular development of the face and not dermatomal nerve distribution, which was previously suspected. The most common mutation in both isolated PWBs and Sturge-Weber syndrome is a somatic activating mutation in *GNAQ*, the gene encoding guanine nucleotide-binding protein G(q) subunit alpha, as detailed in a seminal paper by Shirley, et al. The highest risk area for CNS involvement in Sturge-Weber syndrome is PWB of the forehead region (including from the lateral canthus to the top of the helices of the ear), with hemi-segmental or segmental lesions at highest risk. All patients with eyelid involvement should be referred to ophthalmology for glaucoma surveillance. More than 75% of patients with Sturge-Weber syndrome develop seizures before one year of age, and early referral to neurology are critical components of management. Mutations in *PiK3CA* are known to cause another PWB-associated syndrome, Klippel-Trénaunay syndrome (KTS), which is characterized by PWBs on an extremity associated with limb hypertrophy and underlying lymphatic and/or venous malformations. PWBs can also occur in association with arteriovenous malformations in capillary malformation–arteriovenous malformation syndrome, which can be caused by mutations in *RASA-1* or *EPHB4*, both involved in regulation of the RAS/MAPK signaling pathway.

Treatment

Goals of PWB treatment include decreasing erythema, reducing psychosocial distress, and preventing development of blebs that may bleed or become secondarily infected. In addition, it has been theorized that treating PWBs early may minimize some PWB progression including nodularity later in life. PDL is considered the gold standard for PWB treatment.

Despite the overall effectiveness of PDL, individual patient response is variable. Approximately 80%

of treated patients see a successful decrease in redness or thickness, but only approximately 20% will clear completely. One study found predictors of improved response include small size (less than 20 cm²), location over bony areas (in particular the central forehead), and early treatment. Another study in 49 infants who started laser treatment before 6 months of age demonstrated an impressive average clearance of 88.6% after 1 year. Early treatment may be more beneficial due to thinner and overall smaller lesions, as well as the presence of hemoglobin F (a type of hemoglobin present during gestation and the first year of life) and less dilated vessels in infants. PWBs may darken again after laser therapy, a phenomenon dubbed "re-darkening," hypothesized to occur due to progressive genetic etiology, lack of complete vessel eradication, and suboptimal laser treatment. Still, re-darkened areas remain lighter than their original untreated color.

Treatments are typically performed at 3- to 6-week intervals for 10 or more treatments until a plateau is reached or the lesion clears (Fig. 2.3). When choosing settings, it is advisable to determine the fluence threshold on the darkest portion of the PWB with one or two test pulses. The fluence is adjusted to achieve the desired end point, which in the case of PDL using short pulse durations (e.g., 1.5 ms) is immediate purpura. If instead a gray color appears, the fluence is too high. Careful monitoring for tissue response is essential.

Changing the pulse duration may allow targeting of different sizes of vessels. The ideal pulse duration for PWB treatment has been proposed at 1–10 ms. In practice, treatment often begins at 1.5 ms, or in young children at 0.45 ms. Parameters to consider include 7- to 10-mm spot size, pulse duration of 0.45–6 ms, with appropriate epidermal cooling, such as cryogen spray cooling of 30 ms with a 20- to 30-ms delay. Longer pulse durations may be considered in darker skin types. Treatment should start at a lower energy that can be increased as tolerated. Parameters will vary by device.

As with any laser treatment, complications of PDL may include pigmentary change. When treating darker skin types, the risk of hypopigmentation and hyperpigmentation can be minimized by using appropriate cooling and longer pulse durations. Treatment intervals may need to be longer to allow for any pigmentation changes to resolve before proceeding with additional treatment.

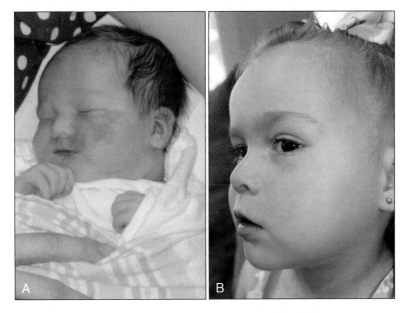

Fig. 2.3 Port-wine birthmark: (A) before and (B) after PDL treatments.

Care must be taken with leg lesions, which are prone to hyperpigmentation.

The alexandrite laser is typically used for PDL-resistant lesions, although it may be implemented as a first-line treatment for more hypertrophic, violaceous PWB in adults (Fig. 2.4). The desired end point in this case is a transient gray color that evolves into a deeper persistent purpura over several minutes, as described by Izikson and Anderson in 2009. Care must be taken not to overlap or "stack" pulses because scarring can occur. Notably, the range of appropriate fluences for alexandrite laser is quite broad.

Nd:YAG laser and combined 595 nm and 1064 nm lasers can also be used for PWBs. Although depth of penetration can be increased, there is a narrow therapeutic window with these devices due to reduced oxyhemoglobin and caution is advised to avoid scarring. Scarring can occur even at low fluences. These devices should only be used by experienced laser surgeons and we prefer to utilize mostly for nodules that develop within PWB.

IPL with appropriate vascular filters can also be used, and some IPL devices have filters to optimize the wavelength range for PWB. As with many lasers, treatment in hair-bearing areas may lead to permanent hair loss. The risk is greater on the eyelashes, given the proximity of follicles to the surface, and on the eyebrows and scalp of young children, particularly those of darker skin types. Hair loss can also occur with any long-pulsed laser treatment of vascular lesions.

Nodules or blebs within PWB can be treated with excision or laser. In the case of PDL, several pulses or intentionally stacked pulses may be required. Given the limited depth of penetration of PDL, deeper penetrating lasers such as alexandrite or Nd:YAG can be used or nodules can be ablated with carbon dioxide (CO_2), or erbium-doped yttrium-aluminum-garnet (Er:YAG) lasers.

Photodynamic therapy (PDT) has been used with some success but is limited by the administration of systemic hematoporphyrin photosensitizers, which result in prolonged photosensitivity over weeks. There is also an increased risk of scarring or pigmentary change when compared to PDL.

Recent research has sought to improve treatment efficacy by combining light-based removal of PWBs with posttreatment antiangiogenic agents, especially rapamycin, which inhibits the mTOR enzyme that regulates cell growth and metabolism. There is no direct mechanistic data to suggest that mutant *GNAQ* or *GNA11* directly impacts mTOR signaling, so rapamycin may not exert a pathway-specific effect. There was initial enthusiasm for

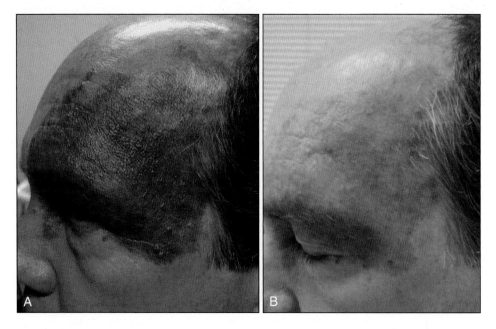

Fig. 2.4 Violaceous, hypertrophic port-wine birthmark: (A) before and (B) after alexandrite laser treatments. Note improvement in color and thickness. (Courtesy of Dr. R. Rox Anderson.)

combined PDL plus rapamycin but in clinical practice, most patients do not achieve significantly enhanced lightening. Other agents are being evaluated for use as adjuvants with laser and this is a promising area of research.

Optical coherence tomography (OCT) is a high-resolution bedside imaging tool that can rapidly characterize the diameter and depth of blood vessels in PWBs to a depth of 1 mm. Dynamic-OCT with matching of laser settings to vessel depth and diameter at each treatment session, may be promising in future clinical practice for more precise laser dosimetry.

PEARL 1

Outline Borders of Pwbs Prior to Treatment

Laser pulses can induce erythema that blurs the border, making it difficult to appreciate the target. Prior to treatment with yellow light lasers such as PDL, lesion edges may be outlined with a yellow highlighter or white pencil to facilitate consistent visualization. This is particularly important prior to general anesthesia as vasodilation of blood vessels often obscure borders of the vascular birthmark.

INFANTILE HEMANGIOMAS

Overview

IH are benign endothelial cell proliferations that represent the most common tumor of infancy, occurring in 4%–10% of infants. Female gender is a notable association, with lesions arising three times as often in female infants. Other risk factors include prematurity, multiple gestation, advanced maternal age, and family history of IH. The relative significance of these risk factors remains under study, and a prospective cohort study on IH in twins suggested the cause is multifactorial. They have been theorized to originate from embolized placental stem cells or as a response to tissue hypoxia. Expression of glucose transporter 1 (GLUT 1), a fetal-type endothelial glucose transporter, distinguishes them histologically from other vascular tumors and vascular malformations. IH may be characterized as localized or segmental and as superficial (clinically red), deep (clinically blue or skin-colored), or mixed. Typical presentation is within the first few weeks of age as a whitish, red, or telangiectatic macule, with 60% arising on the head and neck.

The proliferative period typically lasts until 3 months for superficial IH, although deep IH may proliferate longer, for 6–8 months. Involution then occurs more slowly over years. An often-cited estimation is that approximately 10% of IH are expected to regress with each year of age, with the vast majority having regressed by age 10, although studies suggest this process may occur sooner. After regression, many IH, especially those that were untreated, leave behind residual fibrofatty tissue, atrophy, or telangiectasias.

Uncomplicated IH typically do not require imaging studies. Multiple IH, usually greater than five, or segmental IH may prompt radiologic investigation to assess for possible associated syndromes or visceral involvement. PHACES syndrome must be considered in segmental facial hemangiomas larger than 5 cm and is characterized by *P*osterior fossa malformations, *H*emangiomas, *A*rterial anomalies, *C*oarctation of the aorta, *E*ye abnormalities, and *S*ternal or supraumbilical raphe. The presence of characteristic segmental lumbar IH should prompt evaluation for related syndromes, such as *P*erineal hemangioma, *E*xternal genital malformations, *L*ipomyelomeningocele, *V*esicorenal abnormalities, *I*mperforate anus, and *S*kin tags (PELVIS) or *L*ower body hemangioma, *U*rogenital anomalies or ulceration, *M*yelopathy, *B*ony deformities, *A*norectal malformations and arterial anomalies, and *R*enal anomalies (LUMBAR). Diffuse hemangiomatosis involves multiple skin hemangiomas with risk for visceral involvement, most commonly liver followed by the gastrointestinal tract. Guidelines exist for evaluation, treatment and serial imaging in patients with diffuse hepatic involvement.

Congenital hemangiomas present at birth and are characterized by GLUT1-negative staining. They do not respond to oral propranolol or timolol. They are known to be caused by mosaic mutations in *GNA11* or *GNAQ* but in contrast to PWB are high flow lesions that behave as small vessel arteriovenous malformations. When they rapidly involute due to early infarction, they are termed rapidly involuting congenital hemangiomas (RICHs). When they do not involute, they are called noninvoluting congenital hemangiomas (NICHs). A category of partially involuting congenital hemangiomas (PICHs) has been described in which lesions begin to regress but then plateau and persist. Persistent lesions can produce pain, and these are amenable to embolization by interventional radiology. Laser is most helpful for the visible telangiectasias.

Treatment

Treatment of IH is indicated for functional impairment, as well as for such complications as ulceration, infection, or bleeding. IH can cause functional difficulties when critical anatomic structures are affected, including airway compromise, symptomatic hepatic involvement, visual obstruction, or auditory canal obstruction.

The historic treatment for many IH in the absence of functional difficulties or complications has been watchful waiting or active nonintervention. More recently, it has been recognized that an indication for treatment is prevention of long-term scarring and associated psychosocial distress, especially when lesions involve cosmetically sensitive areas.

Systemic pharmacotherapy with oral propranolol is considered safe and effective first-line treatment for IH, and is FDA approved for treatment as an outpatient in infants 5 weeks and older. A randomized controlled trial on 460 infants, among the largest studies to date, showed propranolol to be effective when given for 6 months. Its mechanism remains unclear and has been speculated to involve promotion of pericyte-mediated vasoconstriction, inhibition of vasculogenesis and catecholamine-mediated angiogenesis, and inactivation of the renin-angiotensin system. Although propranolol is generally well tolerated, infrequent adverse effects include hypoglycemia, bronchospasm, hypotension, and bradycardia.

Topical treatments may be used as therapy for superficial IH. Timolol has emerged as the preferred topical option, although it carries a risk for systemic absorption in deep hemangiomas or in low-birth weight infants. In those patients, propranolol should be utilized first line. In a randomized controlled trial, timolol plus PDL was superior to PDL alone in effecting resolution of IH. Laser options are discussed in further detail below; however, it is important to note that laser treatment is no longer considered first line.

Some studies have suggested early treatment with laser, especially PDL, may halt further growth and facilitate a transition to the plateau or involution phase. Laser treatment may also be beneficial for ulcerated hemangiomas or in areas prone to ulceration, specifically the anogenital area. A study on 78 patients with ulcerated hemangiomas showed that 91% improved after a mean of two PDL treatments. Combined propranolol and PDL may achieve enhanced resolution of ulcerated lesions.

If laser is to be used for proliferating IH, there is a risk of ulceration with treatment and low fluences should be used. Treatment settings to consider for PDL include pulse duration 0.45–1.5 ms, 10- or 7-mm spot, fluence 5–7 J/cm^2, and appropriate cooling. Lower fluences and longer pulse durations are advisable in darker skin types.

Parameters vary by device. Multiple treatments are generally required and may be performed at 2-week intervals for rapidly proliferating lesions or 4- to 6-week intervals for involuting lesions. The main risks of treatment are ulceration and scarring, as well as hypopigmentation. There have been rare reports of serious bleeding after

PDL treatment for hemangiomas, primarily with older lasers without cooling, and one case with a 595-nm laser with cooling, using relatively high fluences.

After involution, hemangiomas can leave behind telangiectasias or residual fibrofatty tissue. Telangiectasias can be treated with the PDL (Fig. 2.5), and texture

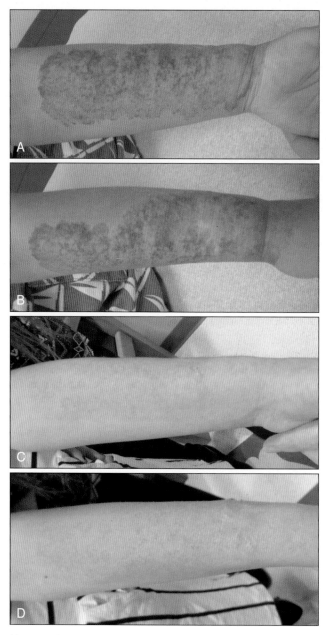

Fig. 2.5 Involuted hemangioma showing progression before (A,B) and after multiple pulsed dye laser treatments (C,D).

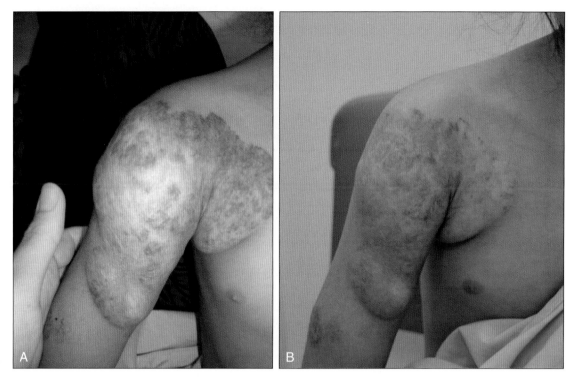

Fig. 2.6 Involuted hemangioma before (A) and after (B) two separate laser treatments: pulsed dye laser to improve the erythema and telangiectasias, and fractionated CO_2 laser to improve the texture and reduce fibrofatty tissue.

changes have been shown to improve with ablative (Fig. 2.6) or nonablative fractional resurfacing.

PEARL 2

1. β-blockers are first-line therapy for infantile hemangiomas.
2. β-blockers may in some cases be combined with laser to achieve faster and more complete resolution.
3. PDL may be useful for healing of ulcerated IH and can be combined with β-blocker treatment.

VENOUS MALFORMATIONS

Venous malformations present clinically as soft, compressible, non-pulsatile blue-violaceous papules or nodules that increase in size with measures that increase venous pressure, such as the dependent position. Vessel walls may exhibit calcifications, and phleboliths are considered pathognomonic. Venous malformations are slow-flow lesions that may be present at birth or present later in life as they progress. Magnetic resonance imaging (MRI) for larger lesions is advised to assess the extent of the lesion.

Laser treatment can be indicated for small and discrete venous malformations, such as those on the lip (Fig. 2.7). The goal is to decrease the size of the lesion. Clinically complete clearance may be achieved, but recurrence is common because venous malformations are associated with genetic mutations in *PiK3CA* or *TEK2*, and residual venules tend to recanalize. For larger lesions, multiple treatment modalities including surgery and sclerotherapy may be used with the option of a preceding laser treatment for debulking. Laser treatment of venous malformations requires a deeper penetrating laser, and the near-infrared lasers, specifically diode or Nd:YAG, are most commonly implemented. Treatment of these lesions is complex and best handled by experienced surgeons. Scherer and Waner noted that the

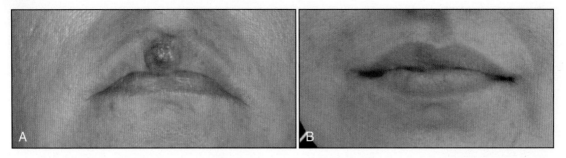

Fig. 2.7 Venous malformation: (A) before and (B) after diode laser treatments. There is significant reduction in size and improvement in color. Patient was undergoing further treatments. (Courtesy of Dr. R. Rox Anderson.)

benefits of Nd:YAG for complex venous malformations include tissue shrinkage, improved color, and induction of dermal fibrosis, thus reducing the risk of skin loss in surgery and sclerotherapy. In their experience, swelling lasted approximately 2 weeks, and blistering, dyspigmentation, and scarring occurred in less than 5% of patients.

VENOUS LAKES

Venous lakes are acquired vascular malformations that consist of ectatic venules in the superficial dermis. Venous lakes appear clinically as compressible violaceous papules, most commonly on the lip. Treatment may be initiated for cosmetic purposes or may be prompted by bleeding.

Laser treatment options include PDL for more superficial lesions. For deeper lesions, a deeper penetrating laser, such as diode, alexandrite, or Nd:YAG, is more effective. Using an 800-nm diode, one report used one or two pulses at 9 mm, 30 ms, and 40 J/cm², with contact cooling via sapphire chill tip held on the skin for 2–3 seconds prior to the laser pulse. The end point is flattening, subtle graying, or deepening of purpura.

LYMPHANGIOMA CIRCUMSCRIPTUM

Lymphangioma circumscriptum is the terminology utilized to describe a microcystic lymphatic malformation characterized by clusters of vesicles that may be clear, yellow, or vascular, sometimes with a verrucous texture. Many are associated with mutations in *PiK3CA*. A common concern for patients is persistent drainage. CO_2 and Er:YAG lasers can be used in an attempt to scar the superficial component and minimize drainage. There

have also been reports of successful treatment with PDL for superficial lesions, although treatments may be limited by depth of penetration and presence of a minimal chromophore target. Serial treatments are required. Laser may be combined with other modalities including oral sirolimus.

ROSACEA AND TELANGIECTASIAS

Rosacea commonly presents in association with chronic photodamage with background facial erythema and telangiectasias, defined as superficial vessels 0.1–1 mm in diameter. Telangiectasias themselves may also be seen in a wide variety of conditions, including connective tissue diseases, various genodermatoses, and hereditary hemorrhagic telangiectasia. Laser treatment of telangiectasias and facial erythema can improve the appearance in many patients, but recurrence is not uncommon. The most commonly used devices include PDL, KTP, and IPL. Near-infrared lasers, specifically diode and Nd:YAG, have been used to treat deeper or larger vessels. Treatment must be tailored to vessel caliber, skin type, and the patient's ability to tolerate purpura. Background erythema may be treated before or after telangiectasias.

Typically, three to four monthly non-purpuric laser treatment sessions with PDL produce a significant reduction in erythema and telangiectasias (Fig. 2.8, Video 2.1). Typical settings include 7- to 12-mm spot, 6- to 10-ms pulse duration, and epidermal cooling. Lower energies are used with larger spot sizes. Lower fluences should be used for patients with intense facial erythema. As always, lower fluences and longer pulse durations are advisable in darker skin types, and

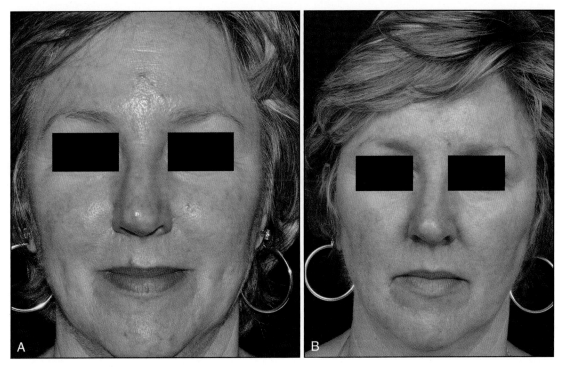

Fig. 2.8 Rosacea: (A) before and (B) after four PDL treatments.

parameters vary by device. Residual telangiectasias can then be treated cautiously in a second pass. The end point for treating vessels is vessel clearance, a transient blue coagulum, or purpura.

Vessels around the nasal ala can be more challenging to treat, and greater efficacy may be achieved with judicious stacking of non-purpuric PDL pulses. Larger-caliber vessels on the nose may require even longer pulse durations and higher fluences. One study on patients with nasal telangiectasias resistant to PDL and KTP showed successful resolution after PDL alone at 40 ms and 3 mm × 10 mm elliptical spot. Nd:YAG may also be used to treat refractory nasal vessels and facial reticular veins, although the risk of scarring is increased.

Patients should be advised that even when treatment successfully reduces erythema and telangiectasias, follow-up treatments will likely be necessary for maintenance.

Poikiloderma of Civatte

Poikiloderma of Civatte presents in chronically photodamaged areas, most commonly on the neck, chest, and lateral cheeks, with mottled red-brown erythema

and associated telangiectasias. IPL may be used for treatment and has the benefits of targeting both pigmentary and vascular components, as well as availability of larger spot sizes to treat larger surface areas. A report of 175 patients treated with IPL showed clearance in more than 80% of patients, with transient side effects in 5%. Scarring or permanent pigmentary change was not observed. PDL has also been implemented to treat the vascular component of poikiloderma of Civatte with good results. Large spot sizes and relatively lower fluences are advised for PDL to limit potential side effects, most commonly a reticulated pattern and hypopigmentation.

Cherry Angiomas

Cherry angiomas are the most common vascular growths of the skin and are benign proliferations that tend to be highly responsive to laser treatment, especially PDL. The clinical end point is purpura (Fig. 2.9). Clearance often occurs with one treatment, but larger lesions may require multiple treatments.

For larger and thicker angiomas, an initial pulse can be delivered while performing diascopy, or compression

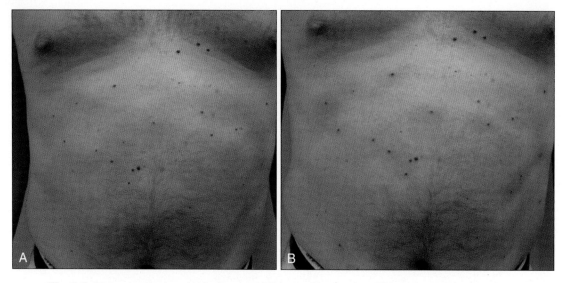

Fig. 2.9 Cherry angiomas: (A) before and (B) immediately after PDL with expected purpura.

with a glass slide, to treat the deeper component. When pulsing through a glass slide there is no cooling of the epidermis. After allowing time for the skin to cool from the initial pulse, a second pulse may be placed to treat the more superficial component, if the lesion has not become purpuric. Spider angiomas can be treated similarly.

For PDL, suggested settings are 5–7 mm, 1.5–6 ms, with appropriate epidermal cooling. Settings may need to be adjusted for patients with darker skin types, and as always, parameters vary by device. Reports have also demonstrated success with KTP, IPL, electrodesiccation, and shave excision.

Angiokeratomas

Angiokeratomas are characterized by ectatic superficial dermal vessels and overlying hyperkeratosis. Lesions are often solitary. Less common variants include multiple angiokeratomas, characteristically found on the lower extremities, angiokeratoma of Fordyce in the genital region, angiokeratoma of Mibelli on the dorsal hands and feet, and angiokeratoma circumscriptum. Lesions may also be seen in association with Fabry disease, an X-linked recessive disorder characterized by a deficiency of α-galactosidase A.

Treatment with vascular lasers, such as PDL, may be initiated to treat the vascular component, although a residual keratotic component may persist. Nd:YAG

or ablative lasers, such as CO_2 or erbium, may also be implemented. Scarring can occur with aggressive treatment and in sensitive areas, so caution is warranted.

APPROACH TO TREATMENT OF VASCULAR LESIONS

A pretreatment consultation is advisable to include a discussion of the amount of improvement expected, number of treatments, expected treatment effects (such as erythema, purpura, and swelling), potential adverse effects, and aftercare required, including sun protection and avoidance of trauma. Photos before each treatment are recommended.

Eye protection is essential during treatment. If the treatment area is on the face but outside the orbital rim, metal goggles should be placed over the patient's eyes. Stick-on laser shields with appropriate wavelength protection can also be used, but complete adherence to the skin must be visually confirmed. Crying creates moisture which may interfere with the adhesive from the laser shields. For younger children, it is advisable to gently but firmly hold gauze over the stick-on laser shields. If the treatment area is within the orbital rim, metal corneal eye shields must be used. These should be placed carefully to avoid a corneal abrasion (Video 2.2).

Many vascular lesion treatments can be performed without anesthesia. Factors to consider include patient age, lesion size, and location. Topical anesthetics can be considered. Manufacturer guidelines for area usage must be followed and ulcerated lesions should be avoided especially in infants where there may be increased absorption and toxic side effects. Deeper or more extensive lesions may require intralesional lidocaine or nerve blocks for patient comfort. For local infiltration, lidocaine without epinephrine is generally used to minimize vasoconstriction.

The approach to using general anesthesia in infants and young children varies widely, a consideration that becomes relevant in light of mounting evidence that early treatment of PWBs may be beneficial, as discussed previously. General anesthesia offers the advantage of avoiding fear and pain in children who will need multiple procedures. However, there are risks of general anesthesia. Studies have documented that in healthy patients with vascular lesions the risk is low; however, advantages and disadvantages need to be considered and discussed with the patient and family.

ADVERSE EFFECTS AND COMPLICATIONS

The risk from laser treatment of vascular lesions primarily consists of scarring and pigmentary changes. Scarring, seen in less than 1% of patients treated with PDL, and can be minimized by performing test pulses and assessing appropriate tissue responses before treating the entire lesion. Persistent gray or white discoloration can be signs of epidermal or dermal injury. The risk of permanent hypopigmentation can be minimized by patient's use of proper sun protection before and after treatment and physician's attention to tailoring laser parameters for individual patients. Darker skin tones carry a greater risk of pigmentary change and scarring due to absorption of laser light by epidermal melanin. Longer pulse durations and lower energies should be considered.

Longer wavelength lasers, including the alexandrite and Nd:YAG, also increase the risk of scarring and ulceration, especially given their narrow therapeutic window and potential need for very high energies in treating vascular lesions. These devices should be used with caution and by experienced physicians.

Swelling after PDL treatment is usually mild and transient, resolving within 24–72 hours. Effects can be more significant with the non-purpuric multiple-pass PDL technique and with deeper penetrating lasers. To reduce swelling, patients should apply ice to the area 1–2 days post treatment and sleep with the treated area elevated if possible.

The use of lasers has truly revolutionized the treatment of vascular lesions in dermatology. Ongoing device development and improved understanding of vascular lesions will continue to optimize treatment options and outcomes.

PEARL 3

The risk of scarring and pigmentary change is increased in patients with darker skin tones. Risks are also increased when using longer wavelength lasers.

FURTHER READING

Anderson RR, Parrish JA. Selective photothermolysis: precise microsurgery by selective absorption of pulsed radiation. *Science.* 1983;220:524–527.

Asilian A, Mokhtari F, Kamali AS, et al. Pulsed dye laser and topical timolol gel versus pulse dye laser in treatment of infantile hemangioma: a double-blind randomized controlled trial. *Adv Biomed Res.* 2015;4:257.

Bagazgoitia L, Torrelo A, Gutiérrez JC, et al. Propranolol for infantile hemangiomas. *Pediatr Dermatol.* 2011;28: 108–114.

Boos MD, Bozarth XL, Sidbury R, et al. Forehead location and large segmental pattern of facial port-wine stains predict risk of Sturge-Weber syndrome. *J Am Acad Dermatol.* 2020;83(4):1110–1117.

Brightman LA, Brauer JA, Terushkin V, et al. Ablative fractional resurfacing for involuted hemangioma residuum. *Arch Dermatol.* 2012;148(11):1294–1298.

Chapas AM, Eickhorst K, Geronemus RG. Efficacy of early treatment of facial port wine stains in newborns: a review of 49 cases. *Lasers Surg Med.* 2007;39:563–568.

Comi A. Current therapeutic options in Sturge-Weber syndrome. *Semin Pediatr Neurol.* 2015;22(4):295–301.

David LR, Malek M, Argenta LC. Efficacy of pulse dye laser therapy for the treatment of ulcerated hemangiomas: a review of 78 patients. *Br J Plast Surg.* 2003;56: 317–327.

Dutkiewicz AS, Ezzedine K, Mazereeuw-Hautier J, et al. A prospective study of risk for Sturge-Weber syndrome in children with upper facial port-wine stain. *J Am Acad Dermatol.* 2015;72(3):473–480.

Huikeshoven M, Koster PH, de Borgie CA, et al. Redarkening of port-wine stains 10 years after pulsed-dye-laser treatment. *N Engl J Med.* 2007;356(12):1235–1240.

Izikson L, Nelson JS, Anderson RR. Treatment of hypertrophic and resistant port wine stains with a 755 nm laser: a case series of 20 patients. *Lasers Surg Med.* 2009;41:427–432.

Krowchuk DP, Frieden IJ, Mancini AJ, et al. Clinical practice guideline for the management of infantile hemangiomas. *Pediatrics.* 2019;143(1):e20183475.

Laubach HJ, Anderson RR, Luger T, Manstein D. Fractional photothermolysis for involuted infantile hemangioma. *Arch Dermatol.* 2009;145(7):748–750.

Léauté-Labrèze C, Hoeger P, Mazereeuw-Hautier J, et al. A randomized, controlled trial of oral propranolol in infantile hemangioma. *N Engl J Med.* 2015;372(8):735–746.

Madan V, Ferguson F. Using the ultra-long pulse width pulsed dye laser and elliptical spot to treat resistant nasal telangiectasia. *Lasers Med Sci.* 2010;25:151–154.

Moy WJ, Yakel JD, Osorio OC, et al. Targeted narrowband intense pulsed light on cutaneous vasculature. *Lasers Surg Med.* 2015;47(8):651–657.

Nasseri E, Piram M, McCuaig CC, et al. Partially involuting congenital hemangiomas: a report of 8 cases and review of the literature. *J Am Acad Dermatol.* 2014;70(1):75–79.

Nguyen CM, Yohn JJ, Weston WL, Weston WL, Morelli JG. Facial port wine stains in childhood: prediction of the rate of improvement as a function of age of the patient, size, and location of the port wine stain and the number of treatments with the pulsed dye (585 nm) laser. *Br J Dermatol.* 1998;138:821–825.

Rusciani A, Motta A, Fino P, Menichini G. Treatment of poikiloderma of civatte using intense pulsed light source: 7 years of experience. *Dermatol Surg.* 2008;34:314–319.

Sabeti S, Ball KL, Burkhart C, et al. Consensus statement for the management and treatment of port-wine birthmarks in Sturge-Weber syndrome. *JAMA Dermatology.* 2021;157(1):98–104.

Scherer K, Waner M. Nd:YAG lasers (1064 nm) in the treatment of venous malformations of the face and neck: challenges and benefits. *Lasers Med Sci.* 2007;22:119–126.

Shirley MD, Tang H, Gallione CJ, et al. Sturge-Weber syndrome and port-wine stains caused by somatic mutation in GNAQ. *N Engl J Med.* 2013;368(21):1971–1979.

Su W, Ke Y, Xue J. Beneficial effects of early treatment of infantile hemangiomas with a long-pulse Alexandrite laser. *Lasers Surg Med.* 2014;46(3):173–179.

Waelchli R, Aylett S, Robinson K, Chong W, Martinez A, Kinsler V. New vascular classification of port-wine stains: improving prediction of Sturge–Weber risk. *Br J Dermatol.* 2014;171(4):861–867.

Wall TL, Grassi AM, Avram MM. Clearance of multiple venous lakes with an 800-nm diode laser: a novel approach. *Dermatol Surg.* 2007;33:100–103.

3

Laser Treatment of Pigmented Lesions and Tattoos

Kerry Heitmiller, Thomas E. Rohrer, and Mona Sadeghpour

SUMMARY AND KEY FEATURES

- Advances in pigment-specific lasers have allowed for the safe and effective treatment of various benign pigmented lesions and tattoos.
- Picosecond (PS) lasers are the newest additions with current studies suggesting a superior efficacy and safety profile for treating pigmented lesions and tattoos compared with nanosecond domain quality-switched (QS) lasers.
- The pigment-specific lasers most commonly used for benign pigmented lesions and tattoos include the PS alexandrite 755 nm, PS Nd:YAG 532 nm, QS ruby 694 nm, QS alexandrite 755 nm and QS Nd:YAG (532 nm and 1064 nm).
- PS lasers are now considered to be the laser of choice for tattoo removal and for Nevus of Ota/Ito lesions.
- Fractional photothermolysis is often optimal for treating diffuse skin pigmentation in photodamaged skin as the entire cosmetic subunits can be treated although multiple treatments are often needed and there are greater associated adverse effects.
- Patients with Fitzpatrick skin types I to III generally have the best outcomes compared to darker skinned

patients. Caution should be taken in patients with Fitzpatrick skin types IV to VI due to risk of postinflammatory dyspigmentation.
- Black tattoos respond the best to laser therapy, while multi-colored tattoos are often more difficult to treat.
- Caution should be taken when utilizing QS or PS lasers to treated cosmetic tattoos containing white or red ink due to the risk of paradoxical darkening. Test spots should be performed prior to treatment.
- Proper patient and lesion selection and evaluation is crucial prior to performing laser therapy for optimal outcomes. Informed consent and pre-procedural photographs should always be obtained prior to initiating therapy.
- Adverse effects of laser therapy of pigmented lesions and tattoos include hypopigmentation, hyperpigmentation, textural change, and scarring.
- Postoperative care following laser therapy includes gentle cleansing, the use of a bland emollient and strict sun protection.

INTRODUCTION

Advances in laser technology over the last two decades have led to greater efficacy and safety for the treatment of a variety of medical and cosmetic indications including benign pigmented lesions and tattoo removal.

Tattooing is an increasingly popular practice. Based on a survey conducted in 2015, 29% of the United States adults have at least one tattoo, an increase of 8% from

4 years earlier, and nearly half of millennials report having at least one tattoo. However, data demonstrates that almost 25% of people with tattoos regret getting them.

In this chapter, we will discuss the use of laser therapy to treat benign pigmented lesions and tattoos, including important patient considerations, recommendations for optimizing outcomes, and postoperative care. While the target of both lesions is pigment, the techniques utilized to lighten and/or remove these lesions are distinct.

25

PRINCIPLES OF PIGMENT REMOVAL WITH LASER THERAPY

Early lasers (including the argon and CO_2 lasers) used for treatment of pigmented lesions and tattoo removal were not pigment-specific and often associated with significant side effects such as dyspigmentation and scarring. In 1980 Drs. Anderson and Parrish first described the theory of selective photothermolysis, which led to a paradigm shift in laser therapy. According to this theory, use of the appropriate wavelength can allow light energy to be preferentially absorbed by a specific chromophore within the skin (i.e., melanin, tattoo ink particles) and transferred into heat energy. Different chromophores within the skin preferentially absorb specific wavelengths of light. In the case of benign pigmented lesions, the chromophore is melanin within melanocytes, keratinocytes, or dermal macrophages. In tattoos, the target chromophore is exogenously placed ink found within macrophages or extracellularly throughout the dermis. Selection of a laser with a wavelength of light that is preferentially absorbed by a certain chromophore and penetrates to the appropriate depth allows for the selective heating and destruction of the targeted chromophore.

While the wavelength will selectively target a specific chromophore, the pulse duration, or the time that the laser is fired, is also important to limit the damage to the chromophore and surrounding tissue. The pulse duration should ideally be less than or equal to the target chromophore's thermal relaxation time (TRT), or the time required for the target to lose 50% of heat to the surrounding tissue. If the pulse duration exceeds the TRT, the heat will likely spread to the surrounding tissue, causing damage that can lead to adverse effects including scarring. Therefore, selection of the appropriate wavelength and pulse duration allows for target destruction of a specific chromophore with minimal damage to surrounding structures. Melanosomes containing melanin are small structures, about 0.5 micrometers in diameter and, therefore, have very short TRTs, estimated to be approximately 250–1000 nanoseconds. Lasers with extremely short pulse durations in the nanosecond (NS) or picosecond (PS) range are ideal to target this chromophore. Quality switched or "Q-switched" (QS) lasers emit pulses in the NS range, and PS lasers emit pulses in the PS range. In tattoos, the exogenous pigment particles are much smaller than melanosomes with correspondingly smaller TRTs.

Therefore, while both QS lasers with pulse durations in the NS domain and PS lasers can be used, PS lasers provide a pulse duration with a better match to the TRT of the tattoo particles. Ho and colleagues found a pulse duration range of 10–100 PS allows for effective pigment destruction and clearance with little collateral damage to surrounding tissue. QS lasers produce rapid, pulsed bursts of energy in the NS range having both photothermal and photoacoustic effects to aid in breaking up of the pigment particles. PS lasers deliver ultrashort bursts of energy in the PS range, creating a rapid rise in temperature that results in a greater photomechanical effect with fragmentation of pigment particles. The rupture of pigment-containing cells triggers phagocytosis and the removal of pigment fragments via lymphatic drainage and scavenging by dermal macrophages. Unique histologic findings have been observed with the use of newer handpieces that fractionate the PS laser energy which may help to explain the added benefits for photorejuvenation, wrinkles and acne scars (discussed below). Tanghetti identified vacuoles, referred to as laser-induced optical breakdown (LIOB), through histologic and confocal imaging following PS laser treatment with a fractional lens array handpiece and believed these vacuoles to be responsible for stimulating repair mechanisms.

Over the past two decades, QS lasers have been the mainstay for treatment of pigmented lesions and tattoos. QS lasers used for pigmented lesions include the QS 694 nm ruby, the QS 755 nm alexandrite, and the QS Nd:YAG at 532 and 1064 nm. Melanin has a broad absorption spectrum throughout the ultraviolet, visible and near-infrared light range. Optimal wavelengths used to treat pigmented lesions would be those that are preferentially absorbed by melanin over oxyhemoglobin, another chromophore within the skin, and reach the targeted depth. Notably, absorption for melanin decreases and depth of penetration increases as the wavelength increases. Therefore, superficial pigmented lesions can be effectively treated with shorter wavelengths, while longer wavelengths are used for lesions with pigment deeper in the dermis. Longer wavelengths are also preferentially used in patients of darker skin types to decrease risk of post-procedural dyschromia as they have less epidermal damage. Likewise, for tattoos, given the location of the ink particles within the dermis, longer wavelengths are often preferred, although the appropriate wavelength also depends on the ink particle color.

Shorter wavelength long-pulsed lasers (millisecond domain) including the potassium-titanyl-phosphate (KTP) (532 nm) and the pulsed-dye laser (PDL) (585–595 nm) can also be used for superficial pigmented lesions because of their melanin absorption. They deliver laser energy over a longer pulse duration, in the millisecond range, with the same wavelengths as their QS counterparts. While the longer pulse duration may cause unacceptable nonselective thermal damage to deeper structures, they may be safely used for epidermal pigmented lesions. Longer wavelength long-pulsed lasers (millisecond domain) including ruby, alexandrite, and Nd:YAG lasers may also be used to treat larger pigmented targets in the dermis such as hair. Epidermal cooling is essential with these devices in order to protect the epidermis and dermal epidermal junction. One should not employ a millisecond domain long-pulsed laser to treat dermal pigment such as nevus of Ota or tattoo pigment.

In 2012, the US Food and Drug Administration (FDA) approved the use of the PS alexandrite laser for laser tattoo removal and the treatment of benign pigmented lesions. PS lasers have recently emerged as an even more targeted method of treating these lesions in comparison to the traditional NS domain QS lasers. The PS lasers with their incredibly short pulse duration, have a greater photomechanical effect as opposed to a photothermal effect within treated tissue, limiting collateral thermal damage to surrounding tissue. This is thought to allow for more efficient removal of pigment particles with decreased risk of post-procedural dyspigmentation. There is growing evidence that fewer treatments are required to achieve tattoo clearance with the PS lasers than with QS lasers. In addition, lower energies are used which help decrease the risk of epidermal and dermal-epidermal junction injury. Since the approval of the PS 755 nm alexandrite laser, a PS Nd:YAG (1064 nm and frequency-doubled 532 nm) has also been made available for commercial use. These new wavelengths allow for the treatment of the full spectrum of tattoo colors as well as a variety of epidermal and dermal pigmented lesions and are often the laser of choice for treating solar lentigines, melasma, dermal melanocytoses, amongst other pigmented lesions. PS lasers have been shown to be safe when used in patients with skin types III to VI; however, there remains a risk of post-procedural hypopigmentation and rebound hyperpigmentation with treatment,

so caution should be taken whenever treating patients with darker skin types.

Recently, a variety of innovative optical attachments for PS lasers including the diffractive lens array (DLA) and the holographic microlens array (MLA) have been introduced that fractionate the laser beam by redistributing energy into multiple tiny high-density high fluence fractionated zones. These zones account for about 10% of the total treatment area, ensuring a significant safety profile. The DLA is often used for improving dyspigmentation (including melasma), skin texture, and fine wrinkles and is currently FDA approved for the treatment of fine wrinkles and acne scars. Similarly, the MLA has demonstrated efficacy for the treatment of fine wrinkles, atrophic acne scars, and rejuvenation based on recent studies.

Nonselective lasers can also be used to treat pigmented lesions. These include fully ablative lasers such as the 10,600 nm carbon dioxide (CO_2) laser, the 2940 nm erbium:yttrium-aluminum-garnet (Er:YAG) laser, and the 2740 nm yttrium-scandium-gallium-garnet (YSGG) laser. These lasers ablate or damage the epidermis and secondarily remove pigmented epidermal processes with the removal of epidermal melanocytes. While treatment with these lasers can produce excellent results, fully ablative laser resurfacing is often operator and technique dependent and the risk of postprocedural adverse effects including erythema, infection, dyspigmentation and scarring is higher than that of nonablative laser modalities. The 2940 nm Er:YAG laser has a greater absorption coefficient for water resulting in more superficial epidermal damage; therefore, leading to a better safety profile and shorter downtime than that associated with the CO_2 laser.

Fractional lasers (both ablative and nonablative) have also been used for the treatment of various pigmented lesions. Fractional photothermolysis, originally introduced in 2004 by Manstein and Anderson, involves the fractional emission of infrared light into microscopic treatment zones (MTZ) creating small columns of focal thermal injury within the skin. Each MTZ is surrounded by normal, undamaged tissue. Within each MTZ there is epidermal and dermal damage that stimulates collagen production and elastin formation. The degenerated dermal material results in the formation of microscopic epidermal necrotic debris (MENDs), which is then exfoliated. MENDs appear to serve as the transport medium for epidermal and dermal pigment across the epidermis, allowing for localized, controlled melanin release following fractional photothermolysis. Due to the presence of surrounding undamaged tissue that can aid in healing of the MTZ, there is a shorter associated downtime and decreased risk of adverse events compared to traditional ablative laser resurfacing. However, given the smaller degree (or percentage of surface area) of injury, a greater number of treatments are often required to achieve the desired results. Fractional photothermolysis has increasingly been used to treat a variety of pigmented conditions including melasma, solar lentigines, nevus of Ota, and postinflammatory hyperpigmentation (PIH). While fractional photothermolysis has shown benefit for many of these conditions, caution must be taken for deeper, dermal pigmentary processes due to the potential risk for rebound or worsening hyperpigmentation following treatment, especially in patients with darker skin types.

Intense pulse light (IPL) is a light-based device that emits filtered polychromatic light with wavelengths ranging from visible to near infrared (500–1200 nm), and therefore can also be used successfully to treat a variety of superficial benign pigmented lesions. These devices have pulse durations in the millisecond domain and therefore should be used with caution in patients with darker skin types due to increased risk of post-procedural pigmentary alterations and should not be used for tattoo removal due to increased risk of scarring. As these devices are not true lasers, they will not be discussed further in this chapter.

⏵   Check online Video 3.1

PREOPERATIVE CONSIDERATIONS

Patient Evaluation and Selection

Prior to treatment of any pigmented lesion, it is important to obtain a thorough and detailed medical history including current medical conditions, allergies to anesthetics, and a current list of medications. If a patient is currently taking isotretinoin, laser therapy (especially those involving tissue ablation) should be delayed until the course of treatment has been completed due to potential risk of increased scarring and delayed wound healing. A history of isotretinoin use in the past 6 months, poor wound healing, PIH, keloid formation or bleeding diathesis would require caution during treatment due

to the increased risk of prolonged recovery or scarring in any of these settings. A history of prior gold or silver use should be elucidated, as treatment with QS or PS lasers is contraindicated in this setting given the risk of chrysiasis—immediate and often irreversible darkening of gold-containing skin. Antiviral prophylaxis is appropriate in patients with a history of herpes simplex virus if treating near an outbreak site, especially if using ablative resurfacing lasers. A personal and/or family history of dysplastic nevi or melanoma should also raise caution prior to treatment of any pigmented lesion.

It is important to consider the patient's skin type when treating pigmented lesions with laser devices. Patients should not be tanned when treated. Patients with darker skin types may be at increased risk of complications, particularly posttreatment dyschromia, and should be counseled appropriately. Lower fluences and longer wavelengths are preferred in patients with darker skin types to decrease the risk of subsequent hypo- and hyperpigmentation. In patients with darker skin types, pretreatment with hydroquinone 4% cream to hyperpigmented areas for 1 month and ceasing treatment 1 week prior to laser therapy is recommended. Topical corticosteroids for 3–4 days posttreatment can be used to prevent any pigmentary alteration secondary to the treatment-induced inflammation.

Realistic expectations regarding number of treatment sessions and treatment outcomes should also be established. Solar lentigines can often be successfully treated with just a few treatments; however, other pigmented lesions, like melasma, PIH, and nevus of Ota and Ito tend to be more difficult to treat, requiring multiple treatments and are associated with higher risks of incomplete clearance and rebound hyperpigmentation. Prior to tattoo removal, Kirby and colleagues published a scale to help physicians approximate the number of treatment sessions required for tattoo removal to help guide patients through the treatment process. Based on the scale, numerical values are assigned to six parameters: (1) Fitzpatrick skin type, (2) tattoo location, (3) tattoo color, (4) amount of ink in the tattoo, (5) scarring or tissue change, and (6) ink layering. The sum of the points for each parameter equate to the number of treatment sessions needed to successfully remove the tattoo, plus or minus 2.5. For patients seeking tattoo removal, it is also important to alert the patient that some tattoo pigment may remain after treatment and that hypopigmentation may occur in the treated area, creating a negative image of the original tattoo. Patients with skin types IV to VI and patients with a tan are at particularly increased risk for this outcome. The ideal patient for tattoo removal is an untanned patient with skin type I or II with a dark blue or black tattoo present for at least 1 year. Patients should be appropriately counseled regarding potential complications and adverse effects associated with treatment including post-procedural dyspigmentation, erythema, textural changes, and scarring. Pre-procedural photographs should be obtained prior to initiating therapy so that progress may be monitored during treatment.

TABLE 3.1	Pigment Sources for Various Tattoo Colors
Tattoo Color	**Pigment Source**
Black	Iron oxide, carbon, india ink, lead, gunpowder
Blue	Cobalt
Green	Chromium oxide, malachite green
Violet	Manganese violet
Yellow	Cadmium sulfide, ochre
Red	Mercuric sulfide (cinnabar), azo dyes, cadmium selenide, sienna
White	Titanium dioxide, zinc oxide
Brown	Ochre

PEARL 1

Prior to use of a QS or PS laser, a history of gold or silver use should be elucidated, as treatment with QS or PS lasers is contraindicated in this setting given the risk of chrysiasis—immediate and often irreversible darkening of gold-containing skin.

Lesion Selection

Appropriate evaluation of the lesion to be treated is just as important as the patient evaluation. Evaluation of a pigmented lesion using a Wood's lamp may be helpful to determine the depth of the pigment (i.e., epidermal, dermal, or mixed), as this will guide laser selection and provide implications for treatment outcomes. Prior to treatment of any pigmented lesion, it is critical that the lesion be accurately diagnosed. If any question or doubt exists regarding the nature of the lesion, a biopsy should be performed to confirm the diagnosis and to evaluate for and rule out malignancy. Lasers should never be used to treat any lesion concerning for melanoma or melanoma in situ. Additionally, the removal of dysplastic nevi with laser therapy is not recommended, despite studies showing no evidence of malignant transformation in laser-treated nevi.

Prior to treating any tattoo with a laser device, it is important to classify the tattoo as different types of tattoos have implications for the appropriate laser device as well as the number of treatments required. Tattoos can be classified as amateur, professional, cosmetic, medical, or traumatic. Amateur tattoos often contain lower concentrations of pigment and are located in various levels of the dermis. Professional tattoos generally contain dense pigment at the junction of the papillary and reticular dermis. Amateur tattoos typically contain pigment of unknown sources including ash, coal, or india ink, while professional tattoos are often composed of several ink pigments mixed together to create unique colors and shading. Commonly used pigments include cinnabar and cadmium red (red), cadmium sulfide (yellow), chromium salts (green), cobalt salts (dark blue), titanium dioxide (white), and iron oxide (red-brown or rust-colored) (Table 3.1). Professional tattoos are often more difficult to remove with laser therapy due to the deeper and denser placement of the pigment and greater number of ink colors mixed together. Therefore, multiple laser modalities and several treatment sessions may be required for optimal clearance. Cosmetic tattoos, created using skin-colored tones typically contain iron oxide or titanium dioxide, are important to distinguish because of the unique risk of paradoxical darkening after QS or PS laser treatment (discussed below). Medical tattoos like those used as radiation markers are also important to distinguish. Traumatic tattoos are those that occur following a trauma or injury. It is important to understand the nature of the injury, so that the type of material implanted into the skin can be identified prior to laser therapy. Treatment of traumatic tattoos caused by fireworks with QS or PS lasers is contraindicated due to the rare risk of microexplosions of the remaining particles upon laser impact leading to cavitation and potentially atrophic scarring.

In addition to identifying the type of tattoo, it is essential to evaluate the ink colors within the tattoo, as there are optimal wavelengths for different tattoo ink colors (Table 3.2). Depending on the colors within a

TABLE 3.2   Optimal Laser and Wavelength for Specific Tattoo Colors

Laser and Wavelength	Black	Blue	Red	Green	Yellow
QS 694 nm ruby	X	X		X	
QS 1064 nm Nd:YAG	X	X		X	
QS 650 nm Nd:YAG				X	
QS and PS 755 nm alexandrite	X	X		X	
QS and PS 532 nm Nd:YAG			X		X

tattoo, several devices with different wavelengths may be required to effectively treat the entire tattoo. Additional aspects that are important to consider include size and age of the tattoo. Smaller tattoos will typically require fewer treatment sessions to achieve clinical improvement. Older tattoos often require fewer treatments due to a degree of ink migration and clearance via lymphatics that has already occurred over time. Treatment should be delayed in the setting of inflamed tattoos, the presence of overlying infection or a concomitant active dermatologic disorder. Treatment in these situations may worsen the underlying condition, resulting in slow postoperative healing or increasing the risk of scarring.

Laser Safety

Ocular safety is a primary concern with the use of all laser systems, including pigment-specific lasers, due to the risk of iris and retinal injury. Laser light in the visible to near infrared spectrum (400–1400 nm) are part of the "retinal hazard region" and all personnel in the room during treatment must wear protective goggles. Regardless of the location on the body being treated, the patient should be given fully protective wrap-around goggles with the appropriate optical density and wavelength ranges of protection for the given laser wavelength to be worn throughout the entirety of the procedure. Laser aids, disposable adhesive eye protectors, can alternatively be utilized during treatment with nonselective, nonablative fractional lasers, which cover predominantly the upper eyelid while allowing access to the brow and infraorbital region. Additional precautions must be taken if treatment of the periorbital area near the eyelid margins or on the eyelid itself is anticipated. In these settings, a metal corneoscleral protective lens shield must be placed prior to treatment and all pulses should be fired in a direction away from the eye. It is important to note that ocular protection devices do not eliminate risk of injury. A recent review reported that eye injury occurred in 33% of cases in which eye protection including metal corneal shields were provided, likely associated with overheating of the metal corneal shields during the procedure. Therefore, other preventative measures including pulling the infraorbital skin away from the orbit during treatment and directing the laser away from the eye should also be employed to minimize complication risk. In addition, sufficient cooling of the treated area between pulses should be ensured during treatment to prevent overheating of the metal corneal shields and subsequent thermal injury.

Additionally, reflective surfaces and windows should be covered and access to the procedure room should be limited during treatment. Potentially flammable materials should be removed. Since QS and PS lasers may cause some tissue and blood splatter, protective plastic cones attached to the handpiece can be used to protect against any potential splatter.

PEARL 2

Ocular safety is paramount for all personnel and patients in the room during laser therapy given QS and PS lasers can cause permanent retinal damage with vision loss without proper eye protection. The laser goggles used must have lenses with an optical density (OD) that block the specific wavelength being used. The lenses should provide an OD of at least 6.

Patient Preparation

The area to be treated should be thoroughly cleaned and free of any make-up, personal care products or topical anesthetics, as these products can cause scatter of the light energy and prevent optimal delivery of the laser energy to the target. Additionally, various topical products remaining on the skin surface may contain ingredients with the potential to ignite when combined with the laser energy. If alcohol is used to clean the treatment area, it must be completely dried and no longer present prior to treatment.

Typically, laser devices utilized for the treatment of pigmented lesions are well-tolerated and neither infiltrative nor topical anesthesia is required. However, the location, size and depth of the lesion as well as the individual patient's pain threshold should be taken into account when determining the need for pre-procedural anesthesia. Removal of pigmented lesions and tattoos can be quite painful, especially if a large treatment area is anticipated. In the authors' practices, neither topical nor infiltrative anesthesia is routinely used for the treatment of lentigines and photodamage with QS or PS lasers. Local anesthesia is recommended prior to the treatment of larger tattoos or lesions with significant amounts of dermal pigment, or when ablative or nonablative fractional lasers are used. Compounded topical anesthesia offers a highly effective vehicle for pain management. Commonly used formulations include BLT (betacaine, lidocaine, and tetracaine at 7% concentrations), commercial preparations, such as LMX-4 or EMLA, 30% topical lidocaine, or mixture of 23% lidocaine/7% tetracaine. A thin layer of product is spread evenly over the treatment area and left in place for 45–60 minutes. Occlusion or the application of warm towels over the area can be used with lower-strength topical formulations to enhance the penetration of the anesthetic. However, extreme caution should be taken if the area

is large, or if more potent (higher concentration) formulations are used as topical anesthetics can produce systemic toxicity. The applied anesthetic should always be completely removed prior to treatment. For medium and large tattoos, the area is often injected with 1% lidocaine with epinephrine.

Prior to treatment informed consent must be obtained after a thorough discussion of the procedure and its associated potential adverse effects. Preprocedural photographs should be obtained prior to initiating therapy so that progress may be monitored during treatment.

TREATMENT TECHNIQUES

Basic Principles

When using an NS or PS laser for the treatment of pigmented lesions or tattoos, the initial desired endpoint is immediate tissue whitening or graying, which reflects cavitation of melanin or pigment particles and heat-induced gas bubble formation. The gas bubbles scatter visible light creating a white color, which may be less vivid after treatment of dermal pigmented lesions. The immediate skin whitening blocks most light from penetrating through it and gradually resolves over 20–30 minutes leaving mild residual erythema. If immediate tissue whitening is not observed following laser therapy, the laser exposure or treatment settings (i.e., laser fluence) were likely not sufficient for effective clearing of the treated pigmented lesion. At fluences below threshold, paradoxical hyperpigmentation may occur due to stimulation of melanocytes. At fluences above threshold, thermal burns with tissue sloughing, prolonged wound healing, hypopigmentation, hyperpigmentation, textural changes, and scarring can result.

Darker skin has a lower threshold for tissue whitening and a greater risk of dyschromia following laser therapy. Therefore test spots with lower fluences in darker skinned patients are recommended prior to treatment of pigmented lesions or tattoos to evaluate for hypopigmentation and hyperpigmentation. Treatments are typically performed at 4- to 6-week intervals or 6- to 8-week intervals for pigmented lesions and tattoos, respectively, although shorter intervals depending on the lesion treated may be effective. The number of treatment sessions required varies based on the lesion to be treated.

Benign Pigmented Lesions

Pigmented lesions may vary in the amount, depth, and density of melanin distribution. These variations can affect the efficacy of certain laser devices and response to treatment. Lesions can be classified based on the distribution of melanin within the epidermis or dermis, which is important to consider when selecting the appropriate laser modality for treatment.

Epidermal Lesions

Epidermal lesions contain pigment primarily within the epidermis. In addition to NS and PS lasers that specifically target pigment, any modality that damages or removes the epidermis such as the ablative CO_2 or Er:YAG lasers will lead to removal or improvement of these lesions. Fractional laser resurfacing, both ablative and nonablative, has also been shown to improve epidermal processes (i.e., photodamage, lentigines).

Lentigo Simplex, Solar Lentigines, Ephelides. Lentigo simplex is an evenly pigmented, tan to brown macule that can occur on both cutaneous and mucosal surfaces. These lesions are not associated with sun exposure and often occur in children. They can also occur in the setting of specific syndromes including LEOPARD syndrome, Carney complex, Peutz-Jeghers syndrome, and Laugier-Hunziker syndrome. Solar lentigines present as tan macules or patches often on the face, shoulders, dorsal forearms and hands of adults in the setting of chronic sun exposure. Ephelides, or freckles, are tan to brown macules occurring on sun-exposed sites and often present early in childhood. These lesions are most prominent during the summer months and fade during the winter months. While physical modalities including chemical peels and cryotherapy treatments are used in clinical practice, laser therapy has been shown to be more effective than both of these modalities. Any laser that damages the epidermis will lead to improvement in epidermal pigmented lesions with one or two treatment sessions. The mainstay lasers for these lesions are pigment-selective QS or PS lasers including the QS or PS 755 nm alexandrite, QS or PS 532 nm Nd:YAG, and QS 694 nm ruby lasers. Millisecond domain lasers and IPL devices can also be very effective in removing epidermal pigmented lesions.

NS domain QS lasers have been used to treat pigmented epidermal lesions for decades. Lasers with shorter wavelengths appear to more effectively treat epidermal lesions due to their high absorption of melanin. The QS 532 nm Nd:YAG, the QS 694 nm ruby laser, and the QS 755 nm alexandrite laser have consistently demonstrated efficacy in treating solar lentigines and lentigo simplex (Fig. 3.1). While studies are more limited when evaluating the use of these devices for ephelides, the QS 755 nm alexandrite and QS 532 nm Nd:YAG lasers have demonstrated efficacy for these lesions with only one to three treatment sessions required. However, treatment outcomes for ephelides tend to be unpredictable. QS lasers have been shown to be relatively safe in most patients, although, there may be a slightly increased risk of PIH, especially in patients with darker skin types.

PS lasers have relatively greater photomechanical effects as opposed to the purely photothermal effects of NS domain lasers, resulting in lower energy fluences and reduced number of treatment sessions required compared to NS laser for similar clinical outcomes and possibly better safety profiles. Through histologic evaluation of laser treated skin, Negishi and colleagues observed destroyed melanosomes with surrounding structural damage after QS Nd:YAG laser treatment, whereas no surrounding structural damage was observed in PS laser treated skin samples. These same investigators treated 20 Asian females (skin types III–IV) with the 532 nm frequency-doubled PS Nd:YAG laser for lentigines and observed 93% of lesions achieved over 75% clearance after a single treatment. PIH was observed in only 4.65% of subjects. Similar studies have demonstrated low rates of postprocedural dyschromia (0.8%) following PS laser therapy. In a retrospective review, Levin and colleagues compared the safety and efficacy of the QS 694 nm ruby and the QS (532 and 1064 nm) Nd:YAG lasers with the PS 755 nm alexandrite for the treatment of pigmentary disorders including solar lentigines in patients with skin of color. All eight patients treated with the PS laser achieved 50% clearance and all associated adverse effects were mild and transient. Permanent dyspigmentation was noted in several subjects that underwent QS NS laser treatments. The PS alexandrite laser with the DLA has also demonstrated efficacy and safety, most notably for photoaging and solar lentigines, even when shorter treatment intervals were used (Fig. 3.2). Novel PS lasers including the 730 and 785 nm PS lasers have similarly demonstrated efficacy for epidermal pigmented lesions,

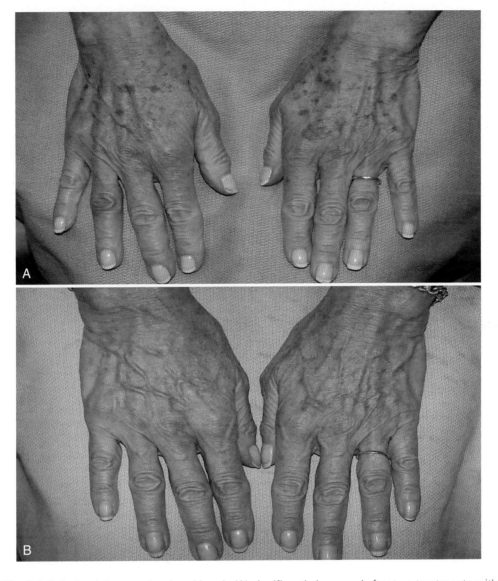

Fig. 3.1 Solar lentigines on the dorsal hands (A) significantly improved after two treatments with the 532 nm Q-switched device (B).

although studies are limited, and these devices are not yet widely available.

Long-pulsed lasers including the long-pulsed 755 nm alexandrite, long-pulsed PDL, long-pulsed 532 nm Nd:YAG, have also been used to effectively treat epidermal pigmented lesions and are proposed to be safe even in patients with skin of color. In a comparative study, Chan and colleagues utilized QS and long-pulsed 532 nm Nd:YAG lasers for treating lentigines in Asian skin, with both modalities demonstrating similar efficacy. However, treatment with QS lasers was associated with a significantly higher risk of PIH compared to long-pulsed lasers. Similarly, Ho and colleagues found no statistically significant difference in the efficacy of QS

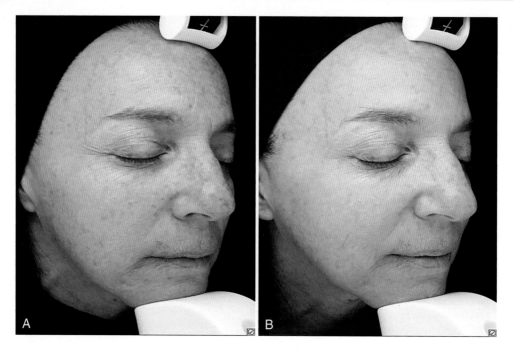

Fig. 3.2 Solar lentigines and photodamage of the face seen at baseline (A) and 1 month after four treatments with the 755 nm picosecond device (B).

compared to the long-pulsed alexandrite laser, although PIH was found to be higher in Asian skin after QS laser therapy (22% for QS vs. 6% for long pulsed).

Fractional photothermolysis can be considered for these conditions if lesions are widespread, as in the case of photodamage. Ablative fractional resurfacing has demonstrated significant improvement in solar lentigines and photodamage. However, the significant clinical improvement comes with a greater risk of adverse effects and a longer downtime when compared to fractional nonablative resurfacing or pigment-selective laser therapy. The nonablative 1550 nm fractional erbium-doped fiber laser and the 1927 nm thulium fiber laser have both demonstrated efficacy in improving pigmented epidermal lesions and photodamage. The 1927 nm thulium fiber laser has a 10 times greater absorption coefficient for water and is therefore absorbed more superficially and has a greater ability to target epidermal processes. In 2010, consensus recommendations were established for the use of the 1550 nm fractional nonablative laser. The panel recommended three to five treatment sessions at 1-month intervals using fluences of 10–20 mJ and treatment levels of 7–11 for lighter skin and 4–7 for darker

skin. In general, fractional nonablative laser resurfacing can lead to significant improvement in pigmented epidermal lesions with a shorter downtime and decreased risk of adverse effects when compared to ablative laser resurfacing. However, multiple treatments are typically required for optimal outcomes. There are limited studies on the use of fractional photothermolysis for the treatment of ephelides.

Overall, solar lentigines appear to be very effectively treated with millisecond, NS, and PS lasers, often only requiring one or two treatment sessions. These devices are typically preferred for significant, larger, and discrete lentigines. Darker lesions have more target for absorption and have greater clearance and lower fluences can be used with shorter pulse durations and no cryogen cooling. Recent studies suggest that PS lasers may be a safer alternative, especially in darker skinned patients. When treating multiple lesions or large areas, treating a full cosmetic unit with a fractionated laser is often beneficial. In clinical practice, lesions that achieve complete clearance with treatment rarely recur, although, new lesions may appear, and partially treated lesions may darken after UV exposure. Counseling the patient on diligent sun protection and proper skin care following the procedure are important for optimal long-term results.

Labial Melanotic Macules. Melanotic macules of the vermilion lip are most commonly seen in young women, but can also be seen as a feature of physiologic racial pigmentation, Carney complex, Peutz-Jeghers syndrome, and Laugier-Hunziker syndrome. As these lesions are superficial, they can be effectively treated using all of the devices listed in the preceding section including the QS 694 nm ruby laser, QS or PS 755 nm alexandrite laser, and the frequency-doubled 532 nm QS or PS Nd:YAG laser (Fig. 3.3). In the setting of an associated underlying syndrome patients should be counseled that new lesions may develop over time requiring additional treatments.

Café-au-lait Macules and Nevus Spilus. Café-au-lait macules (CALMs) are tan evenly pigmented patches found in about 10%–28% of the general population. Nevus spilus are benign, congenital lesions that can resemble CALMs except that darker brown to blue macules or papules occur within the tan patch. Prior to treatment, a thorough physical exam and history should be obtained to rule out underlying neurofibromatosis, especially if multiple CALMs are present. Lasers described to treat these lesions include the QS and PS 532 nm Nd:YAG, QS 694 nm ruby laser, QS and PS 755 nm alexandrite lasers. Ablative and nonablative fractional resurfacing lasers have also been used.

While multiple studies have demonstrated efficacy of QS lasers in achieving clinical improvement of CALMs and nevus spilus, clinical results are variable and there is significant risk of repigmentation, often spotty in nature. A recent retrospective study however did demonstrate success of the QS 755 nm alexandrite for the treatment of CALMs with 54% of 48 patient achieving good to excellent results and recurrence rate of only 10.4%. Similarly, Kagami and colleagues observed greater than 50% clearance in 32.1% of 28 Japanese patients with CALMs and nevus spilus after at least one treatment with the QS 755 nm alexandrite laser.

PS lasers have also shown improvement in CALMs and nevus spilus with a potentially more favorable risk profile than QS lasers. Specifically, the PS 532 nm Nd:YAG was shown to have superior clearance rates and fewer adverse effects when compared to QS lasers as none of the 16 treated patients in a recent study experienced post-procedural dyspigmentation. The recurrence rate in the study was also relatively low. Additional studies evaluating the PS 532 nm Nd:YAG laser and the PS 755 nm alexandrite laser have similarly demonstrated significant improvement in treated lesions after one to seven treatment sessions with minimal adverse events and no recurrences within the specified follow-up period (about 6 months).

Ablative and nonablative fractional resurfacing lasers have also been used for the treatment of CALMs, typically in the setting of recalcitrant lesions. Successful

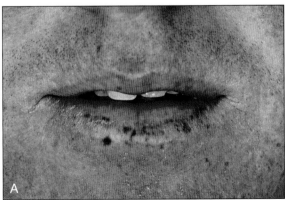 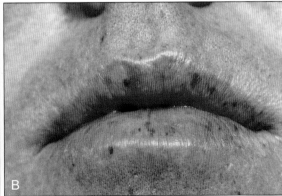

Fig. 3.3 Multiple small lentigines of the mucosal lip vermilion seen with Peutz-Jeghers syndrome seen (A) preoperatively and (B) 6 weeks after three treatments with the Q-switched ruby laser, showing excellent fading without scarring.

treatment of recalcitrant CALMs has been reported utilizing the 2940 nm Er:YAG and the 1927 nm fractional thulium-doped fiber laser.

Overall responses to laser therapy have been variable across studies with incomplete pigment removal, residual spotty hyperpigmentation, and recurrence being commonly observed. Patients with darker skin types are at particularly increased risk for PIH and hypopigmentation, which can be very problematic. Lighter skin patients are better candidates for CALM treatment because of a lower risk of post-procedural dyspigmentation. Interestingly, according to a recent study, CALM morphology appears to influence response to laser therapy. CALMs with jagged edges, referred to as "Coast of Maine," appear to have a better response to laser treatment compared to lesions with smooth borders, referred to as "Coast of California". As emphasized earlier, patients must be made aware of all potential risks prior to treatment and appropriate expectations should be managed. Treatment sessions are spaced at least 8 weeks apart and clearance typically requires at least two to four treatment sessions.

Seborrheic Keratoses and Dermatosis Papulosa Nigra. Seborrheic keratoses are benign lesions that often present as tan to brown to black, waxy, stuck-on appearing papules or plaques mainly on the trunk and extremities of adults and typically increase in number over time. Dermatosis papulosa nigra are considered variants of SKs that occur in darker skinned patients, especially on the face in the periorbital area. While these lesions are benign, they are often cosmetically bothersome to patients, prompting them to seek treatment. Nonselective laser modalities that destroy the epidermis including the ablative CO_2 laser and Er:YAG lasers, a 532 nm diode laser, and nonablative fractional lasers have all been shown to be safe and effective in the treatment of SKs and DPNs with low rates of recurrence. In addition, pigment-selective lasers including the long-pulsed 755 nm alexandrite laser, the long-pulsed 1064 nm Nd:YAG, 532 nm KTP laser, and various QS lasers have also been shown to improve these lesions. Limited studies have suggested efficacy of PS lasers in the treatment of seborrheic keratoses and dermatosis papulosa nigra. Unfortunately, as these lesions are often thick and do not always contain melanin, clinical results with these lasers have been extremely variable and generally disappointing.

It is important to recognize that given dermatosis papulosa nigra typically occur in patients with darker skin types, caution must be taken when utilizing laser therapy for the treatment of these lesions given the risk of post-procedural dyspigmentation in this patient population. Selection of the proper laser modality, use of the appropriate treatment settings, and using test-spots will help minimize risk.

Dermoepidermal Lesions

Dermoepidermal lesions contain pigment within both the epidermis and dermis. Examples of commonly treated dermoepidermal lesions include Becker's nevus, melasma, PIH, drug-induced hyperpigmentation and melanocytic nevi. Laser devices with both shorter and longer wavelengths or a combination of resurfacing lasers and pigment-specific lasers have been utilized to target the pigment in the superficial and deep locations within the tissue.

Becker Melanosis (Nevus). Becker melanosis or Becker's nevus is a unilateral, hyperpigmented and often hypertrichotic patch or slightly elevated plaque most commonly on the shoulder of males with onset in adolescence. Laser therapy has been reported to be effective in treating both the pigmented portion of the lesion as well as the overlying hypertrichosis. The pigmented areas of a Becker's nevus have shown improvement with the PS 755 nm alexandrite, QS 694 nm ruby laser, QS Nd:YAG laser, the 1550 nm erbium-doped fiber laser, and the 2940 nm Er:YAG laser. However, according to a recent multicenter retrospective study evaluating laser treatment of epidermal nevi, QS lasers failed to show any degree of improvement in almost all patients with Becker's nevi. Additionally, although the risk profile is much higher, studies have demonstrated superior efficacy of ablative laser resurfacing over QS laser therapy. The terminal hairs within the lesion can be removed with hair removal lasers using long-pulse durations. While ablative and nonablative laser resurfacing may be superior for the pigmented areas of Becker's nevi, these modalities are not beneficial for treating any overlying hypertrichosis and have a significant risk of scarring and postprocedural dyspigmentation. Regardless of device used, lightening is often incomplete and patchy and most avoid treatment of these lesions with lasers.

Melanocytic Nevi. Melanocytic nevi are pink to tan to brown macules or papules that may be congenital, appear near or at birth, or acquired during childhood or puberty. Controversy exists over the use of laser therapy for the treatment of melanocytic nevi; and the risk of malignant transformation after laser therapy, while theoretically extremely low, remains difficult to prove. Overall, surgical excision is the treatment of choice for complete removal of melanocytic nevi and laser therapy is reserved for use in very large nevi which cannot be excised and those in cosmetically sensitive areas which have been shown to be benign.

In vitro studies of melanoma cells treated with QS lasers have revealed changes in cell surface integrin expression with associated alteration in cell migration. Another in vitro study found a significant increase in p16INK4a in p16-positive cell lines following treatment with a QS laser and suggested that DNA damage secondary to sublethal laser exposure may lead to increased p16 expression. Additionally, recurrence of benign-appearing nevi following laser therapy demonstrating new clinical and histological atypia, referred to as pseudomelanoma, has been reported. However, no markers for malignant transformation have been seen and there has never been a report of proven malignant transformation of a benign pigmented lesion following laser treatment.

A variety of laser modalities including QS lasers, PS lasers, long-pulsed lasers, ablative lasers (CO_2 and Er:YAG lasers) or a combination of QS lasers and ablative laser resurfacing have been successfully used to treat melanotic nevi. However, multiple treatments are often needed, and a high recurrence rate is typical. Thicker lesions are often more resistant to treatment, especially in the setting of congenital nevi with nevus cells involving the deeper dermis and the surrounding adnexal structures. QS lasers appear to demonstrate the best results when treating thinner lesions. Long-pulsed lasers may be more effective for compound melanocytic nevi and thicker congenital nevi, likely due to greater depth of penetration to facilitate clearance of the lesion. Ablative lasers have been recommended for the treatment of melanocytic nevi as these lasers remove both the pigment and hyperplastic tissue of the lesion. Some studies suggest that combination therapy with QS lasers and ablative resurfacing may be associated with superior clearance rates and lower rates of repigmentation compared to either modality alone. However, ablative laser resurfacing may be associated with greater risks of adverse events including scarring. Horner and colleagues treated 12 congenital nevi with the CO_2 laser with 6 of the 12 patients developing subsequent hypertrophic scarring. Based on current studies, hypertrophic scarring appears to be more likely after treatment of congenital nevi on the anterior trunk, flanks or upper extremities and, thus, special caution should be taken when treating lesions at these locations.

In general, most studies evaluating the use of laser therapy for the treatment of melanocytic nevi have been performed in children with congenital nevi rather than adults. Currently, the definitive value of laser therapy for the removal of melanocytic nevi has yet to be established given high rates of repigmentation and incomplete clearance.

Melasma. Melasma often presents as reticulated brown hyperpigmentation of the forehead, lateral cheeks and upper lip in adult females. It is exacerbated by UV exposure and may be associated with hormonal changes or medication use (i.e., pregnancy, oral contraceptives). Treatment is difficult as melasma is frequently refractory to therapy, and recurrence is common. While topical lightening agents and diligent sun protection remain the gold standards and staples of any treatment, laser therapy can be considered as second-line after initial treatment has failed. The QS 694 nm ruby, QS 755 nm alexandrite, QS 1064 nm Nd:YAG, 2940 nm Er:YAG, 1550 nm fractionated erbium-doped fiber laser and fractional CO_2 laser have all been reported as successful treatment modalities for melasma; however, the risk of recurrence is high and laser therapy may even worsen hyperpigmentation.

Very low fluence protocols with the QS 1064 nm Nd:YAG laser have emerged as a potentially safer and more effective treatment of choice for melasma. It is hypothesized that due to subcellular-selective photothermolysis, melanin is selectively destroyed while melanocytes remain intact. This would theoretically decrease the risk of adverse events including PIH, especially in patients of darker skin types. Recent systematic reviews of melasma therapies have placed low fluence QS Nd:YAG laser therapy as one of the best options for laser treatment of melasma, particularly in darker skin types. However, results of studies are inconsistent. Recent studies of new pulse modes of QS lasers including the quickly-pulse-to-pulse (Q-PTP) mode, suggest a benefit for the treatment of melasma with greater patient satisfaction, less procedural pain and a shorter duration of erythema despite similar clearance efficacy when compared to the traditional single pulse QS 1064 nm Nd:YAG laser. However, studies are limited.

PS lasers have increasingly demonstrated safety and efficacy for the treatment of melasma and recent studies suggest a slight superiority of the PS 755 nm

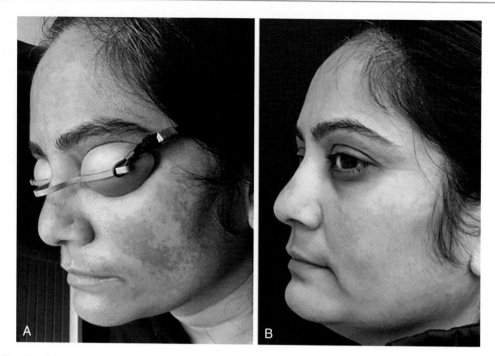

Fig. 3.4 Melasma of the bilateral cheeks seen at baseline (A) and 6 months after one treatment with the 755 nm picosecond laser in combination with oral tranexamic acid (B).

alexandrite laser over the QS Nd:YAG laser (Fig. 3.4). In a split-face study performed by Lee and colleagues, 12 patients received treatment with the PS alexandrite laser to one hemiface and the QS 1064 nm Nd:YAG laser on the other hemiface. The side treated with the PS laser demonstrated a faster rate of clearance and a greater overall improvement in pigmentation at 3 months posttreatment. The PS alexandrite laser with the fractionated DLA handpiece has similarly demonstrated benefit for melasma and appears to be non-inferior to topical therapy with minimal associated adverse effects. While data remains limited by few studies, small sample sizes and short follow-up periods, results of current studies suggest the PS laser may be an effective treatment modality for melasma with a potentially decreased risk of recurrence and adverse events.

Fractionated resurfacing lasers, both ablative and nonablative, have also been investigated for the treatment of melasma. In 2005, the FDA approved the nonablative fractional 1550/1540 nm laser for the treatment of melasma. However, studies evaluating the efficacy of these devices are limited and have demonstrated mild to moderate efficacy comparable to topical therapy with relatively high recurrence rates and a high risk of PIH. Recent studies evaluating the efficacy of low fluence 1927 nm fractional thulium-doped fiber laser show that this device may be more effective for the treatment of melasma with less discomfort and associated adverse events compared to the 1550, 1540, or 1440 nm devices, albeit with similarly high recurrence rates. However, there have been no studies directly comparing the efficacy and safety of all the devices for the treatment of melasma, and studies thus far have been limited by small sample sizes and short follow-up periods.

The ablative fractional CO_2 lasers and the Er:YAG laser have demonstrated minimal to modest benefit for melasma, even when used in combination with additional treatment modalities including QS lasers or topical lightening agents. These devices seem to be associated with a high risk of PIH and high rates of recurrence, especially when used as monotherapy and therefore should be avoided or used with caution in patients, especially those with darker skin types. Additionally, these treatment modalities have not been shown to be significantly more efficacious than topical therapy alone.

Traditionally, treatments for melasma have focused on targeting melanin; however, recently, there has been emerging evidence suggesting a role of increased vasculature in the pathophysiology of melasma, as lesional skin has been found to have increased density of dermal blood vessels compared to normal perilesional skin. As a result, vascular lasers have been also investigated as potential treatment modalities for melasma. Results of current studies evaluating the efficacy of vascular lasers for the treatment of melasma have been mixed. Vascular lasers, including the PDL, are often associated with a high risk of PIH due to the shorter laser wavelength, which may also target melanin in addition to hemoglobin. Passeron and colleagues performed a randomized, single-blinded, split-face trial comparing PDL plus triple-combination therapy (TCC) (hydroquinone 4%, tretinoin 0.05%, and fluocinolone acetonide 0.01% [Tri-Luma Cream; Galderma Laboratories LP, Fort Worth, TX]) daily to TCC daily alone and observed a significant decrease in pigmentation on the combination therapy side with continued improvement during the follow-up period and decreased recurrence rates. However, these improvements were only observed in patients with Fitzpatrick's skin types II and III, and about half of the patients with darker skin types developed PIH on the PDL-treated side. Additional studies evaluating the use of other vascular lasers including the copper bromide laser demonstrated inferiority compared to topical lightening agents (Kligman's formula).

In general, laser therapy has limited efficacy as monotherapy and appears to offer optimal results when used in combination with other modalities including diligent sunscreen used, topical lightening agents such as hydroquinone cream or Kligman's formula (5% hydroquinone, 0.1% tretinoin, 0.1% dexamethasone), oral tranexamic acid or chemical peels. Topical lightening agents and strict photoprotection using broad-spectrum sunscreen (with protection against UVA, UVB, and visible light) should be continued as part of a maintenance regimen between and after laser treatments. Treatment sessions should be spaced 4–8 weeks apart and four to eight sessions are typically required for significant clinical improvement.

PEARL 4

While laser therapy can prove to be an effective second or third line, adjunctive treatment for melasma, strict sun protection and topical lightening agents should always be employed in combination. Triple combination lightening agents containing hydroquinone remain the gold standard, although controversy exists regarding the long-term use of hydroquinone due to risk of exogenous ochronosis. Hydroquinone-free over-the-counter products are available to patients for maintenance after laser therapy. These products contain ingredients including kojic acid, anisic acid, arbutin, niacinamide, tranexamic acid, ascorbic acid, glycolic acid, cysteamine, and *Rumex occidentalis*.

Postinflammatory Hyperpigmentation. PIH occurs due to inflammation with subsequent hemosiderin and/or melanin deposition. Regardless of the etiology, it is often difficult to treat and recalcitrant to therapy. Laser therapy is not often used due to unpredictable response and risk of worsening hyperpigmentation, as PIH is often an adverse effect of laser therapy, especially in patients with darker skin types. There are limited case reports and small studies demonstrating some benefit with the use of the 1550 nm erbium-doped nonablative fractional laser and low fluence QS 1064 nm Nd:YAG; however, studies are sparse and results are inconsistent. PIH following sclerotherapy can occur due to hemosiderin deposition and can be effectively treated with the QS ruby, alexandrite, or Nd:YAG laser. While data is currently limited and somewhat inconsistent, there has been recent anecdotal improvement of both hemosiderosis and melanin-induced PIH reported with the use of fractionated handpieces of the PS lasers. However, more studies are needed to evaluate the true safety and efficacy of laser therapy for PIH. If laser therapy is considered, test spots are recommended prior to treating large areas. Prior to the use of lasers for treatment of PIH, all patients should be instructed to prepare the affected skin using topical hydroquinone 4% cream twice daily (or other topical therapy known to suppress tyrosinase activity) along with vigilant use of broad-spectrum sunscreen before and after treatment.

Periorbital Hyperpigmentation. Periorbital hyperpigmentation is often seen more commonly in certain ethnicities. It may result from dermal melanin pigmentation, chronic dermatitis, chronic edema, or prominent superficial blood vessels. When due to melanin deposition, laser therapy with the QS 694 nm ruby laser, the QS 755 nm alexandrite laser following CO_2 laser treatment, and the 1550 nm fractionated erbium-doped fiber laser have demonstrated efficacy in improving the hyperpigmentation in case reports. Recently, the PS 755 nm alexandrite with the fractionated DLA handpiece demonstrated efficacy in improving infraorbital hyperpigmentation in a patient with skin type IV after one treatment session. The DLA handpiece of PS 1064 Nd:YAG laser is another potentially useful modality for treatment of periorbital hyperpigmentation, which needs to be further studied.

Dermal Lesions

Dermal lesions contain pigment primarily in the deeper dermis. Examples of dermal lesions include nevus of Ota, nevus of Ito, acquired nevus of Ota-like lesions (Hori's nevi), congenital dermal melanocytosis, blue nevi, drug-induced pigmentation, argyria, and amalgam tattoos. In general, laser devices with longer wavelengths are most effective for deeper penetration into the tissue and optimal clearance of the pigment.

Nevus of Ota, Ito, and Hori's Nevus. Nevus of Ota presents as a blue to blue-gray patch involving the temple, periorbital, and malar areas usually often with scleral involvement in a unilateral distribution that develops shortly after birth or at puberty. Nevus of Ito is a related lesion that appears clinically similar but occurs on the shoulder or scapular area. Hori's nevus,

or acquired bilateral nevus of Ota, presents clinically similar to nevus of Ota except that there is no associated scleral involvement and occurs more commonly in young Asian females around puberty.

Traditionally, the QS 1064 nm Nd:YAG laser has been considered the gold standard for treatment of these lesions and is the safest laser to use in patients with darker skin types. In patients with lighter skin types, the QS 694 nm ruby laser and the QS 755 nm alexandrite laser have been successfully used (Fig. 3.5). Combination therapy with various laser modalities may provide superior results, although may also be associated with proportionally increased risk of adverse effects. Adjunctive topical hydroquinone has also been used in combination with QS lasers with improvement. Additionally, studies suggest that different colored nevi of Ota may have varying responses to QS laser therapy. Ueda and colleagues treated different colored nevi of Ota with the QS 694 nm ruby laser and observed 81%, 69%, 80%, and 67% of patients having greater than 75% improvement of brown, brown-violet, violet-blue, and blue-green lesions, respectively. Complete clearance of a nevus of Ota has also been reported following the use of a fractionated 1440 nm Nd:YAG laser and the 1550 erbium laser.

Most recently, PS lasers have emerged as a potentially superior treatment modality for nevus of Ota, Ito and Hori's nevi. Studies suggest that fewer treatments may be required to achieve significant clinical improvement or clearance with more favorable safety profiles using PS lasers compared to QS lasers. According to

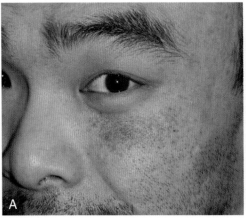 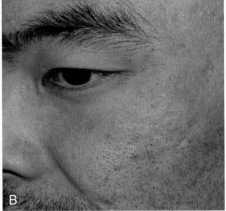

Fig. 3.5 Nevus of Ota seen preoperatively (A) and following two treatments with the Q-switched 755 nm alexandrite laser, showing significant improvement (B).

a recent retrospective review, PS lasers may even be considered first-line treatment for these lesions. Ge and colleagues conducted a randomized, double-blind split lesion trial comparing a 750 nm PS alexandrite laser and a 70 NS alexandrite laser for nevus of Ota in 56 patients, each receiving six treatments at 12-week intervals. At 3-months follow-up, clinical clearance rates and patient satisfaction were superior for PS laser. Similarly, Yu and colleagues performed a split-face randomized controlled trial comparing the PS 755 nm alexandrite laser with the QS 755 nm alexandrite laser in 33 patients with Hori's nevi. All patients underwent three treatment sessions over 6 months with the PS-treated side demonstrating 97% good to excellent improvement compared to 46% on the NS-treated side. The PS laser was also associated with less pain, decreased healing time, and reduced rate of PIH compared to the NS laser. In a retrospective review, Oshiro and Sasaki evaluated the PS 755 nm laser and the PS 1064 nm Nd:YAG laser in 10 patients for the treatment of nevus of Ota (n = 6) and Mongolian spots (n = 4). Seven patients were treated with the 755 nm PS laser and three patients were treated with the 1064 nm PS Nd:YAG laser. After three treatment sessions, the 1064 nm laser and the 755 nm laser were equally effective in achieving 50%–94% improvement at 3-months follow-up. Adverse effects reported included transient hyperpigmentation in the 755-nm treated group and transient erythema and edema without pigmentary alteration in the 1064-nm treated group. Limited studies have also reported efficacy of the 532 and 755 nm PS lasers for treatment of recalcitrant nevi of Ota that have not responded to prior treatments.

In general, longer wavelengths, lower fluences, and PS pulse widths are preferred when treating patients with darker skin types. Treatments are typically spaced 3–4 months apart with up to 10 treatment sessions needed for clearance with QS lasers. Fewer sessions are likely needed with PS lasers. Patients should be made aware that the pigment on the cheek and temple responds better to laser therapy compared to pigment on the upper and lower eyelid. Patients should also be informed that the scleral component is not amenable to laser therapy.

Congenital Dermal Melanocytosis. Congenital dermal melanocytosis, also known as a Mongolian spot, often appears at birth as a blue-gray macule or patch of various sizes in the sacrococcygeal region with gradual resolution in childhood, although some lesions may persist into adulthood. Clinical improvement has been achieved with PS 755 nm alexandrite, QS 755 nm alexandrite, QS 694 nm ruby, and QS 1064 nm Nd:YAG lasers. PIH is a risk, especially given patients who commonly present with these lesions have darker skin types. Sacral lesions appear to be less responsive to laser therapy compared to extrasacral lesions and initiating treatment at a younger age often leads to better results.

Blue Nevi. Blue nevi present as blue to blue-gray homogenous macules or papules typically on the extremities, face or scalp, arising in childhood or adolescence. Histologically they are characterized by aggregates of dendritic, heavily pigmented melanocytes within the dermis. As with melanocytic nevi, it is important to rule out malignancy prior to considering laser therapy. Few studies have evaluated the use of laser therapy for the treatment of blue nevi. Although, based on the current literature, QS lasers may be effective. Milgraum and colleagues reported the use of the QS 694 nm ruby laser in two patients with complete clearance of both lesions. However, given the limited data based on small case reports, the true efficacy of laser therapy for the treatment of blue nevi is not well known. Similar to congenital melanocytic nevi, these lesions are likely difficult to treat with laser therapy alone given the deep dermal aggregates of dendritic melanocytes. Therefore, blue nevi may be better managed with surgical excision.

Drug-Induced Hyperpigmentation. Several medications can lead to abnormal pigmentation of the skin including minocycline, amiodarone, zidovudine (AZT), antimalarials, clofazimine, and imipramine. The gray-blue, gray-brown, or brown pigmentation typically resolves following medication cessation; however, resolution can take months to years. Laser therapy may hasten clearance and QS lasers have been most frequently used to successfully treat the hyperpigmentation. Minocycline-induced hyperpigmentation (occuring after long-term use of this antibiotic) is most commonly encountered by dermatologists. Successful clearance of minocycline-induced hyperpigmentation has been reported following QS or PS 755 nm alexandrite laser as well as QS Nd:YAG laser (Fig. 3.6). Limited studies have also documented efficacy of fractional photothermolysis for minocycline hyperpigmentation.

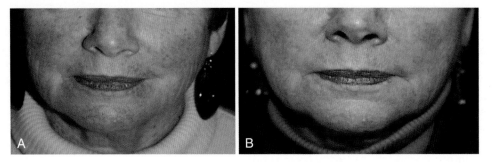

Fig. 3.6 Minocycline pigmentation (A) successfully treated with one treatment using the Q-switched 755 nm alexandrite device (B).

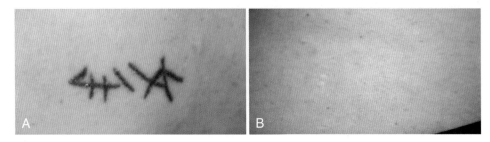

Fig. 3.7 Black tattoo (A) treated with 755 nm picosecond device demonstrating excellent clearance without dyspigmentation or scarring (B).

Chronic use of topical hydroquinone can lead to blue-black to gray blue pigmentation known as exogenous ochronosis. While difficult to treat, improvement with the QS 755 nm alexandrite and the QS 1064 nm Nd:YAG laser has been reported. Multiple treatment sessions are typically required. Additionally, ablative fractional lasers have demonstrated improvement.

Argyria. Argyria is a rare skin disease due to chronic exposure to silver including in settings of occupational exposure, use of alternative medications or systemic absorption from use of silver sulfadiazine on extensive burns or wounds. Histologically, silver granules can be found in the basement membrane of eccrine glands, attached to elastic fibers or around hair follicles and arrector pili muscles within the skin. Studies have shown successful treatment with the QS 1064 nm Nd:YAG laser and, recently, case reports have demonstrated clinical improvement to complete clearance with the use of PS lasers. Caution should be taken when treating these lesions with QS or PS lasers given the risk of darkening similar to the risk of chrysiasis with gold ingestion.

Amalgam Tattoos. Amalgam tattoos can occur on the gingival or buccal mucosa secondary to iatrogenic implantation of dental amalgam. These lesions can be successfully removed with the QS 694 nm ruby or QS 755 nm alexandrite laser.

Tattoos

QS and PS lasers are both effective in lightening or clearing most tattoos, although response and number of treatments required is variable and dependent on a variety of factors. Based on recent studies and retrospective reviews, PS lasers are now considered the gold standard for the treatment of tattoos of almost any color. Long-pulsed lasers and IPL should never be used for tattoo removal due to the unacceptable risk of scarring.

Dark Blue or Black Tattoos

Dark blue or black tattoos are often the most responsive to laser therapy. The QS and PS 755 nm alexandrite laser, the QS 694 nm ruby, and the QS and PS 1064 nm Nd:YAG can all be used to successfully remove or lighten dark blue and black tattoos (Fig. 3.7). The laser

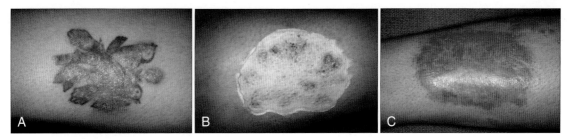

Fig. 3.8 Tattoo granulomas from an allergic reaction to the *red* (cinnabar or mercury tattoo ink) color in a multicolored tattoo seen (A) preoperatively, (B) immediately after removal of the tattoo and all granulomas with the vaporizational mode of the CO_2 laser, and (C) 3 months later showing the residual erythematous permanent scar.

modality of choice should be based on the patient's skin type to limit risk of adverse effects. In lighter-skinned patients, any of the previously listed lasers can be safely used to effectively remove the tattoo. In darker skinned patients, lasers with longer wavelengths (1064 nm Nd:YAG) are safer because they are more gentle on the epidermis and have a lower risk of PIH or hypopigmentation. Recent studies suggest that the PS lasers may be superior in safety and efficacy with fewer treatments required.

Treatment of black traumatic tattoos requires knowledge of the etiology of trauma because in some settings, such as gun powder tattoos and fireworks tattoos, these tattoos can undergo microexplosions after QS or PS laser treatment, potentially leading to atrophic scarring. To eliminate this risk, ablative or fractionally ablative lasers may be the treatment of choice in this setting as these lasers do not ignite incendiary particles.

Red and Yellow Tattoos

While the optimal wavelength for removal is the PS or QS 532 nm frequency-doubled Nd:YAG, red and yellow tattoo ink can be challenging to treat. Caution should be taken when using the 532 nm wavelength in darker skin patients given an increased risk of post-procedural pigmentary alteration due to greater epidermal melanin absorption at the shorter wavelength. However, limited studies have suggested that with the appropriate treatment settings, the PS frequency doubled 532 nm Nd:YAG may be safe in these patients.

Dermatologists should also be aware that red tattoo ink is a common culprit of allergic and granulomatous reactions associated with tattoo placement (Figs. 3.8 and 3.9). In these settings, laser treatment of the red tattoo

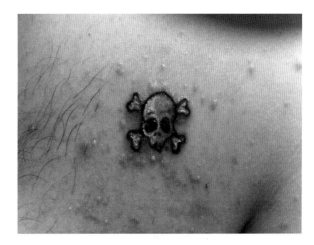

Fig. 3.9 Multicolored tattoo showing allergy to yellow ink. The area was successfully treated with class I topical corticosteroids, thus avoiding the need to remove the tattoos with laser.

can result in dispersion of the antigen with a subsequent urticarial reaction or systemic allergic reaction including anaphylaxis. The use of QS or PS lasers in this situation should be avoided, or done with great caution (to include premedication with ssytemic corticosteroids and antihistamines). Alternatively, ablative or fractionally ablative CO_2 or Er:YAG lasers can be used to vaporize the tattoo, or surgical excision, (depending on the size and location of the tattoo) can be performed.

Green Tattoos

The QS 694 nm ruby laser has been considered the wavelength of choice for the treatment of green tattoo ink. The QS and, more recently, the PS 755 nm alexandrite lasers are also significantly effective for the removal of green tattoos. In a case series of 10 patients, Brauer and colleagues treated 12 blue and/or green tattoos with the PS 755 nm alexandrite laser. Eleven of twelve patients had greater than 75% clearance with one or two treatments at 1-month follow-up. The PS 1064 nm Nd:YAG has also demonstrated efficacy in lightening green tattoo ink as well as the QS 650 nm Nd:YAG laser. If the QS 694 nm ruby laser is used, caution should be taken in patients with darker skin types due to the greater absorption of melanin at this wavelength and increased risk of PIH or hypopigmentation.

Cosmetic Tattoos

Cosmetic tattoos can present a treatment challenge due to the risk of paradoxical darkening with the use of QS or PS lasers. Cosmetic tattoos often contain iron oxide (rust-colored) or titanium dioxide (white), which can undergo reduction reactions (i.e., rust-colored ferric oxide to jet black ferrous oxide) after laser treatment resulting in immediate and permanent tattoo darkening. This darkening often becomes apparent once the immediate whitening has faded. Prior to any treatment of a cosmetic tattoo, a test spot should be performed to evaluate for this reaction. While paradoxical darkening can be improved with repeated QS or PS lasers, multiple treatment sessions are required. Therefore some recommend treating cosmetic tattoos with ablative lasers to eliminate risk of paradoxical darkening. Ablative lasers do have a greater risk of adverse effects and prolonged recovery time, which should be discussed with the patient prior to treatment.

> **PEARL 5**
>
> Test spots should be performed prior to treating cosmetic tattoos with QS or PS lasers due to the risk of paradoxical darkening. If a test spot darkens, ablative and/or fractional resurfacing or surgical excision should be considered for treatment.

Multi-Colored Tattoos

When treating tattoos containing multiple colors, more than one laser is often required for optimal clearance. In these settings, the individual ink colors should be treated with the optimal corresponding wavelength as discussed in the prior sections (Fig. 3.10). The black outline of the tattoo can be first treated with the QS or PS 1064 nm Nd:YAG laser. After clearance of the black pigment, the QS or PS 532 nm frequency-doubled Nd:YAG can be used to treat any red or yellow ink within the tattoo. If green tattoo ink is present, the QS 694 nm ruby laser or the QS or PS 755 nm alexandrite laser can be used. Alternatively, the QS Nd:YAG with a 650 nm wavelength dye-containing handpiece can be used. If prominent immediate whitening of the tattoo ink is noted after treatment, that laser wavelength will typically effectively lighten that color.

It is important to avoid overlapping treatment pulses as much as possible by matching the size of the laser beam to the size of the area containing the targeted tattoo pigment. With this technique, it is often possible to treat an entire multi-colored tattoo during a single treatment session, resulting in more rapid resolution than if each color were treated individually at separate visits.

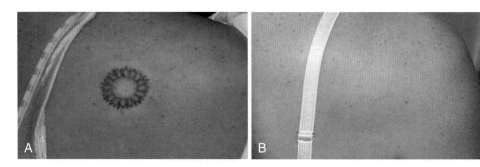

Fig. 3.10 Multi-colored tattoo seen preoperatively (A) and after three treatments with 532 nm, 755 nm, and 1064 nm Q-switched devices (B) demonstrating essentially complete clearance without scarring.

Enhancing Tattoo Removal Outcomes

Increasing fluences are often required with subsequent treatment as ink particle density decreases. One pass over the treatment area with minimal overlap (<10%) minimizes untreated areas and the development of "honey-combing." Recently, newer treatment methods allow for multiple laser passes to be performed per treatment session. Typically, the gas bubble formation that occurs from the rapid tissue heating and mechanical dissolution of ink particles after laser therapy temporarily reduces the visibility of the remaining ink particles. This typically resolves in about 20 minutes. The R20 method, initially introduced by Kossida and colleagues, includes four consecutive passes separated by 20 minutes to allow time for the gas bubbles to resolve. This method has been shown to be safe and more effective than a single-pass treatment session. However, this method is not time-efficient, especially in a busy practice. The R0 method addresses this issue by applying a topical liquid fluorocarbon, perfluorodecalin, which immediately resolves the ash-white tissue response, allowing for subsequent treatment passes immediately in tandem (Fig. 3.11). It has been shown to be faster and just as effective as the R20 method. Recently, the rapid acoustic pulse (RAP) device has been introduced, which generates acoustic shock wave pulses that clear epidermal and dermal vacuoles created by QS or PS laser treatment to allow for multiple passes in a single laser tattoo removal session. Early studies have demonstrated superior tattoo clearance when the RAP device is used in combination with a QS laser compared to a single pass QS laser treatment. Monthly treatments are typically performed to allow for adequate clearance of ink particles and skin healing.

PEARL 6

When treating tattoos, the desired clinical endpoint is tissue whitening, lasting about 10–20 minutes. If this endpoint is not reached, the laser fluence or wavelength used will likely not lead to lightening of the treated area.

POSTOPERATIVE CARE

After treatment with a QS or PS laser, cool compresses, emollient application, and/or the use of occlusive dressings can be soothing and provide pain relief. No specific wound care is generally needed after treatment of epidermal lesions. A subtle crusting over the treated area may form and slough off within the first 7–10 days after treatment. Patients should be instructed to gently clean the treated areas daily followed by application of occlusive emollients to hasten healing. Crusts should be allowed to slough off on their own. After treatment of dermal lesions or tattoos, the treated area may appear abraded or vesiculation or bullae may develop due to the more aggressive treatment settings required for these lesions.

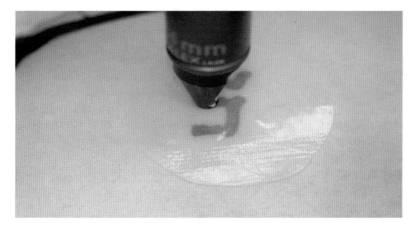

Fig. 3.11 Laser treatment of a tattoo utilizing a perfluorodecalin gel pad, allowing for subsequent treatment passes immediately in tandem.

An occlusive emollient or petrolatum beneath a dressing of nonstick gauze and paper tape or hydrocolloid dressing can be used. Patients should be instructed to change the dressing daily after cleansing the area with soap and water—a process that should be continued until reepithelialization occurs. The treated area generally heals within 5–14 days.

After ablative laser resurfacing, an occlusive dressing should be applied for the first few days postoperatively, followed by daily cleansing, gentle soaks and emollient application until the area has reepithelialized. After fractional nonablative laser resurfacing, a gentle emollient or non-comedogenic moisturizer should be applied for up to 1 week.

Regardless of laser device used, patients should be advised to perform strict sun avoidance and to apply broad-spectrum sunscreen to minimize the risk of post-procedural dyspigmentation.

> ### PEARL 7
>
> After laser therapy of any benign pigmented lesion or tattoo, it is important for the patient to practice strict sun protection to prevent recurrence of pigmentation or postinflammatory hyperpigmentation. Mineral sunscreens including those with iron oxide as they provide broad spectrum coverage against UVA, UVB, and visible light.

SIDE EFFECTS AND COMPLICATIONS

Even after taking appropriate precautions, dyspigmentation may still occur following laser therapy of benign pigmented lesions or tattoos. Hyperpigmentation often improves spontaneously over time or with the use of topical lightening agents including 4%–5% hydroquinone cream or Kligman's formula. Hypopigmentation is more difficult to treat, commonly with incomplete resolution despite multiple treatments of excimer laser or narrow-band ultraviolet light. Patients with darker skin types are at increased risk of post-procedural dyspigmentation, especially when undergoing laser tattoo removal. As mentioned earlier, test spots evaluated at 6–8 weeks are recommended prior to treatment to anticipate and potentially minimize this complication.

If a patient with an unknown history of gold therapy is treated with a QS or PS laser, immediate darkening of the treated skin can occur due to darkening of the gold particles within the skin. While the pigmentation is considered to be permanent, effective clearance has been reported with the use of the long-pulsed 694 nm ruby or 755 nm alexandrite laser.

Textural changes and scarring can also occur secondary to the thermal injury induced by the laser treatment. While these are rare complications if the appropriate treatment techniques and settings are utilized, the risk is slightly higher when treating tattoos. Avoidance of excessive fluences or pulse stacking, and the use of larger spot sizes and appropriate spacing of treatment sessions at 6- to 8-week intervals can minimize the risk of these complications. These complications may occur more frequently with treatments on the chest, outer upper arm, and ankle. Proper daily wound care with normal saline cleansing and application of an occlusive emollient under a nonstick gauze dressing may help to prevent infection, which could subsequently result in scarring. If scarring does occur, various treatment modalities including a series of PDL or fractional photothermolysis treatments, intralesional low-dose triamcinolone acetonide with or without 5-fluorouracil injections and topical application of silicone gel sheeting with scar message may help to improve the appearance of the scar. A slight cobblestone texture developing 2 weeks after treatment may be a sign of impending scar formation and can often be reversed with twice daily application of class I topical corticosteroids.

▌ CONCLUSIONS

Various benign pigmented lesions and tattoos can be effectively and safely treated with lasers. Proper patient selection and a thorough preoperative evaluation are paramount. Proper skin preparation before treatment using topical therapies that suppress melanocyte activity along with strict photo-protection, as well as the use of appropriate treatment parameters and the adjustment of settings to achieve desired treatment endpoints will optimize outcomes and minimize the risk of adverse events. Continued advancements in laser technology will likely further improvements in the treatment of pigmented lesions.

FURTHER READING

Alabdulrazzaq H, Brauer JA, Bae YS, Geronemus RG. Clearance of yellow tattoo ink with a novel 532-nm picosecond laser. *Lasers Surg Med.* 2015;47(4):285–288.

Alkhalifah A, Fransen F, Le Duff F, Lacour J-P, et al. Laser treatment of epidermal nevi: a multicenter retrospective study with long-term follow-up. *J Am Acad Dermatol.* 2020;83(6):1606–1615.

Alora MB, Arndt KA. Treatment of a café-au-lait macule with the erbium:YAG laser. *J Am Acad Dermatol.* 2001;45(4): 566–568.

Alster TS, Williams CM. Café-au-lait macule in type V skin: successful treatment with a 510 nm pulsed dye laser. *J Am Acad Dermatol.* 1995;33(6):1042–1043.

Alster TS, Williams CM. Treatment of nevus of Ota by the Q-switched alexandrite laser. *Dermatol Surg.* 1995;21(7):592–596.

Alster TS. Complete elimination of large café-au-lait birthmarks by the 510-nm pulsed dye laser. *Plast Reconstr Surg.* 1995;96(7):1600–1604.

Anderson RR, Parrish JA. Selective photothermolysis: precise microsurgery by selective absorption of pulsed radiation. *Science.* 1983;220(4596):524–527.

Angsuwarangsee S, Polnikorn N. Combined ultrapulse CO_2 laser and Q-switched alexandrite laser compared with Q-switched alexandrite laser alone for refractory melasma: split-face design. *Dermatol Surg.* 2003;29(1):59–64.

Artzi O, Mehrabi JN, Koren A, Niv R, Lapidoth M, Levi A. Picosecond 532-nm neodymium-doped yttrium aluminium garnet laser—a novel and promising modality for the treatment of café-au-lait macules. *Lasers Med Sci.* 2018;33(4):693–697.

Ashinoff R, Tanenbaum D. Treatment of an amalgam tattoo with the Q-switched ruby laser. *Cutis.* 1994;54(4):269–270.

Bae YS, Alabdulrazzaq H, Brauer J, Geronemus R. Successful treatment of paradoxical darkening. *Lasers Surg Med.* 2016;48(5):471–473.

Balaraman B, Ravanfar-Jordan P, Friedman PM. Novel use of non-ablative fractional photothermolysis for café-au-lait macules in darker skin types. *Lasers Surg Med.* 2017; 49(1):84–87.

Belkin DA, Neckman JP, Jeon H, Friedman P, Geronemus RG. Response to laser treatment of café au lait macules based on morphologic features. *JAMA Dermatol.* 2017;153(11): 1158–1161.

Bellew SG, Alster TS. Treatment of exogenous ochronosis with a Q- switched alexandrite (755 nm) laser. *Dermatol Surg.* 2004;30(4 Pt 1):555–558.

Bernstein EF, Schomacker KT, Basilavecchio LD, Plugis JM, et al. A novel dual-wavelength, Nd:YAG, picosecond-domain laser safely and effectively removes multicolor tattoos. *Lasers Surg Med.* 2015;47(7):542–548.

Brauer JA, Reddy KK, Anolik R, Weiss ET, et al. Successful and rapid treatment of blue and green tattoo pigment with a novel picosecond laser. *Arch Dermatol.* 2012;148(7):820–823.

Chalermchai T, Rummaneethorn P. Effects of a fractional picosecond 1,064 nm laser for the treatment of dermal and mixed type melasma. *J Cosmet Laser Ther.* 2018;20(3): 134–139.

Chan HH, Fung WK, Ying SY, et al. An in vivo trial comparing the use of different types of 532 nm Nd:YAG lasers in the treatment of facial lentigines in Oriental patients. *Dermatol Surg.* 2000;26(8):743–749.

Chan HH, Leung RS, Ying SY, Lai CF, et al. A retrospective analysis of complications in the treatment of nevus of Ota with the Q-switched alexandrite and Q-switched Nd:YAG lasers. *Dermatol Surg.* 2000;26(11):1000–1006.

Chan HH, Xiang L, Leung JC, et al. In vitro study examining the effect of sub-lethal QS 755 nm lasers on the expression of p16INK4a on melanoma cell lines. *Lasers Surg Med.* 2003; 32(2):88–93.

Chan JC, Shek SY, Kono T, Yeung CK, et al. A retrospective analysis on the management of pigmented lesions using a picosecond 755-nm alexandrite laser in Asians. *Lasers Surg Med.* 2016;48(1):23–29.

Chan MWM, Shek SY-N, Yeung CK, Chan HH-L. A prospective study in the treatment of lentigines in Asian skin using 532 nm picosecond Nd:YAG laser. *Lasers Surg Med.* 2019;51(9):767–773.

Chen H, Diebold G. Chemical generation of acoustic waves: a giant photoacoustic effect. *Science.* 1995;270(5238): 963–966.

Chesnut C, Diehl J, Lask G. Treatment of nevus of Ota with a picosecond 755-nm alexandrite laser. *Dermatol Surg.* 2015;41(4):508–510.

Cho SB, Park SJ, Kim MJ, Bu TS. Treatment of acquired bilateral nevus of Ota-like macules (Hori's nevus) using 1,064-nm Q-switched Nd:YAG laser with low fluence. *Int J Dermatol.* 2009;48(12):1308–1312.

Choi JE, Kim JW, Seo SH, Son SW, et al. Treatment of Becker's nevi with a long-pulsed alexandrite laser. *Dermatol Surg.* 2009;35(7):1105–1108.

Choi YJ, Nam JH, Kim JY, Min JH, et al. A prospective, randomized, multicenter, split-face, 2% hydroquinone cream-controlled clinical trial. *Lasers Surg Med.* 2017;49(10): 899–907.

Chong SJ, Jeong E, Park HJ, Lee JY, Cho BK. Treatment of congenital nevomelanocytic nevi with the CO_2 and Q-switched alexandrite lasers. *Dermatol Surg.* 2005;31(5):518–521.

Chung HJ, McGee JS, Lee SJ. Successful treatment of ephelides in Asian skin using the picosecond 785-nm laser. *J Cosmet Dermatol.* 2020;19(8):1990–1992.

Chung BY, Han SS, Moon HR, Lee MW, Chang SE. Treatment with the pinhole technique using erbium-doped yttrium aluminum garnet laser for a café au lait macule and carbon dioxide laser for facial telangiectasia. *Ann Dermatol*. 2014;26(5):657–659.

Culbertson GR. 532-nm diode laser treatment of seborrheic keratoses with color enhancement. *Dermatol Surg*. 2008; 34(4):525–528.

DiGiorgio CM, Wu DC, Goldman MP. Successful treatment of argyria using the picosecond alexandrite laser. *Dermatol Surg*. 2016;42(3):431–433.

Dover JS, Margolis RJ, Polla LL, et al. Pigmented guinea pig skin irradiated with Q-switched ruby laser pulses. Morphologic and histologic findings. *Arch Dermatol*. 1989;125(1):43–49.

Dover JS, Smoller BR, Stern RS, et al. Low-fluence carbon dioxide laser irradiation of lentigines. *Arch Dermatol*. 1988;124(8):1219–1224.

Dummer R, Kempf W, Burg G. Pseudo-melanoma after laser therapy. *Dermatology*. 1998;197(1):71–73.

Ee HL, Goh CL, Khoo LS, Chan ES, et al. Treatment of acquired bilateral nevus of Ota-like macules (Hori's nevus) with a combi- nation of the 532 nm Q-Switched Nd:YAG laser followed by the 1,064 nm Q-switched Nd:YAG is more effective: prospective study. *Dermatol Surg*. 2006;32(1):34–40.

Eggen CAM, Lommerts JE, van Zuuren EJ, Limpens J, Pasmans SGMA, Wolkerstorfer A. Laser treatment of congenital melanocytic naevi: a systematic review. *Br J Dermatol*. 2018;178(2):369–383.

Fitzpatrick RE, Goldman MP. Tattoo removal using the alexandrite laser. *Arch Dermatol*. 1994;130(12):1508–1514.

Fitzpatrick RE, Goldman MP, Ruiz-Esparza J. Clinical advantage of the CO_2 laser superpulsed mode. Treatment of verruca vulgaris, seborrheic keratoses, lentigines, and actinic cheilitis. *J Dermatol Surg Oncol*. 1994;20(7):449–456.

Freedman JR, Kaufman J, Metelitsa AI, et al. Picosecond lasers: the next generation of short-pulsed lasers. *Semin Cutan Med Surg*. 2014;33(4):164–168.

Friedman DJ. Successful treatment of a red and black professional tattoo in skin type VI with a picosecond dual-wavelength, neodymium-doped yttrium aluminum garnet laser. *Dermatol Surg*. 2016;42(9):1121–1123.

Ge Y, Yang Y, Guo L, et al. Comparison of a picosecond alexandrite laser versus a Q-switched alexandrite laser for the treatment of nevus of Ota: A randomized, split-lesion, controlled trial. *J Am Acad Dermatol*. 2020;83(2):397–403.

Geronemus RG. Q-switched ruby laser therapy of nevus of Ota. *Arch Dermatol*. 1992;128(12):1618–1622.

Glaich AS, Goldberg LH, Dai T, Kunishige JH, Friedman PM. Fractional resurfacing: a new therapeutic modality for Becker's nevus. *Arch Dermatol*. 2007;143(12):1488–1490.

Goldberg DJ, Stampien T. Q-switched ruby laser treatment of congenital nevi. *Arch Dermatol*. 1995;131(5):621–623.

Goldberg DJ, Nychay SG. Q-switched ruby laser treatment of nevus of Ota. *J Dermatol Surg Oncol*. 1992;18(9):817–821.

Goldman L, Wilson RG, Hornby P, Meyer RG. Radiation from a Q-switched ruby laser. Effect of repeated impacts of power output of 10 megawatts on a tattoo of a man. *J Invest Dermatol*. 1965;44:69–71.

Green D, Friedman KJ. Treatment of minocycline-induced cutaneous pigmentation with the Q-switched alexandrite laser and a review of the literature. *J Am Acad Dermatol*. 2001;44(2 suppl):342–347.

Grevelink JM, van Leeuwen RL, Anderson RR, Byers HR. Clinical and histological responses of congenital melanocytic nevi after single treatment with Q-switched lasers. *Arch Dermatol*. 1997;133(3):349–353.

Grevelink JM, Gonza lez S, Bonoan R, Vibhagool C, et al. Treatment of nevus spilus with the Q-switched ruby laser. *Dermatol Surg*. 1997;23:365–369.

Guss L, Goldman MP, Wu DC. Picosecond 532nm neodymium-doped yttrium aluminum garnet laser for the treatment of solar lentigines in darker skin types: safety and efficacy. *Dermatol Surg*. 2017;43(3):456–459.

Guo X, Cai X, Jin Y, Zhang T, et al. Q-PTP is an optimized technology of 1064-nm Q-switched neodymium-doped yttrium aluminum garnet laser in the laser therapy of melasma: a prospective split-face study. *Oncol Lett*. 2019;18(4):4136–4143.

Haimovic A, Brauer JA, Cindy Bae YS, Geronemus RG. Safety of a picosecond laser with diffractive lens array (DLA) in the treatment of Fitzpatrick skin types IV to VI: a retrospective review. *J Am Acad Dermatol*. 2016;74(5):931–936.

Hammami Ghorbel H, Boukari F, Fontas E, et al. Copper bromide laser vs triple-combination cream for the treatment of melasma: a randomized clinical trial. *JAMA Dermatol*. 2015;151(7):791–792.

Hantash BM, Bedi VP, Sudireddy V, Struck SK, Herron GS, Chan KF. Laser-induced transepidermal elimination of dermal content by fractional photothermolysis. *J Biomed Opt*. 2006;11(4):041115.

Herd RM, Alora MB, Smoller B, Arndt KA, et al. A clinical and histologic prospective controlled comparative study of the picosecond titanium:sapphire (795 nm) laser versus the Q-switched alexandrite (752 nm) laser for removing tattoo pigment. *J Am Acad Dermatol*. 1999;40(4):603–606.

Ho DD, London R, Zimmerman GB, Young DA. Laser-tattoo removal—a study of the mechanism and the optimal treatment strategy via computer simulations. *Lasers Surg Med*. 2002;30(5):389–397.

Ho SG, Goh CL. Laser tattoo removal: a clinical update. *J Cutan Aesthet Surg*. 2015;8(1):9–15.

Ho SG, Yeung CK, Chan NP, et al. A comparison of Q-switched and long-pulsed alexandrite laser for the treatment of freckles and lentigines in oriental patients. *Lasers Surg Med.* 2011;43(2):108–113.

Hofbauer Parra CA, Careta MF, Valente NYS, de Sanches Osório NEG, Torezan LAR. Clinical and histopathologic assessment of facial melasma after low fluence Q-switched neodymium-doped yttrium aluminum garnet laser. *Dermatol Surg.* 2016;42(4):507–512.

Horner BM, El-Muttardi NS, Mayo BJ. Treatment of congenital melanocytic nevi with CO_2 laser. *Ann Plast Surg.* 2005;55(3):276–280.

Huang A, Phillips A, Adar T, Hui A. Ocular injury in cosmetic laser treatments of the face. *J Clin Aesthet Dermatol.* 2018;11(2):15–18.

Hwang K, Lee WJ, Lee SI, et al. Pseudomelanoma after laser therapy. *Ann Plast Surg.* 2002;48(5):562–564.

Imhof L, Dummer R, Dreier J, Kolm I, Barysch MJ. A prospective trial comparing q-switched ruby laser and a triple combination skin-lightening cream in the treatment of solar lentigines. *Dermatol Surg.* 2016;42(7):853–857.

Izikson L, Farinelli W, Sakamoto F, Tannous Z, et al. Safety and effectiveness of black tattoo clearance in a pig model after a single treatment with a novel 758 nm 500 picosecond laser: a pilot study. *Lasers Surg Med.* 2010;42(7):640–646.

Izikson L, Anderson RR. Resolution of blue minocycline pigmentation of the face after fractional photothermolysis. *Lasers Surg Med.* 2008;40(6):399–401.

Jang KA, Chung EC, Choi JH, Sung KJ, Moon KC, Koh JK. Successful removal of freckles in Asian skin with a Q-switched alexandrite laser. *Dermatol Surg.* 2000;26(3):231–234.

Jeong SY, Shin JB, Yeo UC, Kim WS, Kim IH. Low-fluence Q-switched neodymium-doped yttrium aluminum garnet laser for melasma with pre-or post-treatment triple combination cream. *Dermatol Surg.* 2010;36(6):909–918.

Kagami S, Asahina A, Watanabe R, et al. Treatment of 153 Japanese patients with Q-switched alexandrite laser. *Lasers Med Sci.* 2007;22(3):159–163.

Kaminer MS, Capelli CC, Sadeghpour M, Ibrahim O, Honda LL, Robertson DW. Increased tattoo fading in a single laser tattoo removal session enabled by a rapid acoustic pulse device: a prospective clinical trial. *Lasers Surg Med.* 2020;52(1):70–76.

Kanechorn-Na-Ayuthaya P, Niumphradit N, Aunhachoke K, Nakakes A, Sittiwangkul R, Srisuttiyakorn C. Effect of combination of 1064 nm Q-switched Nd:YAG and fractional carbon dioxide lasers for treating exogenous ochronosis. *J Cosmet Laser Ther.* 2013;15(1):42–45.

Katz TK, Goldberg LH, Friedman PM. Dermatosis papulosa nigra treatment with fractional photothermolysis. *Dermatol Surg.* 2009;35(11):1840–1843.

Katz TM, Goldberg LH, Firoz BF, Friedman PM. Fractional photothermolysis for the treatment of postinflammatory hyperpigmentation. *Dermatol Surg.* 2009;35(11):1844–1848.

Kent KM, Graber EM. Laser tattoo removal: a review. *Dermatol Surg.* 2012;38(1):1–13.

Khetarpal S, Desai S, Kruter L, Prather H, et al. Picosecond laser with specialized optic for facial rejuvenation using a compressed treatment interval. *Lasers Surg Med.* 2016;48(8):723–726.

Kilmer SL, Wheeland RG, Goldberg DJ, Anderson RR. Treatment of epidermal pigmented lesions with the frequency- doubled Q-switched Nd:YAG laser. A controlled, single-impact, dose-response, multicenter trial. *Arch Dermatol.* 1994;130(12):1515–1519.

Kim jH, Kim H, Park HC, Kim IH. Subcellular selective photothermolysis of melanosomes in adult zebrafish skin following 1064-nm Q-switched Nd:YAG laser irradiation. *J Invest Dermatol.* 2010;130(9):2333–2335.

Kim EH, Kim YC, Lee ES, Kang HY. The vascular characteristics of melasma. *J Dermatol Sci.* 2007;46(2):111–116.

Kim S, Cho KH. Treatment of facial postinflammatory hyperpigmentation with facial acne in Asian patients using Q-switched neodymium-doped yttrium aluminum garnet laser. *Dermatol Surg.* 2010;36(9):1374–1380.

Kirby W, Desai A, Desaei T, Kartono F, Patel G. The Kirby-Desai scale: a proposed scale to assess tattoo-removal treatments. *J Clin Aesthetic Dermatol.* 2009;2(3):32–37.

Kono T, Nozaki M, Chan HH, Mikashima Y. A retrospective study looking at the long-term complications of Q-switched ruby laser in the treatment of nevus of Ota. *Lasers Surg Med.* 2001;29(2):156–159.

Kono T, Chan HH, Erçöçen AR, et al. Use of Q-switched ruby laser in the treatment of nevus of Ota in different age groups. *Lasers Surg Med.* 2003;32(5):391–395.

Kossida T, Farinelli W, Flotte T. Mechanism of immediate whitening during tattoo removal. *Lasers Surg Med.* 2006;18:70.

Kossida T, Rigopoulos D, Katsambas A, Anderson RR. Optimal tattoo removal in a single laser session based on the method of repeated exposures. *J Am Acad Dermatol.* 2012;66(2):271–277.

Kouba DJ, Fincher EF, Moy RL, et al. Nevus of Ota successfully treated by fractional photothermolysis using a fractionated 1440-nm Nd:YAG laser. *Arch Dermatol.* 2008;144(2):156–158.

Kroon MW, Wind BS, Beek JF, et al. Nonablative 1550-nm fractional laser therapy versus triple topical therapy for the treatment of melasma: a randomized controlled pilot study. *J Am Acad Dermatol.* 2011;64(3):516–523.

Kundu RV, Joshi SS, Suh KY, Boone SL, et al. Comparison of electrodesiccation and potassium-titanyl-phosphate laser for treatment of dermatosis papulosa nigra. *Dermatol Surg.* 2009;35(7):1079–1083.

Kung KY, Shek SY, Yeung CK, Chan HH. Evaluation of the safety and efficacy of the dual wavelength picosecond laser for the treatment of benign pigmented lesions in Asians. *Lasers Surg Med*. 2019;51(1):14–22.

Kwon SH, Hwang YJ, Lee SK, Park KC. Heterogeneous pathology of melasma and its clinical implications. *Int J Mol Sci*. 2016;17(6):824.

Labadie JG, Krunic AL. Long pulsed dye laser with a back-to-back double-pulse technique and compression for the treatment of epidermal pigmented lesions. *Lasers Surg Med*. 2019;51(2):136–140.

Lam AY, Wong DS, Lam LK, Petzoldt D. A retrospective study on the efficacy and complications of Q-switched alexandrite laser in the treatment of acquired bilateral nevus of Ota-like macules. *Dermatol Surg*. 2001;27:937–941.

Larry S. Tattoo takeover: three in ten Americans have tattoos, and most don't stop at just one. Health & Life. The Harris Poll. http://www.theharrispoll.com/health-and-life/Tattoo_Takeover.html. Accessed December 12, 2020.

Lee MW. Combination 532-nm and 1064-nm lasers for noninvasive skin rejuvenation and toning. *Arch Dermatol*. 2003;139(10):1265–1276.

Lee HS, Won CH, Lee DH, An JS, Chang HW, Lee JH, et al. Treatment of melasma in Asian skin using a fractional 1, 550-nm laser: an open clinical study. *Dermatol Surg*. 2009;35(10):1499–1504.

Lee M-C, Lin Y-F, Hu S, Huang Y-L, et al. A split-face study: comparison of picosecond alexandrite laser and Q-switched Nd:YAG laser in the treatment of melasma in Asians. *Lasers Med Sci*. 2018;33(8):1733–1738.

Lee HM, Haw S, Kim JK, Chang SE, Lee MW. Split-face study using a 1, 927-nm thulium fiber fractional laser to treat photoaging and melasma in Asian skin. *Dermatol Surg*. 2013;39(6):879–888.

Lee DB, Suh HS, Choi YS. A comparative study of low-fluence 1, 064 nm Q-Switched Nd: YAG laser with or without chemical peeling using Jessner's solution in melasma patients. *J Cosmet Laser Ther*. 2014;16(6):264–270.

Levin MK, Ng E, Bae YS, Brauer JA, et al. Treatment of pigmentary disorders in patients with skin of color with a novel 755 nm picosecond, Q-switched ruby, and Q-switched Nd:YAG nanosecond lasers: a retrospective photographic review. *Lasers Surg Med*. 2016;48(2):181–187.

Li YT, Yang KC. Comparison of the frequency-doubled Q-switched Nd:YAG laser and 35% trichloroacetic acid for the treatment of face lentigines. *Dermatol Surg*. 1999;25(3):202–204.

Lipp MB, Angra K, Wu DC. Safety and efficacy of a novel 730 nm picosecond titanium sapphire laser for the treatment of benign pigmented lesions. *Lasers Surg Med*. 2021;53(4):429–434.

Lomeo G, Cassuto D, Scrmali L, Sirago P. Er:YAG versus CO_2 ablative fractional resurfacing: a split face study. Abstract

presented at American Society for Laser Medicine and Surgery Conference, Kissimmee F; 2008.

Lomeo G, Cassuto D, Scrimali L, Siragò P. Er:YAG versus CO_2 ablative fractional resurfacing: a split face study. *Lasers Surg Med*. 2008;76:40.

Lou WW, Kauvar ANB, Geronemus RG. Evaluation of long pulsed alexandrite laser and Q-switched ruby laser for the treatment of benign pigmented lesions. *Lasers Surg Med Suppl*. 2000;12:56.

Lowe NJ, Wieder JM, Sawcer D, Burrows P, Chalet M. Nevus of Ota: treatment with high energy fluences of the Q-switched ruby laser. *J Am Acad Dermatol*. 1993;29(6):997–1001.

Lowe NJ, Wieder JM, Shorr N, Boxrud C, Saucer D, Chalet M. Infraorbital pigmented skin. Preliminary observations of laser therapy. *Dermatol Surg*. 1995;21(9):767–770.

Lyons AB, Moy RL, Herrmann JL. A randomized, controlled, split-face study of the efficacy of a picosecond laser in the treatment of melasma. *J Drugs Dermatol*. 2019;18(11):1104–1107.

Manaloto RMP, Alster T. Erbium:YAG laser resurfacing for refractory melasma. *Dermatol Surg*. 1999;25(2):121–123.

Manstein D, Herron GS, Sink RK, Tanner H, et al. Fractional photothermolysis: a new concept of cutaneous remodeling using microscopic patterns of thermal injury. *Lasers Surg Med*. 2004;34(5):426–438.

Manuskiatti W, Sivayathorn A, Leelaudomlipi P, Fitzpatrick RE. Treatment of acquired bilateral nevus of Ota-like macules (Hori's nevus) using a combination of scanned carbon dioxide laser followed by Q-switched ruby laser. *J Am Acad Dermatol*. 2003;48(4):584–591.

Manuskiatti W, Fitzpatrick R, Goldman MP. Treatment of facial skin using combinations of CO2, Q-switched alexandrite, flashlamp- pumped pulsed dye, and Er:YAG lasers in the same treatment session. *Dermatol Surg*. 2000;26(2):114–120.

Masub N, Nguyen JK, Austin E, Jagdeo J. The vascular component of melasma: a systematic review of laboratory, diagnostic, and therapeutic evidence. *Dermatol Surg*. 2020;46(12):1642–1650.

McIlwee BE, Alster TS. Treatment of cosmetic tattoos: a review and case analysis. *Dermatol Surg*. 2018;44(12):1565–1570.

Mehrabi D, Brodell RT. Use of the alexandrite laser for treatment of seborrheic keratoses. *Dermatol Surg*. 2002;28(5):437–439.

Milgraum SS, Cohen ME, Auletta MJ. Treatment of blue nevi with the Q-switched ruby laser. *J Am Acad Dermatol*. 1995;32(2 Pt 2):307–310.

Moody MN, Landau JM, Vergilis-Kalner IJ, et al. 1, 064-nm Q-switched neodymium-doped yttrium aluminum garnet laser and 1, 550-nm fractionated erbium-doped fiber laser for the treatment of nevus of Ota in Fitzpatrick skin type IV. *Dermatol Surg.* 2011;37(8):1163–1167.

Moody MN, Landau JM, Goldberg LH, Friedman PM. Fractionated 1550-nm erbium-doped fiber laser for the treatment of periorbital hyperpigmentation. *Dermatol Surg.* 2012;38(1):139–142.

Moore M, Mishra V, Friedmann DP, Goldman MP. Minocycline- induced postsclerotherapy pigmentation successfully treated with a picosecond alexandrite laser. *Dermatol Surg.* 2016;42(1):133–134.

Mun JY, Jeong SY, Kim JH, Han SS, Kim IH. A low fluence Q-switched Nd:YAG laser modifies the 3d structure of melanocyte and ultrastructure of melanosome by subcellular-selective photothermolysis. *J Electron Microsc (Tokyo).* 2011;60(1):11–18.

Murphy GF, Shepard RS, Paul BS, Menkes A, et al. Organelle-specific injury to melanin-containing cells in human skin by pulsed laser irradiation. *Lab Invest.* 1983;49(6):680–685.

Naga LI, Alster T. Laser tattoo removal: an update. *Am J Clin Dermatol.* 2017;18(1):59–65.

Nanni CA, Alster TS. Treatment of a Becker's nevus using a 694-nm long-pulsed ruby laser. *Dermatol Surg.* 1998;24(9):1032–1034.

Narurkar V, Struck S, Jiang K, England L, et al. Safety and efficacy of a 1, 927-nm non-ablative fractional laser for the facial and non-facial resurfacing in skin types I to V. *Lasers Surg Med.* 2010;42(S22):1–125.

Negishi K, Akita H, Matsunaga Y. Prospective study of removing solar lentigines in Asians using a novel dual-wavelength and dual-pulse width picosecond laser. *Lasers Surg Med.* 2018;50(8):851–858.

Niwa Massaki AB, Eimpunth S, Fabi SG, Guiha I, et al. Treatment of melasma with the 1,927-nm fractional thulium fiber laser: A retrospective analysis of 20 cases with long-term follow-up. *Lasers Surg Med.* 2013;45(2):95–101.

Nouri K, Bowes L, Chartier T, Romagosa R, et al. Combination treatment of melasma with pulsed CO_2 laser followed by Q-switched alexandrite laser: a pilot study. *Dermatol Surg.* 1999;25(6):494–497.

Ohshiro T, Maruyama Y. The ruby and argon lasers in the treatment of naevi. *Ann Acad Med Singap.* 1983;12(suppl. 2):388–395.

Ohshiro T, Ohshiro T, Sasaki K, Kishi K Picosecond pulse duration laser treatment for dermal melanocytosis in Asians: a retrospective review. *Laser Ther.* 2016;25(2):99–104.

Ostertag JU, Quadvlieg PJF, Kerckhoffs FEMJ, Vermeulen AH, et al. Congenital naevi treated with Erbium:YAG laser (Derma K) resurfacing in neonates: clinical results and review of the literature. *Br J Dermatol.* 2006;154(5):889–895.

Park KY, Kim DH, Kim HK, Li K, Seo SJ, Hong CK. A randomized, observer-blinded, comparison of combined 1064-nm Q-switched neodymium-doped yttrium–aluminum–garnet laser plus 30% glycolic acid peel vs. laser monotherapy to treat melasma. *J Clin Exp Dermatol Res.* 2011;36(8):864–870.

Passeron T, Genedy R, Salah L, Fusade T, et al. Laser treatment of hyperpigmented lesions: position statement of the European Society of Laser in Dermatology. *J Eur Acad Dermatol Venereol.* 2019;33(6):987–1005.

Passeron T, Fontas E, Kang HY, Bahadoran P, et al. Melasma treatment with pulsed-dye laser and triple combination cream: a prospective, randomized, single-blind, split-face study. *Arch Dermatol.* 2011;147(9):1106–1108.

Patel PD, Mohan GC, Bhattacharya T, Patel RA, et al. Pediatric laser therapy in pigmented conditions. *Am J Clin Dermatol.* 2019;20(5):647–655.

Polder KD, Bruce S. Treatment of melasma using a novel 1,927-nm fractional thulium fiber laser: a pilot study. *Dermatol Surg.* 2012;38(2):199–206.

Polder KD, Landau JM, Vergilis-Kalner IJ, Goldberg LH, Friedman PM, Bruce S. Laser eradication of pigmented lesions: a review. *Dermatol Surg.* 2011;37(5):572–595.

Poldner KD, Harrison A, Eubanks LE, et al. 1,927-nm fractional thulium fiber laser for the treatment of nonfacial photodamage: a pilot study. *Dermatol Surg.* 2011;37(3):342–348.

Polnikorn N, Tanghetti E. Treatment of refractory melasma in Asians with the picosecond alexandrite laser. *Dermatol Surg.* 2020;46(12):1651–1656.

Polnikorn N, Tanrattanakorn S, Goldberg DJ. Treatment of Hori's nevus with the Q-switched Nd:YAG laser. *Dermatol Surg.* 2000;26(5):477–480.

Rahman Z, Alam M, Dover JS. Fractional laser treatment for pigmentation and texture improvement. *Skin Therapy Lett.* 2006;11(9):7–11.

Rajpar SF, Abdullah A, Lanigan SW. Er:YAG laser resurfacing for inoperable medium-sized facial congenital melanocytic naevi in children. *Clin Exp Dermatol.* 2007;32(2):159–161.

Rashid T, Hussain I, Haider M, Haroon TS. Laser therapy of freckles and lentigines with quasi-continuous frequency doubled, Nd:YAG (532 nm) laser in Fitzpatrick skin type IV: a 24-month follow-up. *J Cosmet Laser Ther.* 2002;4(3-4):81–85.

Redbord KP, Hanke CW. Case reports: clearance of lentigines in Japanese men with the long-pulsed alexandrite laser. *J Drugs Dermatol.* 2007;6(6):653–656.

Reddy KK, Brauer JA, Anolik R, Benstein L, et al. Topical perfluorodecalin resolves immediate whitening reactions and allows rapid effective multiple pass treatment of tattoos. *Lasers Surg Med.* 2013;45:76–80.

Rho N-K. Treatment of café-au-lait Macules using a Q-switched Laser Followed by Serial Fractional thulium Laser treatments. *Med Lasers.* 2017;6(1):41–43.

Rodrigues M, Bekhor P. Treatment of minocycline-induced cutaneous pigmentation with the picosecond alexandrite (755-nm) laser. *Dermatol Surg.* 2015;41(10):1179–1182.

Rokhsar CK, Fitzpatrick RE. The treatment of melasma with fractional photothermolysis: a pilot study. *Dermatol Surg.* 2005;31(12):1645–1650.

Ross EV, Naseef G, Lin C, et al. Comparison of responses of tattoos to picosecond and nanosecond Q-switched neodymium: YAG lasers. *Arch Dermatol.* 1998;134(2):167–171.

Sadighha A, Saatee S, Muhaghegh-Zahed G. Efficacy and adverse effects of Q-switched ruby laser on solar lentigines: a prospective study of 91 patients with Fitzpatrick skin type II, III, and IV. *Dermatol Surg.* 2008;34(11):1465–1468.

Saedi N, Metelitsa A, Petrell K, Arndt KA, et al. Treatment of tattoos with a picosecond alexandrite laser: a prospective trial. *Arch Dermatol.* 2012;148(12):1360–1363.

Schweiger ES, Kwasniak L, Aires DJ. Treatment of dermatosis papulosa nigra with a 1064 nm Nd:YAG laser: report of two cases. *J Cosmet Laser Ther.* 2008;10(2):120–122.

Shah G, Alster TS. Treatment of an amalgam tattoo with a Q-switched alexandrite (755 nm) laser. *Dermatol Surg.* 2002;28(12):1180–1181.

Sherling M, Friedman PM, Adrian R, Burns AJ, et al. Consensus recommendations on the use of an erbium-doped 1, 550-nm fractionated laser and its applications in dermatologic laser surgery. *Dermatol Surg.* 2010;36(4):461–469.

Sheth VM, Pandya AG. Melasma: Comprehensive update: part II. *J Am Acad Dermatol.* 2011;65(4):699–714.

Shin JU, Park J, Oh SH, Lee JH. Oral tranexamic acid enhances the efficacy of low-fluence 1064-nm quality-switched neodymium-doped yttrium aluminum garnet laser treatment for melasma in Koreans: a randomized, prospective trial. *Dermatol Surg.* 2013;39(3 Pt 1):435–442.

Spierings NMK. Melasma: A critical analysis of clinical trials investigating treatment modalities published in the past 10 years. *J Cosmet Dermatol.* 2020;19(6):1284–1289.

Stern RS, Dover JS, Levin JA, Arndt KA. Laser therapy versus cryotherapy of lentigines: a comparative trial. *J Am Acad Dermatol.* 1994;30(6):985–987.

Suh DH, Han KH, Chung JH. The use of Q-switched Nd:YAG laser in the treatment of superficial pigmented lesions in Koreans. *J Dermatol Treat.* 2001;12(2):91–96.

Tan SK. Exogenous ochronosis – successful outcome after treatment with Q-switched Nd:YAG laser. *J Cosmet Laser Ther.* 2013;15(5):274–278.

Tanghetti EA. The histology of skin treated with a picosecond alexandrite laser and a fractional lens array. *Lasers Surg Med.* 2016;48(7):646–652.

Taylor CR, Flotte TJ, Gange RW, Anderson RR. Treatment of nevus of Ota by Q-switched ruby laser. *J Am Acad Dermatol.* 1994;30:743–751.

Taylor CR, Anderson RR. Treatment of benign pigmented epidermal lesions by Q-switched ruby laser. *Int J Dermatol.* 1993;32(12):908–912.

Taylor CR, Anderson RR. Ineffective treatment of refractory melasma and postinflammatory hyperpigmentation by Q-switched ruby laser. *J Dermatol Surg Oncol.* 1994;20(9):592–597.

Todd MM, Rallis TM, Gerwels JW, Hata TR. A comparison of 3 lasers and liquid nitrogen in the treatment of solar lentigines: a randomized, controlled, comparative trial. *Arch Dermatol.* 2000;136(7):841–846.

Torbeck RL, Schilling L, Khorasani H, Dover JS, et al. Evolution of the picosecond laser: a review of the literature. *Dermatol Surg.* 2019;45(2):183–194.

Tourlaki A, Galimberti MG, Pellacani G, Bencini PL. Combination of fractional erbium-glass laser and topical therapy in melasma resistant to triple-combination cream. *J Dermatolog Treat.* 2014;25(3):218–222.

Trafeli JP, Kwan JM, Meehan KJ, et al. Use of a long-pulse alexandrite laser in the treatment of superficial pigmented lesions. *Dermatol Surg.* 2007;33(12):1477–1482.

Trelles MA, Allones I, Moreno-Arias GA, Vélez M. Becker's naevus: a comparative study between erbium: YAG and Q-switched neodymium:YAG; clinical and histopathological findings. *Br J Dermatol.* 2005;152(2):308–313.

Trelles MA, Velez M, Gold MH. The treatment of melasma with topical creams alone, CO_2 fractional ablative resurfacing alone, or a combination of the two: A comparative study. *J Drugs Dermatol.* 2010;9(4):315–322.

Trivedi MK, Yang FC, Cho BK. A review of laser and light therapy in melasma. *Int J Womens Dermatol.* 2017;3(1):11–20.

Tse Y, Levine VJ, McClain SA, Ashinoff R. The removal of cutaneous pigmented lesions with the Q-switched ruby laser and the Q-switched neodymium:yttrium aluminum garnet laser. A comparative study. *J Dermatol Surg Oncol.* 1994;20(12):795–800.

Ueda S, Imayama S. Normal-mode ruby laser for treating congenital nevi. *Arch Dermatol.* 1997;133:355–359.

Ueda S, Isoda M, Imayama S. Response of naevus of Ota to Q-switched ruby laser treatment according to lesion colour. *Br J Dermatol.* 2000;142(1):77–83.

Ungaksornpairote C, Manuskiatti W, Junsuwan N, Wanitphakdeedecha R. A prospective, split-face, randomized study comparing picosecond to Q-switched Nd:YAG laser for treatment of epidermal and dermal pigmented lesions in Asians. *Dermatol Surg.* 2020;46(12):1671–1675.

van Leeuwen RL, Dekker SK, Byers HR, et al. Modulation of alpha 4 beta 1 and alpha 5 beta 1 integrin expression: heterogeneous effects of Q-switched ruby, Nd:YAG, and alexandrite lasers on melanoma cells in vitro. *Lasers Surg Med.* 1996;18(1):63–71.

Vangipuram RK, DeLozier WL, Geddes E, Friedman PM. Complete resolution of minocycline pigmentation following a single treatment with non-ablative 1550-nm fractional resurfacing in combination with the 755-nm Q-switched alexandrite laser. *Lasers Surg Med.* 2016;48(3):234–237.

Wang Y, Qian H, Lu Z. Treatment of café au lait macules in Chinese patients with a Q-switched 755-nm alexandrite laser. *J Dermatolog Treat.* 2012;23(6):431–436.

Wang YJ, Lin ET, Chen YT, et al. Prospective randomized controlled trial comparing treatment efficacy and tolerance of picosecond alexandrite laser with a diffractive lens array and triple combination cream in female Asian patients with melasma. *J Eur Acad Dermatol Venereol.* 2020;34(3):624–632.

Wanitphakdeedecha R, Manuskiatti W, Siriphukpong S, Chen TM. Treatment of melasma using variable square pulse Er:Yag laser resurfacing. *Dermatol Surg.* 2009;35:475–481.

Wanner M, Tanzi EL, Alster TS. Fractional photothermolysis: treatment of facial and nonfacial cutaneous photodamage with a 1,550-nm erbium-doped fiber laser. *Dermatol Surg.* 2007;33(1):23–28.

Watanabe S, Takahashi H. Treatment of nevus of Ota with the Q-switched ruby laser. *N Engl J Med.* 1994;331:1745–1750.

Wattanakrai P, Mornchan R, Eimpunth S. Low-fluence Q-switched neodymium-doped yttrium aluminum garnet (1,064 nm) laser for the treatment of facial melasma in Asians. *Dermatol Surg.* 2010;36(1):76–87.

Westerhoff W, Gamei M. Treatment of acquired junctional me- lanocytic naevi by Q-switched and normal mode ruby laser. *Br J Dermatol.* 2003;148(1):80–85.

Wind BS, Kroon MW, Meesters AA, Beek JF, van der Veen JPW, Nieuweboer-Krobotová L, et al. Non-ablative 1,550 nm fractional laser therapy versus triple topical therapy for the treatment of melasma: A randomized controlled split-face study. *Lasers Surg Med.* 2010;42(7):607–612.

Wu DC, Fletcher L, Guiha I, Goldman MP. Evaluation of the safety and efficacy of the picosecond alexandrite laser with specialized lens array for treatment of the photoaging décolletage. *Lasers Surg Med.* 2016;48(2):188–192.

Wu D, Goldman MP, Wat H, Chan HHL. A systematic review of picosecond laser in dermatology: evidence and recommendations. *Lasers Surg Med.* 2021;53(1):9–49.

Xi Z, Gold MH, Zhong L, Ying L. Efficacy and safety of Q-switched 1, 064-nm neodymium-doped yttrium aluminum garnet laser treatment of melasma. *Dermatol Surg.* 2011;37(7):962–970.

Yoshimura K, Sato K, Aiba-Kojima E, et al. Repeated treatment protocols for melasma and acquired dermal melanocytosis. *Dermatol Surg.* 2006;32(3):365–371.

Yu W, Zhu J, Yu W, Lyu D, Lin X, Zhang Z. A split-face, single- blinded, randomized controlled comparison of alexandrite 755- nm picosecond laser versus alexandrite 755-nm nanosecond laser in the treatment of acquired bilateral nevus of Ota-like macules. *J Am Acad Dermatol.* 2018;79(3):479–486.

Zachary CB, Rofagha R. *Laser therapy. Dermatology.* 3rd ed. Philadelphia, PA: Elsevier Saunders; 2012:2261–2282.

Zeng Y, Ji C, Zhan K, Weng E. Treatment of nasal ala nodular congenital melanocytic naevus with carbon dioxide laser and Q-switched Nd:YAG laser. *Lasers Med Sci.* 2016;31(8):1627–1632.

4

Laser Hair Removal

Omar A. Ibrahimi, Suzanne L. Kilmer, and Farah Moustafa

SUMMARY AND KEY FEATURES

- Laser hair removal (LHR) is the most commonly requested cosmetic procedure in the world.
- The ideal candidate for LHR is fair skinned with dark terminal hair; however, LHR can currently be successfully performed in all skin types.
- Thin hairs and hairs with white, blond, and red color are extremely difficult to treat with LHR devices.
- Wax epilation should be avoided prior to and during LHR treatments.
- Lasers pose a safety risk to both the patient and device operator.

- Informed consent should be reviewed with every patient prior to treatment.
- Wavelength, spot size, pulse duration, and skin cooling are key variables that can be used to tailor laser–tissue interactions for a given patient.
- Approximately 15%–30% of hairs can be removed with each treatment session using ideal parameters. Remaining hairs are often thinner and lighter in color.
- The most common complication is pigmentary alteration, which can be temporary or permanent.

INTRODUCTION

The nonspecific damage of human hair follicles with a laser was noted more than 50 years ago. The theory of selective photothermolysis, first described by Rox Anderson and John Parrish, provided the framework of selectively targeting a particular chromophore based on its absorption spectrum. In 1996, this group also reported the first successful use of a normal-mode ruby laser for long-term and permanent hair removal.

Removing unwanted body hair is popular worldwide, and hair removal using laser or other light-based technology is one of the most highly requested cosmetic procedures. Prior to the advent of laser hair removal (LHR), only temporary methods for removing unwanted hair were available, such as bleaching, plucking, shaving, waxing, and chemical depilatories. In addition to not providing permanent hair removal,

these methods are also inconvenient and tedious. Electrolysis is a technique in which a fine needle is inserted deep into the hair follicle and uses electrical current, thereby destroying the hair follicle and allowing for permanent hair removal of all types of hair. However, this technique is impractical for treating large areas, extremely tedious, operator-dependent, and with variable efficacy in achieving permanent hair removal. Eflornithine (α-difluoromethylornithine [DFMO]) is a topical inhibitor of ornithine decarboxylase that slows the rate of hair growth and is currently US Food and Drug Administration (FDA) cleared for the removal of unwanted facial hair in women. In this chapter, we provide a detailed overview on LHR, including discussion of hair follicle biology, the science behind LHR, key factors in optimizing treatment, and future trends.

BASIC HAIR BIOLOGY

The hair follicle is a hormonally active structure (Fig. 4.1) that is anatomically divided into an infundibulum (hair follicle orifice to insertion of the sebaceous gland), isthmus (insertion of the sebaceous gland to the insertion of the arrector [erector] pili muscle), and bulb (insertion of the arrector pili to the base of the hair follicle) segments. The dermal papilla provides neurovascular support to the base of the follicle and helps to form the hair shaft.

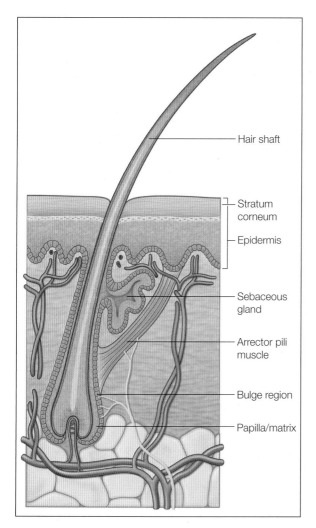

Fig. 4.1 Hair follicle anatomy. *(Reproduced from Tsao SS, Hruza GJ. Laser hair removal. In: Robinson JK, Hanke CW, Sengelmann RD, Siegel DM, eds. Surgery of the Skin. Philadelphia, PA: Elsevier Mosby; 2005:575–588.)*

Every hair follicle is controlled by a programmed cycle that is dependent on the anatomic location. The hair cycle consists of anagen, catagen, and telogen phases. Anagen is characterized by a period of active growth in which the hair shaft lengthens. A catagen transition period follows in which the lower part of the hair follicle undergoes apoptosis. A resting period, telogen, then ensues and regrowth occurs when anagen resumes. Hair regrowth (entry into another anagen cycle) is dependent on stem cells within or near the hair bulb matrix. Slow-cycling stem cells have also been found in the follicular bulge arising off the outer root sheath at the site of the arrector pili muscle attachment.

The main types of hair include lanugo, vellus, and terminal hairs. Lanugo hairs are fine hairs that cover a fetus and are shed in the neonatal period. Vellus hairs are usually nonpigmented and have a diameter of approximately 30–50 µm. Terminal hair shafts range from 150 to 300 µm in diameter. The type of hair produced by an individual follicle is capable of change (e.g., vellus to terminal hair at puberty or terminal to vellus hair in androgenic alopecia).

The amount and type of pigment in the hair shaft determine hair color. Melanocytes produce two types of melanin: eumelanin, a brown-black pigment; and pheomelanin, a red pigment. Melanocytes are located in the upper portion of the hair bulb and outer root sheath of the infundibulum.

Definitions of what constitutes excessive or unwanted body hair depend on cultural norms, but can usually be classified as either hypertrichosis or hirsutism. Hirsutism is the abnormal growth of terminal hair in women in male-pattern (androgen-dependent) sites, such as the face and chest. Hypertrichosis is excess hair growth at any body site that is not androgen-dependent. In addition, the use of grafts and flaps in skin surgery can often introduce hair to an area that causes a displeasing appearance or functional impairment.

MECHANISM OF LASER HAIR REMOVAL

The theory of selective photothermolysis enables precise targeting of pigmented hair follicles by using the melanin of the hair shaft as a chromophore. Melanin has an absorbance spectrum that matches wavelengths in the red and near-infrared (IR) portion of the electromagnetic spectrum (approximately 700–1000 nm). To achieve permanent hair removal, the biologic "target" is the follicular stem cells located in the bulge region and/or dermal papilla. Due to the slight spatial separation of the chromophore and desired target, an extended theory of selective photothermolysis was proposed that requires diffusion of heat from the chromophore to the desired target for destruction. This requires a laser pulse duration that is longer in duration than if the actual chromophore and desired target are identical. Temporary LHR can result when the follicular stem cells are not completely destroyed, primarily through induction of a catagen-like state in pigmented hair follicles. Temporary LHR is much easier to achieve than permanent removal when using lower fluences. Long-term hair removal depends on hair color, skin color, and tolerated fluence. Approximately 15%–30% long-term hair loss may be observed with each treatment when optimal treatment parameters are used (Fig. 4.2). A list of commonly used laser and light devices that are currently commercially available for hair removal is provided in Table 4.1.

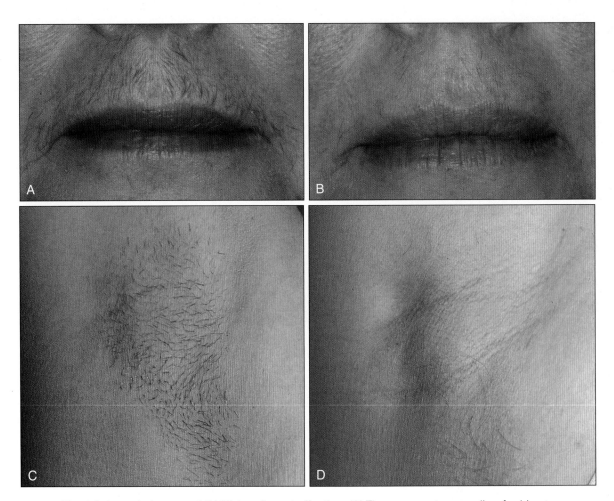

Fig. 4.2 Laser hair removal (LHR) is safe and effective. (A) The upper cutaneous lip of a hirsute female. (B) Appearance of same subject following only three treatments with a long-pulsed 755-nm alexandrite laser used with a 12-mm spot size, 16 J/cm², 3-ms pulse duration, and dynamic cooling device (DCD) setting of 30/30/0. (C) Axilla of an adult female. (D) Following four treatments with a long-pulsed diode laser (LPDL) with a large spot size and vacuum-assisted suction. The fluence used was 12 J/cm² and the pulse duration was 60 ms. Both of the above subjects achieved excellent hair reduction and further benefit would likely be attained with additional treatments.

TABLE 4.1 Commonly Used Commercially Available Lasers and Light Sources for Hair Removal[a]

Laser/Light Source	Wavelength (nm)	System Name	Pulse Duration (ms)	Fluence (J/cm²)	Spot Size (mm)	Other Features
Long-pulsed alexandrite	755	Apogee + (Cynosure, Westford, MA, USA)	0.5–300	2–50	5–18	Cold air or integrated cooling, can add 1064-nm Nd:YAG module (Elite +)
	—	Arion (Alma Laser, Buffalo Grove, IL, USA)	5–140	Up to 40	6–16	Cold air cooling Optional scanner 60 × 65mm
	—	Clarity (Lutronic, Gyeonggi-do, Korea)	0.1–300	Up to 600	2–20	Cryo or air cooling options, available with 1064-nm wavelength
	—	Clarity II (Lutronic, Gyeonggi-do, Korea)	0.1–300	Up to 600	2–25 mm	Cryo or air cooling options, single fiber handpiece with multi-spot cartridges
	—	Elite + (Cynosure, Westford, MA, USA)	0.5–300	Up to 50	3–24	Cold air cooling, available with 1064-nm Nd:YAG, can simultaneously treat with 755-nm alexandrite and 1064-nm Nd:YAG
	—	EpiCare Alex (Light Age, Somerset, NJ, USA)	0.5–300	Up to 2500	1.5–18	Dynamic cooling; can be combined with 1064 in EpiCare Zenith and Epicare Duo systems
	—	Excel HR (Cutera, Brisbane, CA, USA)	3	Up to 100	5–18	Chilled sapphire tip (contact cooling), comes with 1064-nm Nd:YAG
	—	GentleLase Pro (Candela, Wayland, MA, USA) GentleMax Pro (Candela, Wayland, MA, USA)	0.25–300	Up to 400 Up to 400	3–24 3–24	Dynamic cooling, comes with 1064-nm Nd:YAG
		SplendorX (Lumenis, Israel)	3–100	20	2–30 (round) 2 × 2 – 27 × 27 (square)	Cold air cooling and contact cooling, simultaneous emission of 755nm and 1064 nm, built-in plume evacuator
Diode	810, 940 (755 nm with Pro series)	MeDioStar XT (Aesclepion)	3–400	Up to 60	10 × 10 15 × 10 30 × 10 31.5 × 31.5	Contact cooling, can come with 755-nm alexandrite

(Continued)

TABLE 4.1 Commonly Used Commercially Available Lasers and Light Sources for Hair Removal[a]—cont'd

Laser/Light Source	Wavelength (nm)	System Name	Pulse Duration (ms)	Fluence (J/cm²)	Spot Size (mm)	Other Features
	805, 1060	LightSheer Quattro (Lumenis, Israel)	5–400	4.5–100, 4.5–12	9 × 9, 12 × 12, 22 × 35	Chilltip for smaller handpiece, vacuum skin flattening for larger handpiece, 1060 nm wavelength available
	810	Soprano XL (Alma Lasers, Buffalo Grove, IL, USA)	10–1350	Up to 120	12 × 10	Contact cooling
	810	Vectus (Cynosure)	5–300	Up to 100	12 × 12, 22 × 38	Contact cooling
Long-pulsed Nd:YAG	1064	—	—	—	—	—
	—	ClearHairYAG (Sciton)	2–200	Up to 400	3 × 6 30 × 30	Contact cooling
	—	Elite + (Cynosure, Westford, MA, USA)	0.4–300	Up to 300	3–18	Cold air, comes with 755-nm alexandrite
	—	Epicare Nd:YAG (Light Age, Somerset, NJ, USA)	0.5–300	Up to 2500	1.5–18	Contact cooling, can be combined with 1064 in EpiCare Zenith and Epicare Duo systems
	—	Excel HR	0.1–300	Up to 300	3–18	Contact cooling, comes with 755-nm alexandrite
	—	SP and XP Dynamis, XP Focus, XP Max (Fotona)	0.1–50	Up to 300	2–10	N/A
	—	GentleYAG Pro (Syneron-Candela, Wayland, MA, USA)	0.25–300	Up to 400	1.5–24	Dynamic cooling
	—	LightPod Neo (Aerolase, Tarrytown, NY, USA)	0.65–1.5	Up to 312	2, 5, 6	—
	—	SmartEpil (Deka, Italy)	Up to 20	11 J (fluence not available)	2.5, 4, 5, 6	Contact cooling. 2940 nm Er:YAG and 410–1400 nm flashlamp in same device
	—	Synchro_FT (Deka)	2–30	Up to 700	2.5–13	Available with IPL handpiece
	—	Xeo (Cutera, Brisbane, CA, USA)	0.1–300	3–300	3, 5, 7, 10	Contact cooling, comes with IPL

IPL sources					
BBL (Sciton)	420–1400	Up to 200	Up to 30	15 × 45	Built-in cooling system
Ellipse IPL (Syneron-Candela, Wayland, MA, USA)	600–950	2.5–88.5	4–26	10 × 48	Contact cooling. Comes as part of Nordlys system including 1550 nm, 1940 nm, and 1064 nm
Harmony XL SHR Pro (Alma Lasers)	700–950	30–50	Up to 40	30 × 30	Harmony XL platform can include 1064-nm Nd:YAG
Icon MaxR Max Rs (Cynosure, Westford, MA, USA)	650–1200	1–100	Up to 48, Up to 72	16 × 46, 12 × 28	Built in contact-cooling
Med Flash II (General Project, Italy)	390–1200	Up to 100	Up to 45	N/A	Air cooling
MiniSilk_FT (Deka)	500–1200	3–8	Up to 160	48 × 13, 23 × 13	1064-nm Nd:YAG handpiece
Mistral (Radiancy)	400–1200	Up to 80	4–15	25 × 50, 13 × 50, 13 × 35, 12 × 12	Contact cooling
NannoLight MP50 (Sybaritic, Minneapolis, MN, USA)	640–1400	1–30	2.8–50	40 × 8	Nd:YAG handpiece, optional cooling
NaturaLight (Focus Medical, Bethel, CT, USA)	640–1200	Up to 500	Up to 50	10 × 40	—
Solera Opus (Cutera)	750–1100	Auto	3–24	10 × 30	—
V-IPL (Viora, Jersey City, NJ, USA)	415–1200	10–205	Up to 35	6.4 × 6.4, 2.4 × 2.4	Contact cooling
PhotoSilk Plus (Deka)	550–950	3–25	3–32	46 × 10, 46 × 18	Contact cooling, comes with 1064-nm Nd:YAG and nm-2940 Er:YAG
ProWave LX (Cutera)	680–1100	35–90	5–35	10 × 30	Contact cooling, comes with Nd:YAG handpiece in Xeo platform
Quadra Q4 (DermaMed, Lenni, PA, USA)	500–1200	48	10–20	34 × 27	—

(Continued)

TABLE 4.1 Commonly Used Commercially Available Lasers and Light Sources for Hair Removal[a]—cont'd

Laser/Light Source	Wavelength (nm)	System Name	Pulse Duration (ms)	Fluence (J/cm²)	Spot Size (mm)	Other Features
Fluorescent-pulsed light	400–1200	Universal IPL (Lumenis, Israel)	4–20	Up to 56	35 × 15, 15 × 8	Contact cooling, comes as part of Stellar M22 platform with long pulse Nd:YAG, q-switched Nd:YAG, and nonablative fractional 1565 nm
	480–920	OmniLight/NovaLight (American Medical Bio Care, Newport Beach, CA, USA)	2–500	Up to 90	7 × 15, 10 × 20, 30 × 30	Sapphire tip cooling
Diode combined with RF electrical energy	810	Elos Motif Vantage (Candela, Wayland, MA, USA)	Up to 100	4–30 optical; 5–30 j/cm³ RF	33 × 14	Contact cooling
Home-use devices	—		—	—	—	
	—	Lumea (Philips, Amsterdam, Netherlands)	—	—	—	IPL-based system
	—	Silkn SensEpil (Skinnovations, Israel)	—	—	—	IPL-based, devices with finite number of pulses
	—	SmoothSkin (Cyden, Swansea, United Kingdom)	—	—	—	IPL-based device, unlimited number of pulses
	—	Viss IPL (Viss Beauty, Korea)	—	—	—	IPL-based, finite number of pulses
	—	Tria Laser 3.0 (Tria Beauty, Pleasanton, CA, USA)	—	—	—	Diode laser, low, medium, and high fluences
		Touch (Illuminage)				IPL and RF

IPL, Intense-pulsed light; RF, radiofrequency.
[a]This table is intended only as a reference aid. The authors have made every attempt to provide an exhaustive list of available devices for LHR but do not guarantee comprehensiveness.

KEY FACTORS IN OPTIMIZING TREATMENT

LHR has revolutionized the ability to eliminate unwanted hair temporarily and permanently in many individuals of all skin colors. Proper patient selection, preoperative preparation, informed consent, understanding of the principles of laser safety, and laser and light source selection are key to the success of laser treatment. An understanding of hair anatomy, growth, and physiology, together with a thorough understanding of laser–tissue interaction, in particular within the context of choosing optimal laser parameters for effective LHR, should be acquired before using lasers for hair removal.

Patient Selection

A focused medical history, physical examination, and informed consent, including setting realistic expectations and potential risks, should be performed prior to any laser treatment (Box 4.1). Patients with evidence of endocrine or menstrual dysfunction should be appropriately worked up. Similarly, patients with an explosive onset of hypertrichosis should be evaluated for paraneoplastic etiologies. There is not enough data demonstrating safety of laser hair removal in pregnancy, therefore it is generally not recommended. The past medical history should be reviewed to identify patients with photosensitive conditions, such as autoimmune connective tissue disorders, or disorders prone to the Koebner phenomenon. A history of recurrent cutaneous infections at or in the vicinity of the treatment area might warrant the use of prophylactic medications. Any past history of keloid or hypertrophic scar formation should be elicited as well. Previous hair removal methods, including past laser treatments, should be reviewed. Any methods of hair shaft epilation (e.g., waxing or tweezing) that entirely remove the target chromophore render LHR less effective for at least 2 weeks. Although there is little evidence for the time frame a patient must wait after complete epilation of the hair shaft and laser treatment, we recommend a minimum of 6 weeks. Shaving and depilatory creams can be used up to the day of laser treatment because they do not remove the entire hair shaft.

BOX 4.1 Pertinent Medical History for Laser and Pulsed Light Hair Removal

- Presence of conditions that may cause hypertrichosis:
  - Hormonal
  - Familial
  - Drugs (i.e., corticosteroids, hormones, immuno-suppressives, self or spousal use of minoxidil)
  - Tumor
  - History of local or recurrent skin infection
  - History of herpes simplex, especially perioral
  - History of herpes genitalis, important when treating the pubic or bikini area
  - History of keloids/hypertrophic scarring
  - History of koebnerizing skin disorders, such as vitiligo and psoriasis
  - Previous treatment modalities—method, frequency, and date of last treatment, as well as response
  - Recent suntan or exposure to tanning or light cabinet
  - Onset of hair regrowth (recent)
  - Tattoos or nevi present
  - Patient's expectations
  - Patient's hobbies or habits which might interfere with treatment
- Present medications:
  - Photosensitizing medications

CASE STUDY 1

A 27-year-old Hispanic female with Fitzpatrick skin type IV presents to you for hair removal on the "beard area." She has been treated five times with a diode laser over the course of 2 years at a local spa and notes only a minimal reduction of hair. On review of systems, you discover that the patient has had a history of irregular menses and periodically flaring acne. She does not see a gynecologist.

Although it appears that the patient is responding poorly to laser treatment, a thorough history reveals that the patient has clinical and historical evidence of hormonal dysfunction. This imbalance may be driving the conversion of vellus hair to terminal hair and can make it appear that LHR treatments are ineffective, when in reality the patient is responding to treatment but is creating new hair follicles.

Informed Consent

Informed consent requires a review of the potential risks of LHR, which include, but are not limited to, temporary and permanent hypo- or hyperpigmentation, blister formation, scar formation, ulceration, urticaria, bruising, infection, acne flare, and folliculitis. For those patients with Fitzpatrick skin type IV or greater or of Mediterranean, Middle Eastern, Asian, or South Asian

PEARL 1

It is imperative to counsel the patient not to partake in any epilation activities that remove the entire hair shaft. Shaving or using a chemical depilatory prior to treatment is acceptable but waxing or plucking will be counteractive to the laser treatments. A 2-week interval after such procedures is recommended for improved efficacy.

A medication history should be obtained. The use of any photosensitizing medications or over-the-counter supplements should be held before treatment. Topical retinoids used in the treatment area should be discontinued 1–2 days prior to treatment. Finally, the patient's reaction to unprotected sun exposure (Fitzpatrick skin phototype) should be elicited as part of the history.

The physical exam should corroborate the patient's Fitzpatrick skin phototype. This will help to determine which lasers and light sources are safe to use for that patient (see Table 4.1) because epidermal melanin in darkly pigmented patients competes with the melanin within hair follicles as a chromophore. Importantly, every patient should always be evaluated for the presence of a tan and, if present, laser treatment should be delayed, or the treatment parameters appropriately adjusted until the tan has faded. Finally, the patient's hair color should be noted as the chromophore for LHR is melanin. Black and brown terminal hairs typically contain sufficient amount of melanin to serve as a chromophore for LHR. The lack of melanin, paucity of melanin, or presence of pheomelanin in the hair follicle clinically correlates with white, gray, or red/blond hair, respectively. These features are all predictive of a poor response to LHR (Fig. 4.3). For patients with little to no melanin in their hair follicles, attempts have been made to use exogenous chromophores that can be topically delivered to the hair follicles, thereby making the removal of white, gray, red, and blond hair hypothetically possible. This concept was first demonstrated with a topical carbon solution dissolved in mineral oil. More recently, silver gold nanoparticles were also studied. However, these did not show satisfactory results. The coarseness and density of hair are also important to note because these factors will influence parameter settings (see later).

PEARL 2

Treatment on tanned patients should be delayed until the tan fades. Risk of pigmentary alteration is significantly higher in these patients.

PEARL 3

Patients with white, gray, or blond hair are currently not appropriate candidates for LHR. Other methods of epilation should be encouraged.

descent, the low risk of paradoxical hypertrichosis (conversion of vellus hairs to thicker, more obvious terminal hairs), especially when treating the lateral face and jaw, should be reviewed. Patients should be counseled that permanent and complete hair removal is not likely but that, with multiple treatments, significant long-term reduction can be achieved. Hirsute women with hormonal abnormalities, such as polycystic ovarian syndrome, may require continued maintenance therapy and should be advised of this possibility. Procedural pain is expected with LHR but can be minimized with topical anesthetics. Erythema and edema are also expected with treatment and may last up to 1 week. Patients should be

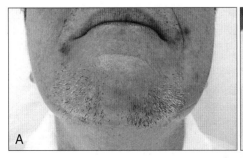
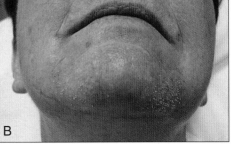

Fig. 4.3 Effective LHR can be obtained for dark, pigmented hairs but not for white hairs: (A) before and (B) after treatment.

aware of the need for strict sun avoidance before and after each treatment.

CASE STUDY 2

A 32-year-old Egyptian female presents for LHR of the lateral preauricular face. On physical exam, she is a Fitzpatrick skin type V with fine, dark vellus hairs in the area of interest.

This patient is a challenge for a variety of reasons (dark skin type, caliber of hair to be treated). Importantly, it is critical for the laser surgeon to also review the rare risk of paradoxical hypertrichosis (see previously). Paradoxical hypertrichosis is a poorly understood phenomenon in which laser stimulates hair growth or a change in hair type from vellus to terminal hairs. This produces an obvious worsening in the appearance of the affected hairs in a cosmetically sensitive area (i.e., the face). Although challenging, these increased hairs can be treated with further hair removal, often with higher fluences and may be more resistant to therapy. Patients may also require electrolysis for hair removal in these cases.

Preoperative Preparation and Laser Safety

The need for topical anesthesia is variable among patients and anatomic sites. Various topical anesthetics, including lidocaine, lidocaine/prilocaine, and other amide/ester anesthetic combinations, can be used to diminish the procedural discomfort and should be applied 30 minutes to 1 hour before treatment under occlusion. Care should be taken when using lidocaine or prilocaine to apply these medications to a limited area to diminish the risk of lidocaine toxicity or methemoglobinemia, respectively. Deaths have resulted from lidocaine toxicity resulting from occlusion of the back, as well as lower extremities, with high concentrations of compounded topical lidocaine. Likewise, systemic toxicity can occur with the use of any topical anesthetic in large amounts. In the authors' experience, topical analgesics is rarely required for laser hair removal.

Device Variables
Wavelength

The chromophore for LHR is melanin. Within the hair follicle, melanin is principally located within the hair shaft, although the outer root sheath and matrix area also contain melanin. Melanin is capable of functioning as a chromophore for wavelengths in the red and near-IR portion of the electromagnetic spectrum, and can be targeted by ruby, alexandrite, diode, and neodymium:yttrium-aluminum-garnet (Nd:YAG) lasers, as well as IPL devices.

PEARL 4

Occlusion increases the absorption of topical medications by at least an order of magnitude. Lidocaine is a cardiotoxic medication, and prilocaine can convert hemoglobin into methemoglobulin. Large areas, such as the back or legs, should have topical anesthesia applied with caution.

Patients should be placed in a room with a treatment chair that makes the desired treatment area easily accessible. The room should be adequately cooled to keep the laser device from overheating and be free of any hanging mirrors or uncovered windows. A fire extinguisher should be readily available. If possible, supplemental oxygen should be turned off when performing laser treatments. Having a vacuum device on hand during treatment can minimize the plume and unpleasant odor created by each laser pulse. Because the retina contains melanin that can be damaged by wavelengths in the red and near-IR range, proper eye protection is absolutely critical for both the patient and laser surgeon. Goggles are not interchangeable between lasers or intense-pulsed light (IPL) devices of different wavelengths. Furthermore, because of the risk of retinal damage from the deeply penetrating wavelengths used for LHR, one should never treat a patient for LHR within the bony orbit.

CASE STUDY 3

A 35-year-old female with Fitzpatrick skin type II and jet-black hair presents to you for LHR. During the consultation, she states her primary concern is that she would like to have her eyebrows shaped permanently. She is inconvenienced by her current regimen of waxing every several weeks.

The patient is an ideal candidate for LHR with her fair skin and dark hair. Almost any hair removal laser would be appropriate for use. The issue of concern in this case is the location of treatment. Caution must be taken when treating near the eye because there is a risk of damage to retinal pigment.

The long-pulsed ruby laser (694 nm) was the first device used to selectively target hair follicles, resulting in long-term hair loss. The long-pulsed ruby laser can be safely used in Fitzpatrick skin phototypes I–III. There are currently no available long-pulsed ruby lasers on the market.

The long-pulsed alexandrite (755 nm) laser has been shown to be effective for long-term hair removal in multiple studies. The long-pulsed alexandrite laser can be safely used in Fitzpatrick skin phototypes I–IV, although some experts limit the use of the long-pulsed alexandrite laser to Fitzpatrick skin phototypes I–III. A few studies have demonstrated the safety of the long-pulsed alexandrite laser in a large cohort of patients with Fitzpatrick skin phototypes IV–VI. There is insufficient data on whether combination treatment of alexandrite and Nd:YAG lasers provides additional benefit over the alexandrite laser alone.

The long-pulsed diode laser (LPDL; 800–810 nm) has also been extensively used for LHR. The diode laser can be safely used in patients with Fitzpatrick skin phototypes I–V and has good long-term efficacy for LHR. A 1060-nm diode laser has also demonstrated long-term efficacy in all Fitzpatrick skin phototypes.

The long-pulsed Nd:YAG laser has been thought to offer the best combination of safety and efficacy for Fitzpatrick skin phototype VI patients. Long-term hair reduction with 18-month follow-up showed 73.6% clearance following four treatments at 2-month intervals.

IPL is composed of polychromatic, noncoherent light ranging from 400 to 1200 nm. Various filters can be used to target particular chromophores, including melanin. One study of patients treated with a single IPL session reported 75% hair removal 1 year after treatment. Two studies providing a head-to-head comparison of IPL versus either the long-pulsed alexandrite laser or Nd:YAG laser both found the IPL to be inferior to laser devices for hair removal. In contrast, a study of hirsute women, some with a diagnosis of polycystic ovarian syndrome, who underwent a split-face treatment with six IPL or LPDL showed statistically equivalent reductions in hair counts at 1 (77% vs. 68%, respectively), 3 (53% vs. 60%, respectively), and 6 months (40% vs. 34%, respectively) after the final treatment.

PEARL 5

One should always evaluate the patient's Fitzpatrick skin type when evaluating a patient for LHR. Darker skin types require longer wavelengths, which pose a lower risk of side effects from the absorption of energy by epidermal melanin. Additionally, longer pulse durations and larger spot sizes confer additional safety when treating darker skin types.

Fluence

Fluence is defined as the amount of energy delivered per unit area and is expressed as J/cm^2. Higher fluences have been correlated with greater permanent hair removal but are also more likely to cause unwanted side effects. Recommended treatment fluences are often provided with each individual laser device for non-experienced operators. However, a more appropriate method of determining the optimal treatment fluence for a given patient is to evaluate for the desired clinical end point of perifollicular erythema and edema seen within a few minutes of treatment (Fig. 4.4). The highest possible tolerated fluence that yields this end point without any adverse effects is the best fluence for treatment. Fluences that result in epidermal disruption are too high and should be reduced.

PEARL 6

When treating a patient for LHR for the first time, it may be prudent to try several test spots at varying fluences to determine the optimal settings. The highest tolerable fluence with desired clinical endpoint of perifollicular erythema and edema without epidermal damage will yield the greatest amount of hair clearance per treatment.

Pulse Duration

Pulse duration is defined as the duration in seconds of laser exposure. The theory of selective photothermolysis enables the laser surgeon to select an optimal pulse duration based on the thermal relaxation time (TRT).

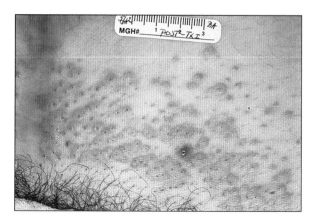

Fig. 4.4 Formation of perifollicular erythema and edema immediately after laser treatment.

Terminal hairs are approximately 300 μm in diameter, and thus the calculated TRT of a terminal hair follicle is approximately 100 ms. However, unlike many other laser applications, the hair follicle is distinct in that there is a spatial separation of the chromophore (melanin) within the hair shaft and the biologic "target" stem cells in the bulge and bulb areas of the follicle. The expanded theory of selective photothermolysis takes this spatial separation into account and proposes a thermal damage time (TDT), which is longer than the TRT. Shorter pulse widths are also capable of removing hair, and it is unclear which is more effective in producing permanent hair removal. Longer pulse widths are likely more selective for melanin within the hair follicle and can minimize epidermal damage as the pulse widths are greater than the TRT of the melanosomes in epidermal keratinocytes and melanocytes.

> ### PEARL 7
> When treating darker Fitzpatrick skin types, a longer pulse duration is preferred because the pulse duration exceeds the TRT of the epidermal melanin and minimizes the risk of epidermal damage.

Spot Size

The spot size is the diameter in millimeters of the laser beam. As photons within a laser beam penetrate the dermis they are scattered by collagen fibers, and those that are scattered outside the area of the laser beam are essentially wasted. Photons are more likely to be scattered outside of the beam area for smaller spot sizes, whereas in a larger spot size the photons are likely to remain within the beam area following scatter. A double-blind, randomized controlled trial of a long-pulsed alexandrite laser for LHR of the axillary region comparing 18- and 12-mm spot sizes at otherwise identical treatment parameters showed a 10% greater reduction in hair counts with the larger spot size. A prospective study using an LPDL with a large 22- × 35-mm handpiece at low fluences, and no skin cooling was shown to have similar long-term hair removal efficacy to published studies of LPDLs with smaller spot sizes, using higher fluences and skin cooling. Thus larger spot sizes are preferable to smaller spot sizes.

> ### PEARL 8
> Using the largest possible spot size allows for optimal penetration and minimizes the number of pulses it takes to cover a treatment area, thereby translating to faster treatment courses.

Skin Cooling

The presence of epidermal melanin, particularly in darker skin types, presents a competing chromophore to hair follicle melanin, which can be damaged during LHR (Fig. 4.5). Cooling of the skin surface is used to minimize epidermal damage as well as pain, while permitting treatment with higher fluences. All of the skin-cooling methods function by acting as a heat sink and removing heat from the skin surface. The least effective type of cooling is the use of an aqueous cold gel, which passively extracts heat from the skin and then is not capable of further skin cooling. Alternatively, cooling with forced chilled air can provide cooling to the skin before, during, and after a laser pulse. Currently, most of the available LHR devices have a built-in skin-cooling system, which consists of either contact cooling or dynamic cooling with a cryogen spray. Contact cooling, usually with a sapphire tip, provides skin cooling just before and during a laser pulse. It is

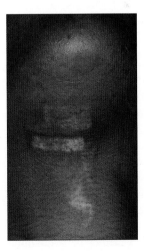

Fig. 4.5 Inadequate contact cooling resulting in postinflammatory hypopigmentation in a patient with type V skin. (*Photograph courtesy of Nathan Uebelhoer.*)

most useful for treatments with longer pulse durations (greater than 10 ms). Dynamic cooling with cryogen liquid spray precools the skin with a millisecond spray of cryogen just before the laser pulse. A second spray can be delivered just after the laser pulse for post cooling, but parallel cooling during the laser pulse is not possible because the cryogen spray interferes with the laser beam. Dynamic cooling is best suited for use with pulse durations shorter than 5 ms. When using LHR devices with dynamic cooling, it is important to ensure the alignment of the cryogen spray with the laser beam. Malalignment can result in crescentic shaped postinflammatory hyperpigmentation in the treatment area and warrants immediate correction.

PEARL 9

Skin cooling is beneficial for minimizing epidermal damage and treatment-associated pain. However, cooling can be overdone and result in pigmentary alterations, particularly with cryogen liquid spray.

Postprocedure Care

It is expected for the patient to have perifollicular erythema and edema in the treatment area following LHR. This generally persists for 2 days but can last for up to 1 week. Ice and application of a topical corticosteroid can be used to shorten the duration of these undesired effects. Patients will often find that a single treatment of LHR with shorter pulse durations results in nearly total epilation of the hair follicles in the treatment area. It is important to counsel the patient that a majority of these hairs will likely regrow, and this is not considered a treatment failure. In general, only approximately 15% of hairs are permanently removed with each laser treatment. On the other hand, LHR treatments with longer pulse durations may leave behind many hairs that appear to "grow" following treatment. It is important to reassure the patient that these "growing" hairs are dislodged from the hair follicle and require 1–2 weeks to be completely shed.

The importance of strict sun precaution following LHR treatments cannot be overemphasized. This can be achieved by the use of topical sunscreens, ultraviolet light impermeable garments, and, most importantly, sun avoidance.

PEARL 10

Beyond sun protection factor 30 (SPF30), higher SPF values do not necessarily correlate with increased protection from the sun. The SPF value of a product only reflects its protection from ultraviolet B (UVB) rays. It is far more important that the product contain broad-spectrum protection, including ultraviolet A (UVA) rays.

Medical Conditions Treated With Laser Hair Removal

In addition to the primary esthetic uses, laser hair removal has a demonstrated benefit as an adjunctive therapy in several dermatologic conditions associated with hair follicular pathology. Further reading reviewing of unconventional uses of laser hair removal is provided at the end of the chapter.

Several studies have demonstrated safety and efficacy of LHR for pseudofolliculitis barbae, a chronic inflammatory skin condition often affecting patients with coarse, curly hair commonly in the beard and neck area as a result of shaving. At least 50% improvement in inflammatory papules can be expected following several sessions of LHR.

Laser hair removal has also demonstrated improvement in pilonidal sinus disease. Sinuses in the sacrococcygeal region can become inflamed and infected over time, leading to painful and debilitating abscesses. Although surgical removal of the sinus tract is the treatment of choice for persistent or complicated disease, adjunctive LHR can decrease disease recurrence and improve quality of life. One study supports 4 sessions of LHR for the best results, with fewer sessions resulting in a higher relapse rate.

Multiple studies support the use of LHR for hidradenitis suppurativa. Although benefit has been reported with diode, Nd:YAG and IPL devices, Nd:YAG is preferred due to deeper tissue penetration. A case-control study examining treated and untreated sites on same patient demonstrated a 32% improvement in the Lesion Area and Severity Index Score for treated areas (2 months after second treatment.)

Reconstruction following head and neck cancer surgery often employs the use of hair-bearing flaps and grafts which can be especially bothersome to patients. Several case reports and case series demonstrate effective hair reduction following LHR for intraoral flaps using alexandrite and Nd:YAG lasers with standard treatment parameters. It is important to note that access to the particular area may be challenging depending on the intraoral location of the flap/graft and the size and shape of the laser handpiece.

Laser hair removal is also an important part of gender affirming surgery and transgender health. Terminal hair distribution on the beard and neck is often treated in male to female transition. Additionally, genital reconstruction may require the use of hair-bearing flap. For transgender women, creation of vaginoplasty with a neovaginal cavity creation requires preoperative hair removal from the penis. LHR is superior to electrolysis for hair removal prior to gender affirming surgery. Preoperative permanent hair removal of skin flap is also required prior to phalloplasty and urethral lengthening for transgender men as skin flap is often harvested from ventral forearm or anterolateral thigh.

Long-Term Efficacy

Permanent hair removal was evident as early as the seminal hair removal trial from the Wellman Center involving a single treatment with the normal mode ruby laser. Seven of the thirteen original subjects were evaluated at 2-year follow-up. Of the seven subjects, four had evidence of persistent permanent hair reduction at 2-year follow-up, whereas three subjects experienced complete regrowth. Follow-up of 18 out of the 50 original study subjects treated with an LPDL showed a 25%–33% and 36%–46% hair reduction at a mean follow-up of 20 months after one or two treatments (9-mm spot size, pulse duration of 5–20 ms, fluences of 15–40 J/cm^2, single or triple pulsed), respectively. A head-to-head trial comparing an LPDL to a long-pulsed alexandrite laser found a 49%–94% hair reduction at 1-year follow-up after four treatments (9-mm spot size, pulse duration of 20 ms, fluences of 12–40 J/cm^2) with the LPDL in 15 subjects. Similar results were achieved with the alexandrite laser used in this study. Fifteen of twenty subjects with Fitzpatrick skin phototypes III–IV treated with a long-pulsed alexandrite laser (12- and 18-mm spot size, 3-ms pulse duration, and fluences of 20 or 40 J/cm^2) or a long-pulsed Nd:YAG laser (12-mm spot size, 3-ms pulse duration, and fluence of 40 J/cm^2) for four sessions at 8-week intervals showed 76%–84% and 74% hair reduction 18 months after the last treatment, respectively. Another head-to-head trial of a high-fluence LPDL

(9-mm spot size, pulse duration of 30 ms, fluences of 20–50 J/cm^2) versus a low-fluence LPDL (12- × 10-mm spot size, pulse duration of 20 ms, fluences of 5–10 J/cm^2) in 22 subjects showed similar, 94% and 90% hair reduction at 18-month follow-up following five treatments spaced 6–8 weeks apart, respectively. Finally, the authors reported statistically significant hair clearance, 54% and 42%, at 6- and 15-month follow-up visits following three monthly treatments using a LPDL with a large handpiece in the largest prospective trial to date. Remaining hairs were found to also grow back less thick and lighter.

Complications

The most common complications of LHR are epidermal damage (Fig. 4.6) and pigmentary alterations, including hyper- and hypopigmentation (Fig. 4.7). This may result from selecting a nonoptimal wavelength, pulse duration, or fluence, using improper epidermal cooling, or treating a tanned patient (Fig. 4.8). Pigmentary alterations may also occur even when optimal treatment parameters are used. These changes are often transient and improve with time, although permanent hypopigmentation can occur (see Fig. 4.7B). Zones of untreated hairs can result from a lack of overlapping between laser pulses (Fig. 4.9). Scarring is an exceedingly rare complication but can occur when an inappropriate wavelength is used on skin of color, excessive fluences, and/or pulse stacking are used.

Treatment of the lateral cheeks and chin area, or less commonly other areas, may result in the induction of

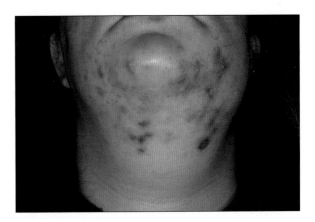

Fig. 4.6 Epidermal damage with focal crusting resulting from excessive laser fluence.

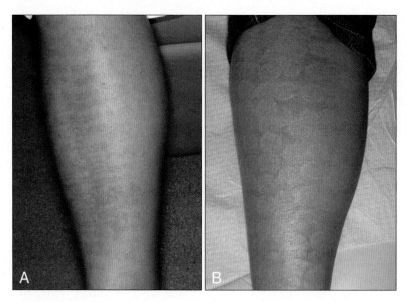

Fig. 4.7 Example of laser hair removal (LHR)-induced hyperpigmentation (A) and permanent hypopigmentation (B).

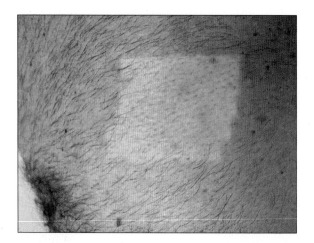

Fig. 4.8 Treatment of recently tanned skin resulted in development of hypopigmentation.

terminal hairs, a phenomenon known as paradoxical hypertrichosis (Fig. 4.10). This has been reported to occur more commonly in females of Mediterranean, Middle Eastern, Asian and South Asian descent. The exact mechanism remains uncharacterized, but it is thought that subtherapeutic laser fluences may lead to the stimulation of hair growth. For patients

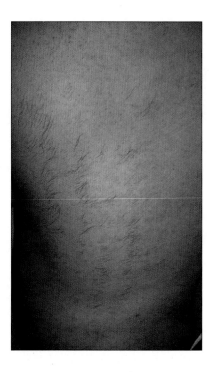

Fig. 4.9 Zones of untreated skin resulting from lack of appropriate overlapping.

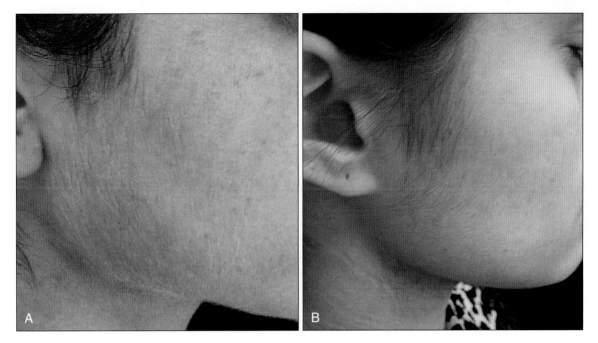

Fig. 4.10 Paradoxical hypertrichosis. Conversion of fine, vellus-like hairs (A) to terminal dark hairs (B) after a single laser hair removal (LHR) treatment.

at increased risk of developing paradoxical hypertrichosis, placement of cold packs surrounding the treatment area may be helpful in mitigating the effect of lower laser fluences on peripheral hair follicles. In patients who develop this despite precautions, treatment options include further treatment with LHR (particularly at higher fluences and using a double pass method—either in the same treatment session or 1 week following, and shorter intervals between sessions), electrolysis, use of eflornithine HCL cream, and possibly the addition of oral spironolactone.

Caution should be exercised to avoid treatment over tattoos and nevi, particularly atypical nevi. Treatment of other dermatologic conditions, such as vascular birthmarks, can cause inadvertent permanent hair reduction because of the overlap in therapeutic window of pulse duration and wavelength for both hemoglobin and melanin.

Laser plume obtained from laser hair removal and analyzed by gas chromatography-mass spectrometry identified at least 13 known or suspected carcinogens and more than 20 known environmental toxins. These findings support the importance of smoke evacuators, properly ventilated rooms, and wearing surgical masks during LHR procedures. A review of legal databases showed that LHR was the most commonly litigated laser procedure among malpractice cases, and that nonphysician operators in the medical spa setting comprised the majority of litigated cases.

FUTURE DIRECTIONS

Advances in Pain Control

A recent technique to reduce LHR-associated pain is pneumatic skin flattening (PSF). PSF works by coupling a vacuum chamber to generate negative pressure and to flatten the skin against the handpiece treatment window. Based on the gate theory of pain transmission, it stimulates pressure receptors in the skin immediately prior to firing of the laser pulse, thereby blocking activation of pain fibers. PSF has been incorporated into commercially available lasers (see Table 4.1). A study of LHR using a LPDL with a large spot size and vacuum-assisted suction showed that the majority of subjects reported feeling no pain at all or up to moderate pain without the use of skin cooling or topical anesthetics. Notably, none of the subjects in the study reported experiencing severe or intolerable pain.

A study of 10 patients undergoing laser hair removal of light-colored hair demonstrated a significant difference in reduction of hair with the application silver nanoparticle solution prior to LHR with 810 diode laser (-18.9% difference between treatments, $P = .04$). This is a promising innovation for treatment of notoriously difficult light (blond and red) hair. These applications have not yet become available for commercial use.

Home-Use Laser and Light Source Devices for Hair Removal

In recent years, a number of devices have been developed that seek to provide patients with the ability to achieve energy-based hair removal at home. These devices are based on IPL, laser, and thermal technologies that target the hair follicle for destruction. Several devices that have 510(k) clearance by the FDA in the United States are listed in Table 4.1. Similar technologies are also being used by a variety of other home-use devices that do not currently have FDA 510(k) clearance.

The evidence behind such devices is scant and limited to small noncontrolled studies. A study demonstrated that a thermally based, home-use device was no better than shaving in removing hair, reducing hair density, or slowing hair regrowth. In addition, the risk for devastating eye injuries with improper use of laser- and IPL-based devices and lack of medical training raises a dilemma of how much autonomy a patient should have with potentially harmful devices. Nonetheless, the appeal of having a personal device to remove unwanted hair in the privacy of one's home without the expense and inconvenience of multiple dermatologist or spa visits will likely drive the development of additional home-use devices.

Alternative Technologies for Hair Removal

Photodynamic therapy (PDT) with aminolevulinic acid (ALA) has been shown in a small pilot study to result in up to 40% hair reduction with a single treatment, although wax epilation was performed prior to treatment in this study.

Electro-optical synergy (ELOS) technology combines electrical (conducted radiofrequency [RF]) and optical (laser/light) energies. A handful of devices based on this technology have been produced (see Table 4.1). The theory behind ELOS is based on the optical component (laser or IPL) heating the hair shaft, which then is thought to concentrate the bipolar RF energy to the surrounding hair follicle. Based on this combination, lower fluences are needed for the optical component, thereby suggesting it might be well tolerated in all Fitzpatrick skin phototypes, and potentially effective in the removal of white and poorly pigmented hair. A study of 40 patients (Fitzpatrick skin phenotypes II–V) with varied facial and nonfacial hair colors were treated with combined IPL/RF ELOS technology. An average clearance of 75% was observed at 18 months following four treatments. No significant adverse sequelae were noted, and there were no treatment differences between patients of varying skin types or hair color. Pretreatment with ALA prior to use of a combined IPL and RF device has been shown to further augment the removal of terminal white hairs. A novel device using Total Reflection Amplification of Spontaneous Emission of Radiation (TRASER) has been shown to produce similar clinical and histopathologic effects as LHR in a small observational study.

CONCLUSIONS

In conclusion, hair removal has made a dramatic shift from an art to science based on the theory of selective photothermolysis. Since the first reports of selective hair removal in 1996 by Anderson and colleagues, there has been a tremendous explosion in the number of devices used for LHR, making LHR the most commonly requested cosmetic procedure in the world. This chapter provides the reader with the fundamentals of hair follicle anatomy and physiology, points for patient selection and preoperative preparation, principles of laser safety, an introduction to the various laser/light devices, and a discussion of laser–tissue interactions that are vital to optimizing treatment efficacy while minimizing complications and side effects.

Check online videos (Video 4.1).

FURTHER READING

Alster TS, Bryan H, Williams CM. Long-pulsed Nd:YAG laser-assisted hair removal in pigmented skin: a clinical and histological evaluation. *Arch Dermatol.* 2001;137(7): 885–889.

Altshuler GB, Anderson RR, Manstein D, Zenzie HH, Smirnov MZ. Extended theory of selective photothermolysis. *Lasers Surg Med.* 2001;29(5):416–432.

Aleem S, Majid I. Unconventional uses of laser hair removal: a review. *J Cutan Aesthet Surg.* 2019;12(1):8–16.

Anderson RR, Parrish JA. Selective photothermolysis: precise microsurgery by selective absorption of pulsed radiation. *Science.* 1983;220(4596):524–527.

Ball K, Gustavsson M, Harris R, Berganza L, Zachary CB. TRASER: acute phase vascular and follicular changes. *Lasers Surg Med.* 2014;46(5):385–388.

Bernstein EF. Hair growth induced by diode laser treatment. *Dermatol Surg.* 2005;31(5):584–586.

Biesman BS. Evaluation of a hot-wire hair removal device compared to razor shaving. *Lasers Surg Med.* 2013;45(5):283–295.

Braun M. Comparison of high-fluence, single-pass diode laser to low-fluence, multiple-pass diode laser for laser hair reduction with 18 months of follow up. *J Drugs Dermatol.* 2011;10(1):62–65.

Campos VB, Dierickx CC, Farinelli WA, et al. Hair removal with an 800-nm pulsed diode laser. *J Am Acad Dermatol.* 2000;43(3):442–447.

Davoudi SM, Behnia F, Gorouhi F, et al. Comparison of long-pulsed alexandrite and Nd:YAG lasers, individually and in combination, for leg hair reduction: an assessor-blinded, randomized trial with 18 months of follow-up. *Arch Dermatol.* 2008;144(10):1323–1327.

Dierickx CC, Grossman MC, Farinelli WA, Anderson RR. Permanent hair removal by normal-mode ruby laser. *Arch Dermatol.* 1998;134(7):837–842.

Eremia S, Li C, Newman N. Laser hair removal with alexandrite versus diode laser using four treatment sessions: 1-year results. *Dermatol Surg.* 2001;27(11):925–929, discussion 929–930.

Garcia C, Alamoudi H, Nakib M, Zimmo S. Alexandrite laser hair removal is safe for Fitzpatrick skin types IV–VI. *Dermatol Surg.* 2000;26(2):130–134.

Gold MH, Bell MW, Foster TD, Street S. One-year follow-up using an intense pulsed light source for long-term hair removal. *J Cutan Laser Ther.* 1999;1(3):167–171.

Goldberg DJ, Littler CM, Wheeland RG. Topical suspension-assisted Q-switched Nd:YAG laser hair removal. *Dermatol Surg.* 1997;23(9):741–745.

Grossman MC, Dierickx C, Farinelli W, Flotte T, Anderson RR. Damage to hair follicles by normal-mode ruby laser pulses. *J Am Acad Dermatol.* 1996;35(6):889–894.

Haak CS, Nymann P, Pedersen AT, et al. Hair removal in hirsute women with normal testosterone levels: a randomized controlled trial of long-pulsed diode laser vs. intense pulsed light. *Br J Dermatol.* 2010;163(5):1007–1013.

Hussain M, Polnikorn N, Goldberg DJ. Laser-assisted hair removal in Asian skin: efficacy, complications, and the effect of single versus multiple treatments. *Dermatol Surg.* 2003;29(3):249–254.

Ibrahimi OA, Avram MM, Hanke CW, Kilmer SL, Anderson RR. Laser hair removal. *Dermatol Ther.* 2011;24(1):94–107.

Ibrahimi OA, Jalian HR, Shofner JD, Anderson RR. Yellow light gone wild: a tale of permanent laser hair removal with a 595-nm pulsed-dye laser. *JAMA Dermatol.* 2013;149(3):376.

Ibrahimi OA, Kilmer SL. Long-term clinical evaluation of a 800 nm long-pulsed diode laser with a large spot size and vacuum-assisted suction for hair removal. *Dermatol Surg.* 2012;38(6):912–917.

Jalian HR, Jalian CA, Avram MM. Increased risk of litigation associated with laser surgery by nonphysician operators. *JAMA Dermatol.* 2014;150(4):407–411.

Khoury JG, Saluja R, Goldman MP. Comparative evaluation of long-pulse alexandrite and long-pulse Nd:YAG laser systems used individually and in combination for axillary hair removal. *Dermatol Surg.* 2008;34(5):665–670, discussion 670–661.

Lask G, Friedman D, Elman M, et al. Pneumatic skin flattening (PSF): a novel technology for marked pain reduction in hair removal with high energy density lasers and IPLs. *J Cosmet Laser Ther.* 2006;8(2):76–81.

Lou WW, Quintana AT, Geronemus RG, Grossman MC. Prospective study of hair reduction by diode laser (800 nm) with long-term follow-up. *Dermatol Surg.* 2000;26(5):428–432.

Nouri K, Chen H, Saghari S, Ricotti CA Jr. Comparing 18- versus 12-mm spot size in hair removal using a gentlease 755-nm alexandrite laser. *Dermatol Surg.* 2004;30(4 Pt 1):494–497.

Rao J, Goldman MP. Prospective, comparative evaluation of three laser systems used individually and in combination for axillary hair removal. *Dermatol Surg.* 2005;31(12):1671–1676, discussion 1677.

Richards RN, Meharg GE. Electrolysis: observations from 13 years and 140, 000 hours of experience. *J Am Acad Dermatol.* 1885;33(4):662–666.

Rohrer TE, Chatrath V, Yamauchi P, Lask G. Can patients treat themselves with a small novel light based hair removal system? *Lasers Surg Med.* 2003;33(1):25–29.

Ross EV, Ibrahimi OA, Kilmer S. Long-term clinical evaluation of hair clearance in darkly pigmented individuals using a novel diode 1060 nm wavelength with multiple treatment handpieces: a prospective analysis with modeling and histological findings. *Lasers Surg Med.* 2018;50(9):893–901.

Zenzie HH, Altshuler GB, Smirnov MZ, Anderson RR. Evaluation of cooling methods for laser dermatology. *Lasers Surg Med.* 2000;26(2):130–144.

5

Treatment of Skin With Intense Pulsed Light Sources

Jeremy Brauer, Karen J. Dover, Jacqueline Watchmaker, and Courtney Gwinn

SUMMARY AND KEY FEATURES

- Intense pulsed light (IPL) devices are highly versatile and can be used for a wide range of esthetic and medical conditions.
- IPL platforms use high-output flash-lamps to produce polychromatic, noncollimated, incoherent (nonlaser) light, with wavelengths ranging from 500 to 1400 nm.
- Benign pigmented lesions, dyschromia, unwanted hair, telangiectasias, facial redness, flushing, Poikiloderma of Civatte, precancerous lesions, and acne can all be effectively treated with IPL.
- While treatment parameters can be adjusted to improve the safety profile of IPL in darker skin types (IV–VI), complications in this patient demographic are not uncommon. IPL should be used with extreme caution in darker skin types and in tanned skin.
- Not all IPL devices are created equally. Differences in the design and optics are significant, translating into huge ranges in efficacy. The device quality seems to correlate almost directly with the price point.
- With thorough understanding of light-tissue interactions and the wide selection of device parameters, experienced practitioners can take advantage of the considerable versatility of high-quality IPL devices.

INTRODUCTION

Intense pulsed light (IPL) treatment is one of the most popular, noninvasive skin procedures performed. IPL devices use filtered, high-intensity, pulsed, nonlaser light of varying wavelengths to treat both esthetic and medical conditions. Current IPL devices contain sophisticated, interchangeable light filters, which allow for versatility and a wide range of treatment options. With appropriate patient selection and practitioner experience, IPL can be highly effective, providing excellent results, typically with little downtime. Inappropriate patient selection, incorrect treatment parameters, or poor technique, however, can lead to significant adverse events. This chapter will provide a brief review of the history and science of IPL, then focus on clinical applications, treatment parameters and technique. In addition, we will share some of our personal treatment pearls, gleaned through years of experience with IPL devices.

HISTORY

In 1992, Dr. Shimon Eckhouse, an aerospace engineer from Israel, conceived the idea of applying a flash-lamp therapeutically to treat leg veins, which was a significant departure from the device's original use as a paint vaporizer for fighter jets. At the time, pulsed-dye lasers, with short pulse durations, were engaged for this purpose, with unsatisfactory results and a high rate of complications. Dr. Eckhouse hypothesized that large vessels could be more uniformly treated with broad-band light, given that shorter, more readily-absorbed wavelengths could heat the superficial part of the vessel, while longer, less-readily absorbed wavelengths would penetrate further to heat the deeper portions of the vessel. Additionally, he theorized that a broad range of wavelengths would more effectively target both oxygenated and deoxygenated hemoglobin. Dr. Eckhouse enlisted the help of Dr. Mitchel Goldman and Dr. Richard Fitzpatrick, and together they developed a prototype IPL device. By 1994, the first commercially available IPL platform, PhotoDerm VL (Lumenis Ltd., Yokneam, Israel), gained FDA approval. Some early IPL devices struggled with efficacy, reproducibility and usability, which contributed to a somewhat controversial reputation in the laser community. By late 1990s and early 2000s, however, newer models addressed many of the initial concerns, and IPL gained popularity for the treatment of epidermal pigmented lesions, vascular lesions and unwanted hair. IPL was also found to be effective for the treatment of acne, and precancerous skin lesions. Over the past 2 decades, further technological developments have allowed for the expansion of treatment indications, decreased the risk of side-effects, and increased the ease of operation. They remain highly operator-dependent procedures, and though often delegated to support staff, the best results are in the hands of experienced, committed clinicians.

INTENSE PULSED LIGHT TERMINOLOGY

The following terms and concepts are important in understanding the science behind IPL devices.
- Intense pulsed light: IPL is polychromatic, noncollimated, incoherent light, with wavelengths ranging from 500 to 1400 nm. This is in contrast to laser light, which is a single wavelength, highly-directional, and coherent in nature.
- Flash-lamp: Flash-lamps are pulsed sources of light, which consist of glass tubing with electrodes at either end. The glass tubing is filled with a gas, typically xenon or krypton. When a power supply triggers an electrical discharge between the two electrodes, the gas ionizes. The ionized gas produces a short burst of high-intensity, broad-band light. IPL devices directly emit this broad-band light. Some lasers also use flash-lamps, but in a different manner; instead of directly emitting the broad-band light, lasers use this light to optically excite the laser medium.
- Selective photothermolysis: Similar to lasers, IPL utilizes the principle of selective photothermolysis, in which there is selective heating of target chromophores with preservation of surrounding tissue. The target chromophores of IPL are primarily melanin, oxyhemoglobin, deoxyhemoglobin and methemoglobin, which have broad, overlapping absorption spectra; the polychromatic nature of IPL thus allows for the treatment of both vascular and pigmented lesions with a single light exposure.
- Pulse duration: Pulse duration represents the length of time over which the light energy is delivered and the duration the tissue is exposed to the light beam. The pulse duration of IPL systems can be set between 0.2 and 100 milliseconds, depending on the device. Pulse duration is guided by thermal relaxation time and thus the size of the target chromophore. Pulse duration is usually set to be shorter than the thermal relaxation time of the target chromophore, to minimize damage to surrounding structures.
- Multiple sequential pulsing and pulse delay: Depending on the IPL device, light can be delivered either as a single-pulse, or as a double- or triple-pulse, separated by short pulse delays in the millisecond range. "Multiple sequential pulsing" is the term used to describe the use of double- or triple-pulses. In theory, and practice, "multiple sequential pulsing" allows for a gentler treatment, given high fluences can be divided into multiple, shorter pulses of lower fluences. "Multiple sequential pulsing" also permits successive heating of large vessels, while still allowing adequate cooling of the epidermis. Some IPL devices also allow adjustment of the pulse duration of each individual pulse and the length of the pulse delay between the pulses. When more epidermal protection is needed, as in the case of tanned skin or darker skin, the pulse delay can be elongated to provide more time for enhanced protection through various means.
- Spectral shift: IPL devices experience a phenomenon known as *spectral shift*, in which a decrease in power causes a relative increase in the amount of energy density emitted at longer wavelengths. Specifically, for a set fluence, when coupled with a longer pulse duration and the accompanying decrease in power, the relative amount of energy density emitted in the

longer wavelengths increases, with a relative decrease at the shorter wavelengths when compared to the same fluence at a shorter pulse duration. The spectral shift phenomenon enhances the effectiveness of IPL devices in treating deeper, darker, and larger vessels, which respond well to longer wavelengths.

EQUIPMENT

There are multiple commercially available IPL devices. This section will provide a broad overview of some of the common components of IPL devices.

- Cut-off filters and absorption filters: Many IPL devices utilize interchangeable, optically-coated, quartz filters, called "cut-off filters." These filters narrow the range of the wavelengths emitted in order to optimize absorption by the desired chromophores. There is a wide range of available cut-off filters, including 515, 550, 560, 590, 615, 645, 690, and 755 nm; filters typically work by blocking the emission of wavelengths of light shorter than the set limit. The Palomar Icon's MaxG hand-piece (Cynosure, Westford, MA) is entirely unique in that it incorporates an absorption filter to allow for dual-spectral output, with two different wavelength ranges, specifically 500–670 nm and 870–1400 nm. This filter absorbs the majority of the wavelengths between 670 and 870 nm, but allows for emission of flanking wavelengths. It is this optimization of the spectral emission that distinguishes this device, and is one of the rationales for its enhanced results. It is known as an OPL, an "Optimized Pulsed Light," for this reason. The BBL (Broad Band light) HERO (High-Energy Rapid Output) device (Sciton, Palo Alto, CA) has seven separate cut-off filters including the 420 nm narrow band blue light filter, the 515, 560, 590, 640, 690 and 800 nm filters. Notably, the BBL is also unique in that it can be used both for facial and nonfacial photodamage of the neck, chest, arms, etc. (Fig. 5.1). This device delivers hundreds of low-energy pulses within minutes in a sweeping motion reducing the risk of stamping

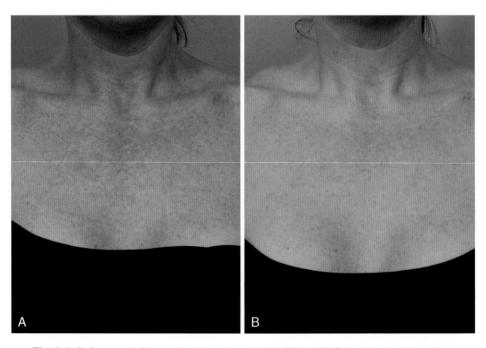

Fig. 5.1 Before and after a single treatment with BBL HERO for chest photoaging.

burns and "zebra stripes" in these high risk areas. The M22 (Lumenis, San Jose, CA) has nine filters including the 515, 560, 590, 615, 640, 695 nm, as well as the "vascular" and "acne" filters. The acne filter is a novel dual-band notch filter delivering wavelengths of 400–600 nm and 800–1200 nm simultaneously that has shown significant promise in clearance of acne. The vascular filter is a dual band notch filter delivering 530–650 nm and 900–1200 nm wavelengths simultaneously designed to targe fine telangiectasias. Most IPL devices (excluding the Palomar Icon) utilize water surrounding the flash-lamp to prevent emission of wavelengths greater than 900 nm.

- IPL hand-piece: Most IPL devices deliver light to the skin through a large, flat, rectangular, sapphire crystal. This large footprint can be advantageous because it allows for rapid coverage, even distribution, and deeper penetration of light. With the large spot-size, however, it can be challenging to achieve uniform skin contact on contoured surfaces, especially around the nose, and it can create difficulty maneuvering in areas of focal treatment. To address these issues, some companies offer compact IPL tips to effectively treat irregular surfaces and discrete lesions. For example, the BBL Hero device has variable sized spot adapters that fit over the sapphire crystal to customize the device footprint. Alternatively, opaque masking devices can be used to effectively convert a large IPL footprint into a smaller one. A sheet of paper with a small, customized, cut-out is also a low-tech, safe, and easy method to decrease the footprint of a device while still allowing adequate and necessary contact cooling. Many IPL platforms integrate "slide-in" or "snap-on" cut-off filters into the device hand-piece, which allows for a single hand-piece to be used for a variety of treatments. Absorption filters, however, require constant cooling to prevent cracking and, thus, require entirely separate hand-pieces for each spectral range.
- Cooling mechanisms: Epidermal cooling significantly decreases side effects and allows for the use of higher fluences. Most high-quality devices utilize integrated, continuous contact-cooling, which is achieved through circulation of chilled water around the IPL crystal. In addition, cooled gel, such as Humatrix, a microclysmic gel, is used in conjunction with IPL devices to (1) diffuse skin surface heat and (2) enhance the optical transmission of light by

decreasing the index of refraction. Added surface cooling with chilling packs can effectively protect the epidermis, applied immediately prepulse and/or posttreatment to minimize or eliminate undesirable issues. Zimmer coolers are another option to quickly and effectively decrease the epidermal temperature, if desired.

- BroadBand Light (BBL): BBL is a marketing term developed by the company Sciton (Palo Alto, CA) to describe their intense-pulsed light devices. The terms "BBL" and "IPL" are sometimes used interchangeably, and have similar meaning.

PEARL 2

Cooled gel, such as Humatrix, is used in conjunction with cooled, sapphire-tipped hand-pieces on IPL devices to (1) diffuse skin surface heat, thus minimizing adverse events, and (2) enhance the optical transmission of light by decreasing the index of refraction, thus increasing efficacy.

PATIENT SELECTION

To maximize benefits and minimize complications, appropriate patient consultation and selection is essential. The clinician should ensure that the patient's skin condition, treatment goals, therapeutic objectives, and skin type are appropriate for IPL therapy. Ideal patients are well-informed, with realistic expectations, presenting with any one or a combination of the following esthetic concerns: diffuse redness, flushing, rosacea, angiomas (spider or cherry), telangiectasias, venous lakes, dyschromia, lentigines, actinic keratosis, and unwanted hair. Regions amenable to therapy include most areas of the body, though treatment parameters must be accommodated accordingly, as the skin responds quite differently from area to area. Patients with conditions less amenable to IPL treatment, such as severe rhytids, without pigmentary or vascular concerns, require counseling on alternative options. While treatment parameters can be adjusted to increase the relative safety of IPL in darker skin types—specifically, lower fluences, longer wavelengths, longer pulse durations, longer pulse delays, and enhanced skin chilling, both pre and postprocedure—complications in this patient demographic are all too common. We, therefore, typically reserve the use of IPL for patients with Fitzpatrick skin types I–III, in which results are predictable and reproducible, and we prefer to use specialized lasers and/or other treatment modalities for patients with darker skin. Even for those with lighter skin, the presence of naturally or artificially tanned skin increases the risk of untoward events, and these patients should be advised to postpone treatment until they are no longer tanned. To assist in the tan assessment, we often compare the skin color of the prospective treatment area to that of the inner forearm or inner upper arm, which are good baselines for untanned skin. Additionally, we typically only treat patients between mid-October and early-June to minimize sun exposure, both before and after treatment. We tend not to rely on the melanin reader devices, such as the Skintel, Melanin Reader, (Cynosure, Westford, MA); though accurate, the recommended treatment ranges can be misleading, in that it is exceedingly wide, and can ultimately translate into under- or over-treatment. We prefer to defer to clinical acumen, which is enhanced with consistent and careful patient follow-up. Combined with a detailed patient history, with particular attention to genotypic and phenotypic ethnicity, a thorough physical exam helps to determine appropriate device settings. A critical component to safe and effective treatments, as with any modality, is high vigilance. Close attention to the intended chromophore targets and the energy-tissue interaction is essential. Accommodation of the parameters as the treatment progresses is quite typical, as the initial settings are simply a starting guide, and good clinical judgement is paramount.

Patients seeking improvement of discrete pigmented lesions require special attention. While dermatologists are educated and trained to recognize abnormal moles and pigmented skin cancers, providers less-trained in skin conditions may be unable to distinguish harmful from benign lesions. If there is any doubt, a skin biopsy should be performed prior to IPL treatment. Additionally, while some studies suggest IPL can be effective for the short-term improvement of melasma, relapse is common and the combination of broad-band light and heat have the potential to flare melasma. For these reasons, we typically do not recommend IPL in melasma and opt for other therapeutic modalities. We also avoid IPL in patients with active connective tissue diseases, such as lupus erythematosus given the potential for exacerbation.

> ### PEARL 3
>
> While treatment parameters can be adjusted to increase the relative safety of IPL in darker skin types—specifically, lower fluences, longer wavelengths, longer pulse durations, longer pulse delays, and enhanced skin chilling, both pre and postprocedure—complications in this patient demographic are all too common. Therefore, IPL is typically reserved for patients with Fitzpatrick skin types I–III.

TREATMENT PROTOCOL

Pretreatment

Once the clinician has deemed the patient a good candidate for IPL therapy and has provided counseling on realistic expectations and potential complications, informed consent can be obtained. IPL treatment is typically well-tolerated without topical anesthesia, however, higher fluences and longer wavelengths can be associated with more pain, in which case application of a topical anesthetic is an option. The treatment area should be thoroughly cleansed immediately pretreatment with gauze and alcohol, to remove any make-up or topical products, which interfere with light transmission. If the patient is undergoing hair removal, the hair should also be shaved prior to treatment.

After cleansing, a thin (2–3 mm), uniform layer of cold gel is applied to the entire treatment area to drop the effective epidermal temperature. Historically, thicker layers of gel were required for earlier versions of IPL that did not have integrated cooling. Some clinicians use ice packs to vigilantly chill the skin before, during, and after the procedure, as needed.

Although the noncollimated nature of IPL theoretically decreases the risk of ocular damage when compared with lasers, ocular injuries can still occur. Therefore, everyone in the treatment room must wear appropriate protective eye gear. Conventional IPL goggles worn by the treating physician were dark green and hindered visibility, newer brown goggles allow for better color recognition. Additionally, flash sensor goggles (Lightspeed, Glendale, Smithfield, RI) are available, which darken only during a flash of light. We prefer to use flash-sensor goggles, given that they provide better real-time feedback of the treatment. Subtle erythema or graying of the skin can be difficult, if not impossible, to appreciate with nonflash sensor goggles. Patients are provided opaque eye protection in the form of adhesive or traditional shields.

Given IPL often results in delayed tissue reactions, preforming a test spot on the same day of treatment can lead to a false sense of security. Additionally, varying anatomic locations can react differently, especially as the target density varies from location to location. A test spot on the lower lateral cheek may not accurately predict the reaction of the skin on the forehead. While the most conservative and safe approach is to perform a test spot prior to the day of treatment, in theory, we often do not find this necessary in practice. For experienced clinicians who are comfortable with their devices, and attuned to the nuances of light-tissue interaction, assessing for potential complications (e.g. excessive pain, graying, imminent blistering, exuberant erythema, and/or edema) after a few pulses in each anatomic location is typically sufficient. If the patient is tolerating the treatment well and the skin is reacting in the expected manner, a full treatment can be performed on the same day.

Treatment Technique

Some prefer to perform multiple passes of a given treatment area, with each pass orientated in a different direction. Others prefer a single pass with or without intentional overlap. Those who overlap usually do so by about 20% between pulses, an amount determined based upon the geometry of the hand-piece tip and the physics of the IPL. Additionally, some providers prefer to use the cooling gel to glide between pulses, while others prefer to lift the sapphire-crystal tip off of the skin between each pulse. Also, for skin types II–III patients, we increase the time between pulses, which allows for more time for cooling between pulses. If the patient is undergoing treatment for a vascular condition, it is beneficial to position the patient in recline, and further increase facial blood flow prior to treatment, either with a Valsalva maneuver, heating the face with a blow-dryer, or a few arm-chair calisthenics, for enhanced therapeutic results.

Determining which part of the face to treat and in what order is up to the individual clinician. Some of us prefer to treat the forehead first, as there is usually less target present, and it is a relatively safe place to assess the tissue-IPL interaction, as well as the patient's tolerance of the pulses. This is typically followed by the upper lateral cheek, sweeping toward the medial cheek, given that the latter is more sensitive, and then continuing inferiorly, where it is tapered along the mandible. Others prefer to start on the medial right cheek, treating first the right cheek then then chin, then the left cheek, followed by the lip, then nose and finally the forehead. Regardless of the technique, it is crucial to frequently communicate with the patient; feedback is critical. If the patient reports intense pain, treatment should be stopped, and the treatment area assessed and addressed accordingly, as this is an indication of incorrect treatment parameters. It is imperative that high vigilance be exercised throughout the treatment. The clinician must look and listen attentively for any and all clues that the treatment is proceeding appropriately (Video 5.1).

Treatment parameters vary, depending upon the types and relative quantity of the target(s), the patient, and the selected device. We often adjust our settings during the treatment to achieve the desired endpoints. Appropriate endpoints include subtle darkening of lentigines, and constriction of the vessels or color conversion from bright red to blue/purple. If a vessel turns blue/purple, which represents a conversion of the intended target from oxyhemoglobin to deoxy- or methemoglobin, we often take advantage of this opportunity and perform a focal second pass with a slightly longer pulse duration, causing an intentional spectral shift to a longer wavelength for better absorption by the deoxy- or methemoglobin. Similarly, if there is an inadequate thermal response, and the vessel still blanches upon compression, implying persistent patency, a second pass focally with increased fluence and/or a shorter pulse duration is performed. Purpura can also be achieved as an endpoint, if so desired, although the esthetic patient population tends to prefer nonpurpuric treatments.

Generally, we start with gentler settings during the first treatment session, when the targets are maximal, and increase treatment intensity at subsequent sessions as the target chromophore(s) become(s) more subtle. The face can tolerate more aggressive settings than the neck and chest, with the extremities typically requiring the gentlest settings. We feather our parameters on the neck, with slightly higher settings, closer to facial settings, on the upper neck, and incrementally decreasing to lower settings on the lower neck, similar to chest settings at the clavicle.

During treatment, it is critical to avoid skip-areas, as well as hair-bearing sites (unless the goal of treatment is hair removal). Skip areas can lead to the undesirable "zebra-stripes," potentially encountered after IPL (Fig. 5.2). Given the imperfect nature of cut-off filters, it

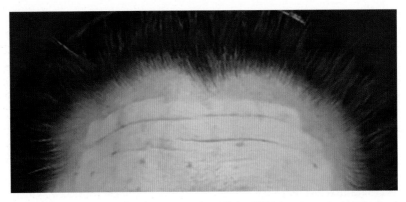

Fig. 5.2 Nonuniform outcome after intense pulsed light (IPL) treatment showing zebra-striping and sharp demarcation between treated and untreated areas. Note patient's background tan.

should always be assumed that the emitted light can and will penetrate deep enough to damage hair and therefore one should avoid treating over, or near, areas such as the eyebrows or hairline.

Additionally, given the rapid beam divergence of intense pulsed light, it is important to maintain the tip of the hand-piece in close and uniform contact with the cool gel on the skin surface. Nonuniform treatment can occur if a pulse is delivered when the treatment tip is either elevated off the skin with irregular contact with the gel and/or skin, or pressed too firmly into the skin, given beam divergence changes effective fluence. Close contact also ensures the cooled sapphire-crystal can provide adequate contact-cooling to the epidermis. For difficult to reach locations, such as the alar groove, applying a thicker layer of cool gel can help ensure adequate contact between the skin, gel and sapphire-crystal. Some of us also advocate for icing before, during and after the procedure. We often ice the treatment area, especially the alar region, immediately prior to treatment to alleviate discomfort and to minimize the potential for redness, swelling, and postinflammatory hyperpigmentation.

Posttreatment

Immediate and liberal posttreatment chilling (not freezing) with ice, a minimum of 10–15 minutes of every waking hour, for the first 24 hours, significantly decreases swelling, redness, and discomfort, and minimizes adverse events, such as postinflammatory pigmentation (PIH). Chilling can be extended to 48 hours posttreatment in the subset of patients who experience

significant post-IPL facial swelling, coupled with advising the patient to sleep with the head elevated on two to three pillows. Scheduling morning appointments for these patients allows for a full day of posttherapeutic cooling and chilling to minimize facial edema.

Once the in-office icing/chilling is complete and the cooling gel is removed from the skin, an application of an anti-redness cream or serum can be immediately soothing, as it cools the skin. Patients should be counseled to keep the skin clean and well-moisturized and to avoid sun exposure after the procedure. If the IPL treatment was for vascular issues (redness, rosacea, telangiectasias), the patient should be counseled to avoid any strenuous activity for 2–3 days after the procedure to minimize dilatation of collapsed or coagulated vessels. If the patient is prone to recurrent herpes labialis, prophylactic antiviral medication is recommended. While recovery time is usually minimal, the presence and duration of erythema, swelling and micro-crust formation varies based on the patient, the anatomical location, the condition addressed and the treatment parameters.

APPLICATIONS

Benign Pigmented Lesions

Given individual melanosomes have a thermal relaxation time in the nanosecond range, IPL devices, which operate in the millisecond domain, are not seemingly optimized for the treatment of epidermal pigment. However, while it is true that Q-switched and picosecond lasers are superior at targeting individual melanosomes,

IPL devices can effectively target aggregated melanosomes and melanocytes, which have longer thermal relaxation times than individual melanosomes. A study by Yamashita et al. elegantly demonstrated this concept with the use of confocal microscopy, by showing that IPL causes denaturation of melanin cap structures containing aggregated melanosomes. Yamashita also proposed that this denaturation triggers accelerated basal keratinocyte differentiation, which leads to the upward transfer of necrotic keratinocytes and melanosomes; this proposal provides a scientific explanation for the microcrusts seen on the skin of patients after IPL treatment of pigmented lesions. These micro-crusts typically last for about 5–10 days on the face, 7–14 days on the chest, or more, and sometimes even longer on the extremities. They naturally flake off or fall off, exposing the desirable, less-pigmented skin layer. Numerous studies have demonstrated the utility of IPL for the treatment of benign pigmented lesions and dyschromia from photoaging (Fig. 5.3). In a study of 18 patients Bjerring et al. showed a 74.2% reduction in solar lentigines after only one IPL treatment. Similarly, Kawada et al. demonstrated an overwhelming majority of patients received a 50%–75% improvement in lentigines and ephelides after three to five IPL treatment sessions. In our own experience, we have had excellent success with IPL for the treatment of epidermal dyspigmentation. We find that darker discrete lentigines typically improve first, after only one or two treatment sessions, followed by improvement in background discoloration and lighter lesions with additional treatment sessions, when fluences are accordingly increased.

While there are very few studies directly comparing IPL to laser treatment, we tend to reserve the use of IPL for benign pigmented lesions in patients with lighter skin, minimal or no tan, and for those who desire minimal downtime. For patients with more constitutive skin pigment, we opt for fractional nonablative thulium, Q-switched or picosecond lasers. Given the larger spot size of IPL devices, Q-switched or picosecond lasers may be more efficient in treating discrete lentigines; however as noted above, IPL devices can be very easily modified to treat individual lesions. Although there have been reports of IPL improving melasma and other pigmentary conditions such as nevus spilus and café au-lait macules, we have had more success and fewer complications with other treatment modalities.

Telangiectasias, Flushing, and Other Vascular Conditions

Numerous studies have demonstrated the success of IPL in the treatment of small telangiectasias often seen in rosacea and photo-damaged skin (Fig. 5.4). One of the main advantages of IPL technology in treating vascular lesions is the effectiveness of the therapy with the lack of postoperative purpura. IPL increases the temperature within blood vessels, causing intravascular coagulation with subsequent destruction and replacement by fibrous granulation. Additionally, IPL can simultaneously target oxyhemoglobin, deoxygenated hemoglobin, and methemoglobin, with peak absorption rates of 418, 542, and 577 respectively. Negishi et al, in a study of 73 patients, demonstrated that over 80% of patients had an 80%–100% improvement in facial telangiectasias after five treatments with IPL. In this study a 560 nm cut-off filter was used and pulse durations ranged from 3.6–5 milliseconds. Similarly, using a 550 or 570 nm cut-off filter, Bitter et al. demonstrated 70% of patients reported 50% or greater improvement in the appearance of telangiectasias after an average of five treatment sessions. Bitter et al. also found that the majority of patients

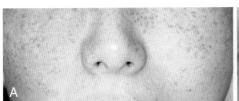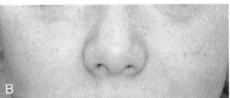

Fig. 5.3 (A) Shows lentigines prior to treatment with intense pulsed light (IPL). (B) Shows improvement in lentigines after one treatment with IPL. (Image published with permission from Cynosure.)

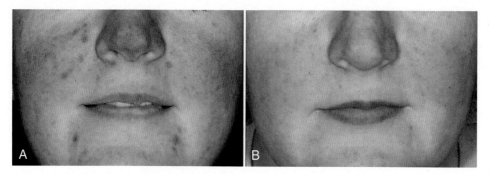

Fig. 5.4 Rosacea improvement after intense pulsed light treatment. (Image published with permission from Cynosure.)

had significant improvement in facial flushing, indicating that IPL helps alleviate symptoms of rosacea. Kassir et al. similarly found that 78% of patients reported reduced flushing after an average of 7.2 treatments. Also of note, Prieto et al. found that IPL can damage Demodex mites, which could correlate with decreased facial inflammation and erythema.

High-powered, randomized studies comparing IPL to PDL for the treatment of telangiectasias are lacking, though one study by Neuhaus et al. compared IPL to nonpurpuric pulsed-dye laser treatment in 29 patients with erythematotelangiectatic rosacea. The study found that both modalities resulted in a significant reduction in erythema, telangiectasias, and rosacea symptoms, and there was no significant difference noted between the two treatment modalities. Similarly, in a split-face study, Tanghetti et al. found IPL resulted in equivalent safety and efficacy outcomes when compared to PDL for the treatment of facial telangiectasias. While we have a tendency to use the pulsed-dye laser as first line for the treatment of telangiectasias and flushing, we often effectively employ IPL for recalcitrant cases. In experienced hands, the IPL is an effective and dependable workhorse for these vascular presentations.

Although IPL was initially created as an alternative option for the treatment of leg veins, clinical success has been inconsistent. It is generally believed that sclerotherapy remains the gold standard for the treatment of leg telangiectasias and IPL and lasers are only indicated for treatment-resistant cases or for small caliber leg telangiectasias. Additionally, although other vascular conditions, such as port-wine stains and infantile

hemangiomas, have been successfully treated with IPL exclusively, we believe hemoglobin-targeting lasers are the preferred treatment modality for these complex conditions.

Poikiloderma of Civatte

IPL can target all three components (erythema, dyspigmentation, and atrophy) of Poikiloderma of Civatte simultaneously. In the largest study examining the use of IPL for this condition, Weiss et al. achieved clearance of more than 75% of telangiectasias and hyperpigmentation after a series of one to five treatment sessions. In many cases, both the patient and physician also noted skin texture improvement.

Rhytids and Collagen Stimulation

Studies have shown that IPL can improve rhytids and skin texture through the stimulation of new collagen formation. Goldberg et al. conducted a study of 30 patients with class I-II rhytids. The subjects were treated with up to four IPL sessions and evaluated 6 months after their last treatment session. Twenty-five of the thirty patients were found to have at least some improvement in rhytids and skin quality. In a study of 73 Asian patients, Negishi et al. demonstrated marked improvements in mild, static wrinkles in the lower eyelids after a series of five or more full face IPL treatments. Efficacy was minimal for dynamic and more severe rhytids. Hernandez-Perez et al. similarly reported moderate to very good improvement in fine lines after five IPL treatments.

Although the wavelengths of light emitted by many IPL devices do not directly target water, (Palomar Icon excluded, which extends to 1400 nm), it is believed that it is the beneficial collateral damage caused by nonselective dermal heating through the transfer of heat from the targeted chromophores which stimulates new collagen synthesis. Given this indirect targeting, studies have shown that, though effective, IPL leads to less impressive wrinkle improvement than ablative and other water-targeting lasers. Our personal findings are similar to those of Negishi et al., with an improvement of fine wrinkling after IPL therapy, but inappreciably so in severe rhytids. Therefore, for patients seeking treatment primarily to address moderate to severe wrinkles or significant textural issues, we prefer ablative or fractional nonablative lasers, with wavelengths better-suited to the absorption spectrum of water.

Hair Reduction

IPL is often used for the treatment of unwanted hair (Fig. 5.5), and many studies have confirmed the efficacy of IPL for this treatment indication. In a study of 48 patients with Fitzpatrick skin types I–V, Weiss et al. found a 33% hair count reduction 6 months after two treatments with IPL. In this study, a 615 nm cut-off filter was used for lighter skin types, and a 645 nm cut-off filter was used for darker skin types. Triple-pulses were delivered with a fluence of 40–42 J/cm^2 and a pulse duration of 2.8–3.2 milliseconds. Sadick et al. had similar success in a study of 67 patients with excess body hair. In this study, varying cut-off filters were used based on patient skin type, with pulse durations ranging from 2.9 to 3.0 milliseconds, and fluences ranging from 40 to 43 J/cm^2. Mean hair reduction after 6 months was 64% after multiple IPL treatment sessions. When IPL is compared to laser treatment for the removal of unwanted hair, the majority of studies find equivalent results.

Although IPL has been studied in all skin types, we typically reserve the use of IPL for patients with skin types I–III and prefer to use long-pulsed Nd:YAG lasers for hair removal in patients with skin types IV–VI.

Dry Eye

While this chapter focuses on the use of IPL for cutaneous conditions, it is interesting to note that IPL has shown promise in the treatment of dry eye disease. Meibomian gland dysfunction (MGD) is one of the most common disorders encountered by ophthalmologists, with a prevalence of 5%–20% in western countries and 45%–70% in Asian populations. Additionally, 80% of patients with skin rosacea suffer from ocular symptoms, with the most common being MGD. MGD and dry eye disease are linked by the triggering of inflammation by skin disorders, eyelid inflammation and microbial infections, leading to increased melting temperatures of meibum, causing blockage and subsequent atrophy of meibomian glands. Ultimately, tear film stability is lost and the cornea is exposed, leading to dry eye disease. Evidence suggests IPL can help restore the function of Meibomian glands through inhibition of inflammatory mediators and restoration of functional meibum. Additionally, it is thought that destruction of vessels can decrease the inflammation that contributes to dry eyes. As mentioned previously, IPL can also damage Demodex mites, which in some patients may exacerbate eye symptoms. Dell et al. conducted a prospective study of 40 subjects (80 eyes) with moderate to severe MGD, with all patients experiencing significant subjective improvement with the proportion of eyes reaching a normal SPEED score (Standard Patient Evaluation of Eye Dryness questionnaire score, which assesses dryness, soreness/irritation, burning/watering,

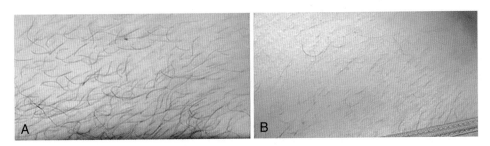

Fig. 5.5 Hair reduction after treatment with intense pulsed light. (Image published with permission from Cynosure.)

and eye fatigue) increased from 22% to 84%. Significant objective improvements in tear film osmolarity, meibomian gland score, and tear break-up time were also seen. Patients were treated with four successive IPL treatments, 3 weeks apart, with each session followed by meibomian gland expression with expresser forceps or two q-tips. It should be noted, the utility and safety of meibomian gland expression after IPL treatment for dry eye disease is controversial and is not advised due to concern for possible damage to the meibomian glands. Treatment was applied horizontally from tragus to tragus then from the maxillary process of the zygomatic bone to the inferior orbital rim, with external disposable eye shields in place for eye protection. For patient comfort, the treatment area was numbed with topical anesthetic (Benzocaine 20%-lidocaine 7%-tetracaine 7% compound gel). It is important to note that treatment with IPL should stay outside the orbital rim given eyelash loss may occur if IPL is applied too close to the eyelid margin.

Intense Pulsed Light and Photodynamic Therapy

The combination of IPL with 5-aminolevulinic acid (5-ALA) has shown promise in the treatment of actinic keratoses, photoaging and inflammatory skin conditions. After 5-ALA is applied to the skin, it is converted to protoporphyrin IX which preferentially accumulates in rapidly-dividing cells and sebaceous glands. Protoporphyrin IX is photosensitive, and thus exposure to light leads to generation of free-radical species and cellular damage. Multiple light sources, including IPL, natural sunlight, and 410-nm blue light, can be used to activate protoporphyrin IX, which has absorption bands at 410, 504, 538, 576 and 630 nm.

In a study by Ruiz-Rodriguez et al. 89% of actinic keratoses cleared following two treatments with 5-ALA and IPL. In this study, 5-ALA was applied under occlusion for 4 hours prior to treatment with IPL and 615 nm cut-off filter was used. A recent study by Michelini et al. similarly showed success with the combination of 5-methylaminolevulinic acid (a photosensitizer similar to 5-ALA) and IPL for the treatment of actinic keratoses. In this study, the photosensitizer was applied for 3 hours prior to IPL treatment with a 640 nm filter. This combination treatment achieved a clearance rate of 95% at 9-month follow-up. When using IPL for the treatment of actinic keratoses, we have had excellent success using a three-treatment-session protocol; for the first

two visits, IPL is performed, without 5-ALA, for background erythema, lentigines, and dyschromia; following an acetone scrub and a 1.5- to 2-hour 5-ALA application and incubation under occlusion, a third treatment IPL is performed.

Regarding photoaging, in a landmark, split-face study of 20 patients, Dover et al. demonstrated a greater improvement in global score for photoaging when 5-ALA was used in combination with IPL compared with IPL alone. In this study, the final investigator cosmetic evaluations, as well as the subject satisfaction scores, were significantly better for the 5-ALA-pretreated side, and there was little difference in the adverse events between the two sides. A previous study by Gold et al. similarly showed greater improvement in photodamage with the combination of 5-ALA and IPL compared with IPL alone. Additionally, given that sebaceous glands preferentially absorb ALA, it is no surprise that inflammatory acne can be improved with the combination of ALA and IPL.

COMPLICATIONS

IPL devices are excellent, versatile devices for skilled practitioners; however, for unskilled or novice practitioners, this versatility can lead to complications. While IPL procedures are often the most delegated light-based treatment in physician offices, we believe they should be one of the last treatments to be delegated, given the high rate of complications in untrained hands.

Pigmentary changes (Fig. 5.2), blistering, persistent erythema, scarring, and undesired hair removal have all been reported. Most side effects and complications can be prevented with assiduous technique. Too high fluence or too short a pulse duration delivered too much energy to quickly increasing the risk of unwanted thermal injury resulting in blistering, crusting and the potential for hyper- and hypopigmentation a patient experiences an exuberant reaction during an IPL treatment, immediate icing and compression of the affected tissue can help minimize subsequent complications. Focal application of a high potency topical corticosteroid immediately after treatment can also be beneficial. In addition, similar to laser hair removal, paradoxical hair growth following IPL is a rare but a possible side effect. For paradoxical hair growth, the use of shorter cut-off filters, higher fluence, or the use of pigment targeting lasers may lead to improvement. Additionally, cooling both the treated area and the surrounding, often moderately-pigmented skin with ice packs during treatment can help to decrease the risk of paradoxical hair growth, while still establishing adequate and effective fluences for therapeutic benefit.

Patients with darker skin types are more prone to side effects with IPL and therefore, we avoid IPL and prefer laser treatment in this patient population. If laser treatment is not available, the use of copious icing, longer wavelengths, lower fluences, longer pulse durations, decreased repetition rate, and prolonged delay times between pulses, and treatments, can improve the safety profile of IPL in darker skin. Appropriate technique, as described above, can help prevent undesirable "zebra" stripes, which occur due to strips of untreated skin remaining between treated areas. Care should be taken to avoid IPL treatment over, or near, tattoos given that the long pulse duration of IPL devices can lead to prolonged heating of tattoo pigment and thermal damage to surrounding tissues. Additionally, after an IPL device is serviced, or replaced, conservative settings should initially be used and extreme caution exercised, given that a "tired" device has a lower output than a new, or newly-serviced, device. In keeping with this concept, comparing settings between two apparently identical devices can also be wrought with disaster, as no two devices are the same. Ultimately, "Know Thy Device!"

NOT ALL INTENSE PULSED LIGHT DEVICES ARE CREATED EQUALLY

There are numerous IPL devices on the market, with a broad range in quality and price. Price differences often reflect a difference in the quality, reliability and safety. Different devices vary in effective fluence, control of spectral emission, pulse profile, and cooling technology. It is therefore very difficult, if not frankly dangerous, to compare treatment parameters and safety profiles amongst various manufacturers. When looking to acquire an IPL device, desirable features include a large capacitor, an external calibration port, minimal spectral jitter, square-shaped pulses, and integrated high-quality contact cooling.

CONCLUSIONS

In conclusion, IPL devices are highly-versatile and extremely effective devices. The wide range of treatment options and settings are advantageous for the experienced clinician. Although some may perceive the IPL as the "ugly stepsister" of lasers, potentially out of fear or ignorance, we know the IPL to be a successful, underestimated "belle of the ball." Excellent outcomes, with minimal side effects, can be achieved with a solid understanding of the science behind the IPL, and a thorough knowledge of dermatologic histology, the physics of the light-tissue interaction, proper technique, and appropriate clinical applications.

FURTHER READING

Babilas P, Schreml S, Szeimies RM, Landthaler M. Intense pulsed light (IPL): a review. *Lasers Surg Med.* 2010;42(2):93–104.

Creadore A, Watchmaker J, Maymone MBC, Pappas L, Vashi NA, Lam C. Cosmetic treatment in patients with autoimmune connective tissue diseases: best practices for patients with lupus erythematosus. *J Am Acad Dermatol.* 2020;83(2):343–363.

DiBernardo BE, Pozner JN. Intense pulsed light therapy for skin rejuvenation. *Clin Plast Surg.* 2016;43(3):535–540.

Dover JS, Bhatia AC, Stewart B, Arndt KA. Topical 5-aminolevulinic acid combined with intense pulsed light in the treatment of photoaging. *Arch Dermatol.* 2005;141(10):12.

Galeckas KJ, Collins M, Ross EV, Uebelhoer NS. Split-face treatment of facial dyschromia: pulsed dye laser with a compression handpiece versus intense pulsed light. *Dermatol Surg.* 2008;34(5):672–680.

Goldman MP, Eckhouse S. Photothermal sclerosis of leg veins. ESC Medical Systems, LTD Photoderm VL Cooperative Study Group. *Dermatol Surg.* 1996;22(4):323–330.

Goldman MP, Weiss RA, Weiss MA. Intense pulsed light as a nonablative approach to photoaging. *Dermatol Surg.* 2005;31(9 Pt 2):1179–1187, discussion 1187.

Kassir R, Kolluru A, Kassir M. Intense pulsed light for the treatment of rosacea and telangiectasias. *J Cosmet Laser Ther.* 2011;13(5):216–222.

Li D, Lin SB, Cheng B. Intense pulsed light: from the past to the future. *Photomed Laser Surg.* 2016;34(10):435–447.

Moreno-Arias GA, Castelo-Branco C, Ferrando J. Side-effects after IPL photodepilation. *Dermatol Surg.* 2002;28(12):1131–1134.

Thaysen-Petersen D, Erlendsson AM, Nash JF, et al. Side effects from intense pulsed light: importance of skin pigmentation, fluence level and ultraviolet radiation—a randomized controlled trial. *Lasers Surg Med.* 2017;49(1):88–96.

Town G, Ash C, Eadie E, Moseley H. Measuring key parameters of intense pulsed light (IPL) devices. *J Cosmet Laser Ther.* 2007;9(3):148–160.

Trivedi MK, Yang FC, Cho BK. A review of laser and light therapy in melasma. *Int J Womens Dermatol.* 2017;3(1):11–20.

Ullmann Y, Elkhatib R, Fodor L. The aesthetic applications of intense pulsed light using the Lumenis M-22 device. *Laser Ther.* 2011;20(1):23–28.

Yi J, Hong T, Zeng H, et al. A meta-analysis-based assessment of intense pulsed light for treatment of melasma. *Aesthetic Plast Surg.* 2020;44(3):947–952.

Yin Y, Liu N, Gong L, Song N. Changes in the meibomian gland after exposure to intense pulsed light in meibomian gland dysfunction (MGD) patients. *Curr Eye Res.* 2018;43(3):308–313.

Nonablative Fractional Laser Skin Rejuvenation

Jacqueline Watchmaker, Jeffrey S. Dover, Bradley S. Bloom, and Leah Spring

SUMMARY AND KEY FEATURES

- Nonablative fractional resurfacing (NAFR) is a safe and effective treatment that has become the cornerstone for facial rejuvenation and acne scarring.
- It is effective in treating a variety of conditions, including scarring, mild-to-moderate photoaging, and some forms of dyspigmentation.
- Nonablative fractional photothermolysis has minimal downtime with almost no restrictions on activity immediately following treatment.
- Erythema and edema are common sequelae after treatment and resolve within a few days. Long-term complications are exceedingly rare.

- All Fitzpatrick skin phototypes can be treated, provided settings are adjusted accordingly.
- The preoperative consultation is a vital component of the treatment regimen to ensure optimal outcomes.
- Fractional picosecond lasers and fractional microneedle radiofrequency devices are newer tools for NAFR.
- Technology in the field is changing rapidly, and the selection of equipment is based on individual preference.

INTRODUCTION

Fractional photothermolysis (FP), a concept introduced in 2004 by Anderson and Manstein, revolutionized the field of skin rejuvenation. Although multiple treatment sessions are required to achieve the desired outcome, advantages of nonablative fractional resurfacing (NAFR) are markedly reduced discomfort compared to ablative resurfacing lasers and minimal recovery period after the procedure—downtime is limited to an average of 3 days of redness and swelling, as opposed to an average of 7–10 days after aggressive nonfractional ablative resurfacing. Combined with an excellent safety profile, NAFR has become the cornerstone of laser skin rejuvenation for the treatment of photoaging, scarring, and a variety of other clinical applications.

PATHOPHYSIOLOGY

In FP, an array of pixelated light energy produced with each scan or stamp of the laser creates microscopic columns of thermally denatured skin called microscopic treatment zones (MTZs) (Fig. 6.1) surrounded by normal unaffected skin. This targeted damage with MTZ is believed to stimulate neocollagenesis and collagen remodeling leading to the clinical improvements seen in scarring and photoaging. Since the discovery of FP, multiple different lasers have been developed to take advantage of this technologic advance. Each laser has parameters that can be modified to alter the density, depth, and size of the vertical columns of MTZs. Additionally, the wavelength of fractional nonablative lasers varies depending on the

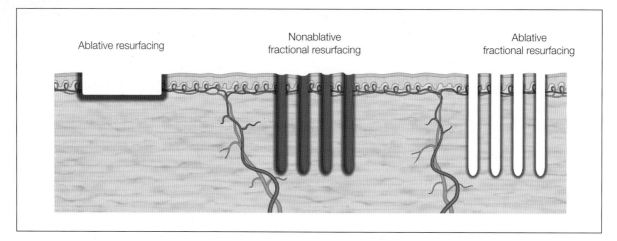

Fig. 6.1 Diagram showing the differences between traditional ablative, nonablative fractional, and ablative fractional resurfacing. With the fractional laser technology, microthermal treatment zones are created with intervening islands of unaffected tissue. Healing time is significantly less, and the energy can safely reach deeper into the dermis.

device which affects the coefficient of absorption and how the laser forms the MTZs.

The histologic changes seen after FP were elegantly described in the original study by Manstein et al. Immediately following treatment, lactate dehydrogenase (LDH) viability staining showed both epidermal and dermal cell necrosis within a sharply defined column correlating with the MTZ. There was continued loss of dermal cell viability 24 hours after treatment, but the epidermal defect was repaired via keratinocyte migration. One week after treatment, individual MTZs were still evident by LDH staining, but after 3 months there was no histologic evidence of loss of cell viability.

Hantash et al. demonstrated a unique mechanism of tissue repair with FP. In 2006, they demonstrated, using an elastin antibody, that damaged dermal content was incorporated into columns of microscopic epidermal necrotic debris (MEND) and shuttled up through the epidermis and extruded in a process of transepidermal elimination. This mechanism, which had not been described with previous laser technologies, explains the elimination of altered collagen in photoaging and scars and was also hypothesized to provide novel treatment strategies for pigmentary disorders, such as melasma, as well as depositional diseases, such as amyloid and mucinoses.

Fractional picosecond lasers are a newer tool in the fractional nonablative resurfacing toolbox. These lasers confine areas of high fluence to microspots with the majority of the treated area receiving low background fluence. The high-energy microspots create areas of laser induced optical breakdown (LIOB) which are epidermal vacuoles with preservation of surrounding epidermis. These LIOBs subsequently trigger collagen remodeling and can improve skin texture and dyspigmentation.

EPIDEMIOLOGY

According to the 2018 American Society of Dermatologic Surgery Annual Survey on Dermatologic Procedures, which provides a comprehensive estimate on the total number of cosmetic procedures performed by dermatologic surgeons in the United States, laser, light, and energy-based treatments have increased by more than 74% since 2012. The majority of laser skin resurfacing procedures are nonablative and performed on women.

EQUIPMENT

As the technology of FB continues to evolve, new devices continually come to market. A list of currently available NAFR systems is given in Table 6.1. The table is not comprehensive and, as one can imagine, subject to change based on market availability. This section will provide a brief description of a few of the more commonly used devices.

The original nonablative fractional resurfacing system described by Manstein and Anderson featured a scanning handpiece with a 1500-nm wavelength. The updated, currently available model, the Fraxel Dual (Solta Medical, a division of Bausch Medical, Bothell, WA), combines a 1550-nm erbium glass laser with a 1927-nm thulium laser in the same platform. The thulium laser provides a more superficial treatment option and better addresses dyspigmentation, whereas the 1550 nm penetrates deeper to stimulate collagen remodeling. The device has tunable settings to adjust the density of the MTZs and energy depending on the treatment. The system increases flexibility, allowing the practitioner to switch between the two lasers to tailor treatment accordingly. Cooling, which helps to minimize procedural discomfort, is built in with the Fraxel Dual.

The Palomar brand of Cynosure (Westford, MA) offers the Icon platform with individual handpieces that attach to a single unit to cover a wide range of uses. The Lux1440 and Lux1540 handpieces provide two wavelength options (1440 and 1540 nm) for fractional nonablative photothermolysis. In addition, the company has developed an XD Microlens for their nonablative laser handpieces which consists of a sapphire window with micro-pins. In their study the company claims that the combination of manual compression and the micro-pins help to compress the dermis and displace interstitial water from the dermal–epidermal junction into the surrounding spaces. With less water to absorb, scattering of the laser light is reduced, enabling increased absorption of the light by deeper targets.

TABLE 6.1 Nonablative Fractional Lasers

Device	Manufacturer	Type	Wavelength(s) (nm)
Clear + Brilliant Original	Solta (Bothell, WA)	Diode	1440
Clear + Brilliant Permea	Solta (Bothell, WA)	Diode	1927
Fraxel Re:Store	Solta (Bothell, WA)	Erbium	1550
Fraxel Dual	Solta (Bothell, WA)	Erbium:Glass + Thulium fiber	1550 + 1927
Halo[a]	Sciton (Palo Alto, CA)	Diode + Erbium:YAG	1470 + 2940
Icon Lux 1440	Palomar, Cynosure (Westford, MA)	Nd:YAG	1440
Icon Lux 1540	Palomar, Cynosure (Westford, MA)	Erbium	1540
Lutronic Ultra	Lutronic (San Jose, CA)	Thulium	1927
Mosaic	Lutronic (San Jose, CA)	Erbium	1550
PicoSure Focus Array	Cynosure (Westford, MA)	Alexandrite	755
PicoWay Resolve	Syneron Candela, Wayland, MA (Irvine, CA)	Nd:YAG	1064 +532
Enlighten PICO Genesis Fx	Cutera (Brisbane, CA)	Nd:YAG	1064

[a]Hybrid fractional nonablative and ablative.

There are quite a few lasers on the market which allow for fractionated delivery of picosecond pulses. These devices include the PicoSure laser with the Focus Lens Array handpiece (Cynosure, Chelmsford, MA), the PicoWay laser with the Resolve handpieces (Syneron Candela, Wayland, MA), and the Enlighten laser with the PICO Genesis FX handpiece (Cutera, Brisbane, CA). The Focus Lens Array handpiece on the PicoSure laser consists of a fixed 6-mm spot size with a fixed fluence. The handpiece fractionates the 750–850-picosecond pulsed 755 nm light so that 70% of the total energy is focused toward only 10% of the total treatment area with the remaining 30% of the energy distributed to 90% of the remaining surface. Similarly, the PicoWay laser (Syneron Candela, Wayland, MA) has beam splitting handpieces for both the 532 and 1064 nm wavelengths which deliver an array of 100 microbeams of 450-picosecond pulses per 6 × 6 mm area. The Enlighten laser (Cutera, Brisbane, CA) has a Micro Lens Array attachment which can be used with the 1064 nm wavelength. This handpiece delivers fractionated laser light through an adjustable spot size with each microbeam fluence approximately 10× higher than the console setting.

APPLICATIONS

Although NAFR is currently approved by the US Food and Drug Administration for the treatment of benign epidermal pigmented lesions, periorbital rhytides, skin resurfacing, melasma, acne and surgical scars, actinic keratoses, and striae, it has been reported to be used in many other clinical settings (Box 6.1).

BOX 6.1   Clinical Indications for Nonablative Fractional Resurfacing

- Photoaging
- Scarring (atrophic, hypertrophic, hypopigmented)
- Disorders of pigmentation (melasma, nevus of Ota, drug-induced pigmentation, idiopathic guttate hypomelanosis)
- Poikiloderma of Civatte
- Premalignant conditions (actinic keratoses, disseminated superficial actinic porokeratosis)
- Striae distensae
- Vascular disorders (but not the treatment of choice) (telangiectatic matting, residual hemangioma)

Photoaging

Photoaging is the process by which ultraviolet radiation induces changes in the skin such as loss of elasticity, dyschromia, and rhytids. Fractional nonablative lasers provide an excellent treatment modality that can address, at least to some degree, nearly every sign of photoaging. While ablative lasers remain the gold standard for skin tightening, NAFR can provide modest improvement as demonstrated by the sentinel study of the prototype fractional 1550-nm laser in 2004. In this study linear shrinkage of 2.1% was measured 3 months after the last treatment and the wrinkle score improved by 18%. This study also demonstrated that the sequence of skin tightening with NAFR appeared to be similar to ablative resurfacing with tightening within the first week after treatment, apparent relaxation at 1 month, and retightening at 3 months (Case Study 1). Another study utilizing rat skin also demonstrated the skin tightening potential of NAFR lasers and showed a 4.3% reduction in surface area of treated skin along with regenerated collagen. Notably, a recent study by Borges et al. demonstrated that patients treated with 1540-nm NAFR had reorganization of collagen type I and II and had signs of fibroblast activation 3 months after treatment.

While the skin tightening effects of fractional nonablative lasers may be modest, improvement of sun-induced pigmentation and lentigines can be more dramatic. Geronemus et al. demonstrated that two treatments with a 1927-nm nonablative fractional thulium laser produced moderate to marked improvement in the treatment of facial sun-induced pigmentation with high patient satisfaction. Similarly, Narurkar et al. demonstrated efficacy in the appearance of photodamage and pigmentation after a series of up to four treatments with 1550 and 1927 nm wavelength lasers. A series of treatments with the 1927-nm nonablative thulium laser is our treatment of choice for photoaging especially when sun-induced pigmentation is prominent.

Fractional picosecond lasers also provide a novel treatment modality to address photoaging. Brauer et al. demonstrated the effectiveness of a fractional 755 nm picosecond laser in treating mild textural changes and pigmentation associated with photoaging. A fractional 532 and 1064 nm picosecond laser improved photoaged skin and significantly decreased elastosis scores in patients with Fitzpatrick skin types I–V treated for facial wrinkles. Additionally, a histological study showed improvement of epidermal and dermal age-related atrophy after treatment with a fractional picosecond laser.

CASE STUDY 1   The Right Patient

A 58-year-old white male with mild rhytides and mild-to-moderate photodamage with scattered facial lentigines presents for consultation. You recommend a series of nonablative fractional resurfacing laser procedures. Six months after the sixth laser procedure, you see the patient back in follow-up. He is delighted with his improvement in both texture and skin tone and subsequently refers a couple of his friends to see you.

This patient is the ideal patient for nonablative fractional resurfacing. These results are typical of the improvement we see in our patients when selected appropriately. Fractional 1927-nm light is best for epidermal dyspigmentation related to photoaging, and the 1550 and 1540 nm wavelengths are best for texture. In this case a combination of wavelengths performed with each visit or alternating devices yields the best possible improvement; 1927-nm NAFR is usually recommended first because of the high degree of rapid improvement in color. Texture is slower to improve.

Subsequent reports have confirmed the efficacy of NAFR beyond just periorbital lines. Wanner et al. showed statistically significant improvement in photodamage of both facial and nonfacial sites, with 73% of patients improving at least 50%. In 2006 Geronemus and colleagues also reported their experience with fractional photothermolysis, finding it to be effective in treating mild-to-moderate rhytides. Figs. 6.2 and 6.3 show typical improvement in rhytides and pigmentation after treatment with nonablative fractional resurfacing. For deeper rhytides, such as the vertical lines of the upper lip, improvement is also seen but not nearly to the same degree as in ablative approaches.

NAFR is also considered to be an effective and safe treatment modality for photoaging off the face, including the neck, chest, scalp, arms, hands (Fig. 6.4), legs, and feet. These body sites are typically very challenging to treat with other treatment modalities, given either increased risks of complications (e.g., scarring) associated with ablative technologies or lack of efficacy that has been previously observed with other nonablative devices. Jih et al. reported statistically significant improvement in pigmentation, roughness, and wrinkling of the hands in 10 patients treated with nonablative fractional resurfacing. In our experience, we have found NAFR on all body sites to be very safe when settings are adjusted accordingly.

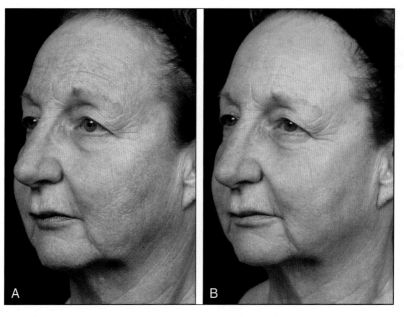

Fig. 6.2 Improvement in moderate rhytides 1 month after two treatments with Fraxel 1927 nm. (Photo courtesy Solta Medical.)

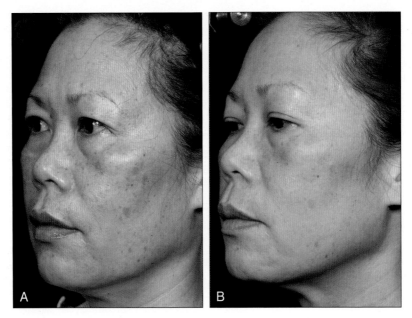

Fig. 6.3 Improvement in rhytides and dyspigmentation 1 month after three treatments with Fraxel re:store. (Photo courtesy Solta Medical.)

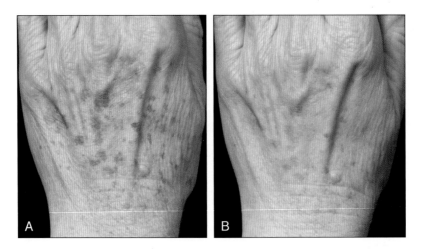

Fig. 6.4 Improvement in rhytides and dyspigmentation of the hands 1 month after two treatments with Fraxel re:store. (Photo courtesy Solta Medical.)

Scarring

Scarring can induce a tremendous psychologic, physical, and cosmetic impact on individuals. Previous therapeutic modalities in scar treatment include surgical punch grafting, subcision, dermabrasion, chemical peeling, dermal fillers, as well as laser resurfacing with ablative and nonablative devices. Published studies have demonstrated that NAFR can be successfully used in the treatment of various forms of scarring with a very favorable safety profile (Fig. 6.5). Mechanistically, FP allows

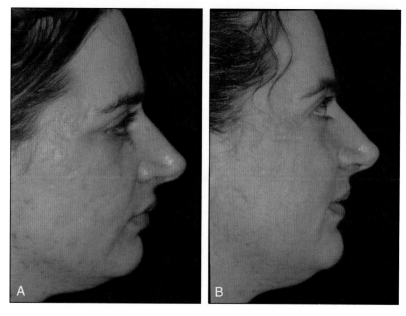

Fig. 6.5 Significant improvement in texture and rolling acne scars 2 months after four treatments with 1550-nm Fraxel.

controlled amounts of high energy to be delivered deep within the dermis, resulting in collagenolysis and neo-collagenesis, which smooths the textural abnormalities of scarring. It has been shown that collagen continues to remodel up to 6 months after NAFR possibly due to laser-induced regulation of matrix metalloprotein (MMP) and interleukin expression. These alterations on gene expression level could play a role for the dermal remodeling, anti-inflammatory effects and increased epidermal differentiation which lead to the improvement of scars.

With such a good efficacy and safety profile, many clinicians, including the authors, prefer NAFR to ablative FP when it comes to treating acne scarring. In a large clinical study, Weiss showed a median 50%–75% improvement of acne scars, using a 1540-nm fractionated laser system after three treatments at 4-week intervals, with 85% of patients rating their skin as improved. Alster showed similarly impressive results in a study of 53 patients with mild-to-moderate acne scarring; 87% of patients who received three treatments at 4-week intervals showed at least 51%–75% improvement in the appearance of their acne scars.

PEARL 1

Patients with deep acne scarring or severe rhytides often require high-energy settings, which correlates with deeper penetration of the laser and subsequent remodeling of collagen deeper in the cutis.

Fractional picosecond lasers provide a new, effective treatment option for acne scarring. A recent split-face study in 25 Asian patients compared treatment with a fractional picosecond 1064-nm laser and fractional carbon dioxide (CO_2) laser for the treatment of acne scars. The authors found that skin texture and atrophy significantly improved with both treatments with no significant difference between the two sides. No patients experienced postinflammatory hyperpigmentation on the fractional picosecond treated side whereas 24% experienced mild PIH on the fractional CO_2 treated side.

NAFR can also be safely used to treat acne scarring in darker-pigmented patients (Fig. 6.6). A study of 27 Korean patients with skin types IV or V that were treated with three to five nonablative fractional resurfacing treatments revealed no significant adverse effects, specifically pigmentary alterations. Furthermore, all

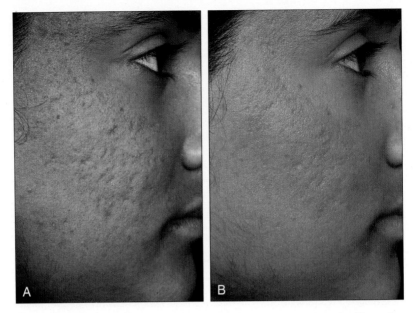

Fig. 6.6 One month after five treatments with 1550-nm Fraxel showing significant improvement in acne scarring in a darkly pigmented patient. (Photo courtesy Solta Medical.)

forms of acne scarring, including ice-pick, boxcar, and rolling scars, improved, with 8 patients (30%) reporting excellent improvement, 16 patients (59%) significant improvement, and 3 patients (11%) moderate improvement. Low density settings appear to reduce the risk of hyperpigmentation in skin of color patients. If hyperpigmentation occurs, it is typically mild and short-lived.

Although there are limited studies, NAFR can also improve contracted and hypertrophic scars. While contracted scars were historically treated with ablative resurfacing, a case study showed both subjective and objective improvement in range of motion in a patient with contracted extremity scars after 1927-nm and 1550-nm NAFR. In a study of eight patients with hypertrophic scarring, all patients had improvement in their scars based on the physician's clinical assessment, with a mean improvement of 25%–50%. Although the flash-lamp-pumped pulsed dye laser (PDL) had long been considered the laser of choice for treating hypertrophic scars, NAFR has shown tremendous promise when compared with PDL. In a study of 15 surgical scars in 12 patients, NAFR outperformed PDL in the improvement of surface pigmentation, texture change, and overall scar

thickness. Although more studies are needed, NAFR should be considered as a therapeutic option to be used in conjunction with or as an alternative to PDL.

Hypopigmentation and Hyperpigmentation

Although the mechanism of pigmentary correction is not fully understood, NAFR has shown success in the treatment of dyspigmentation as well as hypo- and hyperpigmented scars. In regard to hypopigmentation, a pilot study showed a 51%–75% improvement in hypopigmented scars in six of seven patients after 1550-nm NAFR. 1550-nm NAFR also showed promise in the treatment of idiopathic guttate hypomelanosis with normalization of skin color after each treatment as measured by colorimetry. In recent years, clinicians have increasingly combined bimatoprost with NAFR for the treatment of hypopigmentation. NAFR is thought to enhance topical drug delivery and dramatic results have been achieved with this combination treatment (Figs. 6.7 and 6.8).

In addition to hypopigmentation, NAFR also can improve hyperpigmentation and hyperpigmented scars. A retrospective study of 61 patients with Fitzpatrick skin types IV–VI and PIH showed a 43.2% improvement

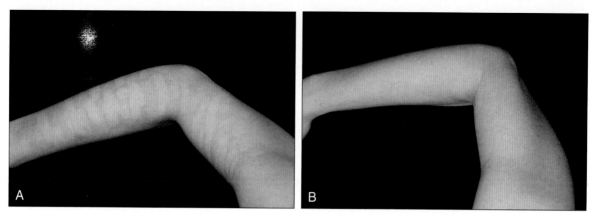

Fig. 6.7 Improvement of hypopigmented scars 1 month after three treatments with Fraxel 1927 nm.

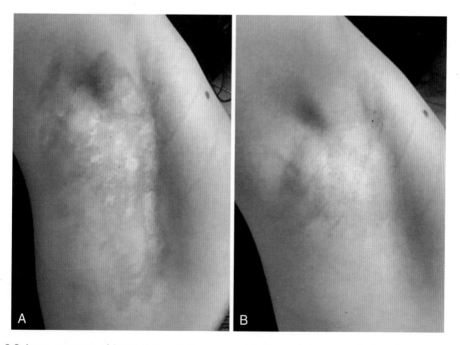

Fig. 6.8 Improvement of hypopigmentation caused by laser hair removal after four treatments with Fraxel 1927-nm NAFR in combination with topical bimatoprost.

in pigmentation after a series of treatments with low energy 1927-nm laser. A series of 1,550-nm NAFR has also proven effective in the treatment of stubborn periorbital hyperpigmentation. In addition to the 1927 and 1550 nm wavelengths, fractional picosecond lasers are being used with increased frequency to address PIH and hyperpigmented scars especially in skin of color owing to their negligible undesirable heat diffusion into surrounding structures and therefore lower risk of dyspigmentation. A recent study of 16 patients demonstrated a considerable decrease in melanin index of hyperpigmented scars after a series of treatments with a fractional 1064 nm picosecond laser with no significant side effects.

Melasma

Successful, yet typically transient, improvement of melasma can be achieved with nonablative fractional lasers. Multiple different wavelengths have been investigated for the treatment of melasma including 1550, 1927, 755, and 1064 nm. It has been proposed that dermal content, such as melanin, may be eliminated through the treatment channels through melanin shuttling.

The initial study looking at NAFR for the treatment of melasma used a 1550-nm laser and demonstrated an astounding 75%–100% clearance of melasma in 60% of the patients at 3 months after four to six sessions. Only one patient developed transient hyperpigmentation, which resolved. Another study by Goldberg et al. showed "good" improvement of melasma in patients with skin type III after treatment with 1550-nm Er:glass laser. In this study they also showed a decrease in melanocytes by electron microscopy and suggested that NAF lasers may delay regimentation due to decreased number of melanocytes noted after three epidermal turnover cycles.

Although early studies showed success using 1550 nm wavelength in the treatment of melasma, more recent studies have reported only modest improvement. A large study of fractional 1550-nm NAFR in 51 patients by Raulin's group in Germany showed the laser treatment to be no better than sunscreen. In addition, a concerning study by Wind et al. showed worsening of hyperpigmentation following NAFR treatments in 9 out of 29 patients in a split-face, randomized trial comparing 1550 nm NAFR laser with triple topical therapy. Not surprisingly, patient satisfaction was significantly lower on the laser-treated side.

Today, 1927 nm is more commonly used than 1550 nm as the wavelength for the treatment of melasma given its superficial depth of penetration corresponds to the general location of epidermal pigment in melasma. Results of studies with 1927-nm NAFR are mixed with some demonstrating significant improvement with lasting results and others demonstrating only modest results with waning improvement; our experience is more consistent with the latter. In a pilot study by Polder and Bruce, a statistically significant 51% reduction in Melasma Area and Severity Index (MASI) score was observed at 1 month after three to four 1927-nm laser treatments. However, the MASI score at 6 months dropped to 34%. A more recent study of 40 patients demonstrated Mottled Pigmentation Area and Severity Index improvement of 50% at posttreatment weeks 4 and 12 after a series of treatments with 1927-nm

NAFR. Further follow-up was not reported. Laser surgeons must use caution when treating melasma with NAFR given aggressive treatments may result in rebound melasma. Given this, the new fractional low-powdered 1927 diode laser (Clear and Brilliant Permea, Solta, Bausch Medical, Bothell, WA) also has been increasingly used although clinical studies are lacking.

Although very few studies have looked at fractional picosecond lasers for the treatment of melasma, these lasers show promise especially in skin of color. Chalermchai et al. compared combination treatment of fractional picosecond 1064-nm laser plus 4% hydroquinone with 4% hydroquinone alone. This study found combination treatment resulted in a significantly better reduction in modified MASI score than hydroquinone alone. In our experience, fractional picosecond lasers provide a safe and effective solution to stubborn pigmentation in darker skinned patients although multiple treatment sessions and maintenance therapy is needed.

In our own practice we favor a combination approach to the treatment of melasma which typically consists of a topical cream containing hydroquinone, stringent sun protection and laser therapy. Regarding laser treatment, we typically use either a fractional 1927-nm laser with gentle settings or a picosecond laser (fractionated if pigment is more epidermal or flat beam if pigment is more dermal). For patients with recalcitrant melasma we also prescribe a 3- to 4-month course of oral tranexamic acid. Laser assisted drug delivery with fractioned lasers (like 1927-nm lasers) and topical tranexamic acid can also be used.

PEARL 2

When treating dyschromia, which is generally more superficial, low energy levels with high-density settings should be used. However, low energy and low-density settings should be used when treating dyspigmentation in darker skin types, and melasma to avoid the risk of postinflammatory hyperpigmentation.

Actinic Keratoses

When treating actinic keratoses, treating the entire surface area of the affected anatomic site, known as field treatment, is preferred to ensure that both clinically visible and microscopic lesions are covered. Initial attempts by Katz et al. to treat these precancerous lesions with fractional 1550-nm laser showed great clinical response, with greater than 73% clearance 1-month posttreatment and 55.6% clearance at 6 months. However, posttreatment biopsies revealed histologic persistence, and as a result, it has been recommended that NAFR not be used as a single treatment modality for actinic keratoses. More recently, fractional 1927-nm thulium laser was approved by the FDA for the treatment of actinic keratosis. Geronemus showed that, after a single treatment with the 1927-nm thulium laser, a mean of 63% of actinic keratoses were cleared and after two treatments, 84% of lesions cleared. Definitive data on histologic clearance are still lacking. Although clinical data are early, our own clinical experience has been positive in treating extensive actinic keratoses on the face and scalp. Further studies are needed, specifically ones with histologic analysis, to prove its efficacy.

PEARL 3

The 1927-nm fractionated thulium laser penetrates less deeply than longer erbium NAFR wavelengths and is useful in treating actinic keratoses. It is especially useful in treating sun-induced lentigines of the face, neck, chest, and hands.

Striae

Although nonablative fractional resurfacing has been FDA approved for the treatment of striae, only a few small studies have examined their effectiveness. Kim et al. performed an early study demonstrating a substantial improvement in the appearance of striae distensae using a 1550-nm NAFR laser in six female subjects. Furthermore, histologic examination showed an increase in epidermal thickness, collagen, and elastic fiber deposition. Other studies have also shown improvement, albeit modest, in striae appearance. One study showed good-to-excellent clinical improvement in 27% of patients, and another study showed a 26%–50% improvement in 63% of patients. Furthermore, large-scale studies need to be performed to more clearly define NAFR's effectiveness in treating striae. In our experience the results, when appreciable, have been only modest. A consensus article recommends performing a large test area before having the patient commit to a series of treatments.

Poikiloderma of Civatte and Neck Dyspigmentation

Poikiloderma of Civatte is characterized by hyperpigmentation and hypopigmentation, atrophy, and telangiectasia. Although PDLs and intense pulse-light sources are considered by many to be the treatments of choice for poikiloderma, fractional nonablative devices at 1550 and 1927 nm are effective in improving overall color and texture of the condition.

Other Conditions

NAFR has also been used to treat a host of other conditions, including nevus of Ota, minocycline-induced hyperpigmentation, matted telangiectasias, residual fibrofatty tissue after hemangioma involution, recalcitrant disseminated superficial actinic porokeratosis, disseminated granuloma annulare, and colloid milium. Although difficult to gauge clinical response in single case reports, these reports provide evidence on the potential applications of this technology.

PATIENT SELECTION

The preoperative consultation is crucial to maximize outcomes while minimizing complications. The clinician should assess the patient expectations and goals for treatment during this encounter. Showing patients before and after photos of a typical result can help to set patient expectations regarding the efficacy of treatment. Even so, the patient must also understand that individual responses can vary.

PEARL 4

Take pretreatment photos prior to treatment to document and assess response.

To achieve satisfactory results with NAFR, a series of two or three treatments is required for 1927-nm treatments, and four to six treatments are required to improve texture with 1540- and 1550-nm devices. Typically, these procedures are spaced out every 4 weeks, and thus an entire treatment regimen may take 6 months or more to complete (Case Study 2). Those patients who prefer to have dramatic results after only one session are not the right candidates for nonablative fractional resurfacing.

Instead, these patients may benefit from fractional ablative resurfacing, which typically requires fewer treatment sessions, but has a much longer recovery. NAFR can be painful, but topical anesthesia and forced-air cooling make the procedure tolerable in most. Redness and swelling last an average of 3 days but is typically less for fractional picosecond lasers. The brown, sandpaper-like feel seen after treating individuals with epidermal dyspigmentation lasts approximately 5 days.

> ### BOX 6.2 Contraindications to Nonablative Fractional Resurfacing
>
> • Pregnancy
> • Active infection (bacterial, viral, or fungal)
> • Patients with unrealistic expectations

CASE STUDY 2 Sometimes More is Better

A 48-year-old male with severe rolling and boxcar acne scars received six nonablative fractional resurfacing treatments with the 1550-nm device. Six months after the last treatment, he comes in wondering what else can be done for his acne scarring. On examination and in comparison with pretreatment photos, you notice improvement in his acne scarring but also some room for further improvement. You recommend another two treatments and see him back 6 months after the eighth treatment. He is extremely pleased and says he noticed significantly more improvement from the final two treatments. This response is predictable because the improvement with nonablative fractional resurfacing is curvilinear. The first two treatments yield very little visible improvement, the next two a bit more, and the final two show the greatest degree of change. Sometimes in patients with bad scarring we perform an additional two treatments but always wait 6 months to see the maximum improvement from the first six before deciding.

NAFR can be performed safely on patients with all Fitzpatrick skin types, but patients with darker skin types should be treated with caution. A study of fractional lasers in the treatment of acne scars by Alajlan and Alsuwaidan and another by Alexis showed a high safety profile in those with skin of color. Although hyperpigmentation was noticed more commonly in darker-skinned patients, particularly when higher fluences and higher densities were used, this effect was usually transient.

It is important to gather a history of prior laser procedures and responses, history of keloids, history of herpes simplex infection, skin phototype, history of PIH, current medications, lidocaine allergy, pain tolerance, and anxiety level. Patients who should not be treated with fractional resurfacing are women who are pregnant or lactating and those with active infection, particularly herpes simplex. A consensus statement from the American Society of Dermatologic Surgery Guidelines Task Force concluded there is insufficient evidence to justify delaying treatment with nonablative fractional lasers for patients currently on or recently exposed to isotretinoin. Furthermore, individuals with unrealistic expectations should not be treated (Box 6.2).

The ideal patient for treatment is a fair-skinned (Fitzpatrick types I–III), motivated patient who desires attainable results with a few days of downtime and has realistic expectations (Case Study 3).

CASE STUDY 3 Just Say No

A 76-year-old female comes for a preoperative consultation for nonablative fractional resurfacing. She has been enjoying her summer on the beach and plans to return to her winter home in a few weeks. On exam, she has significant photodamage, sagging, and deep rhytides on a background of tanned skin with numerous lentigines. During the consultation, she makes it clear that because she is leaving soon, she wants to have one treatment that will improve her lines significantly with as little downtime as possible. She has read on the internet that nonablative fractional resurfacing is a great treatment for her aging face with little recovery time and wants to know when she can start.

This patient is clearly not a suitable candidate for nonablative fractional resurfacing. Patients should be counseled that, although NAFR is a highly effective treatment regimen with little downtime, a series of treatments spaced at least a couple of weeks apart is required to achieve those results. In addition, this patient has a distinct tan making her not ideal for laser treatment because she would be at an increased risk for hyperpigmentation, and more conservative treatment parameters would need to be used. Finally, her sagging skin will not improve with this procedure. She might be a better candidate for ablative fractional resurfacing or nonsurgical or surgical skin tightening.

PRETREATMENT

All patients should wear a broad-spectrum sunscreen (SPF > 30) and should avoid sun exposure before, during, and immediately after their treatments. There is no evidence that treating with topical hydroquinone for 1–2 months prior to nonablative fractional resurfacing decreases the risk of postinflammatory pigmentation in individuals with darker skin types (types IV–VI). Nor is there any scientific proof that topical retinoids need to be discontinued prior to treatment in those with sensitive skin. In spite of this many physicians recommend using hydroquinone and ask patients to discontinue retinoids prior to nonablative fractional resurfacing.

PEARL 5

Topical retinoids do not need to be discontinued prior to nonablative fractional resurfacing. However, for some patients with sensitive skin, doing so may make treatment more tolerable.

Pretreatment with oral antiviral medications is recommended in those with a history of herpes simplex virus (HSV) infection (Box 6.3). We typically recommend patients take 2 grams of Valtrex the morning of the procedure and 2 grams 12 hours later. Although some practitioners advocate the routine use of HSV prophylaxis regardless of previous infection, we do not feel that this is necessary. Firoz et al. reported the first three cases of herpes zoster within the distribution of the trigeminal nerve after NAFR. The patients all had a history of chicken pox, and none had received prophylaxis prior to treatment. Patients with a family history of herpes zoster and who have not had shingles themselves may thus benefit from antiviral treatment prior to treatment. Prophylactic antibiotics are not needed for nonablative fractional resurfacing.

On the day of the first procedure, serial standardized photographs should be taken to allow patients to observe their treatment progress. Topical anesthesia should be applied 1 hour prior to starting the treatment. Several different anesthetic agents are currently available, including 5% lidocaine; 2.5% lidocaine/2.5% prilocaine; 7% lidocaine/7% tetracaine; 23% lidocaine/7% tetracaine; and 30% lidocaine. In our experience, anesthetic agents with tetracaine induce significant erythema,

---

BOX 6.3 Procedural Steps in Nonablative Fractional Photothermolysis

1. Obtain consent and prepare patient:
   a. Review risks and limitations of procedure and answer questions.
   b. Assess patient expectations.
   c. Take preoperative photos.
   d. Start prophylaxis for HSV if patient has a history of cold sores (could consider in patients with a history of varicella zoster without a history of shingles).
2. Wash the area to be treated.
3. Gently cleanse skin with alcohol wipe.
4. Apply topical anesthetic ointment and leave on for 1 h prior to the procedure.
5. Perform procedure:
   a. Use a skin-cooling device.
   b. Apply handpiece perpendicular to skin.
   c. Take precaution not to bulk heat.
6. Prepare patient for discharge:
   a. Apply cold compresses or ice to minimize swelling.
   b. Review posttreatment care.
   c. Schedule follow-up appointment.

---

leading to patient dissatisfaction. We use 30% lidocaine in an adherent ointment base in our practice because it provides the most comfort with the least erythema. To minimize the risk of systemic toxicity from the topical anesthetics, areas no greater than 300–400 cm^2 should be treated during each session. Before the treatment, all of the anesthetic should be thoroughly washed off (Case Study 4). Oral anxiolytics and analgesics may be required in a small fraction of patients who cannot tolerate the procedure with topical anesthesia alone. In those who find the procedure too uncomfortable with topical anesthesia, extend contact time from 60 to 90 minutes, being sure to rub the cream into the skin several times during the 90-minute period to increase percutaneous penetration. It is remarkable how much better the procedure is tolerated with longer application of the topical anesthesia. Should that still not suffice, we first add ketorolac (Toradol). In more anxious or intolerant individuals we have had success with diazepam and intramuscular (IM) meperidine (Demerol). Intravenous (IV) sedation is not needed for this procedure. Although metal eye protection is advised for the patient by some, many practitioners recommend that keeping the eyes closed during the procedure is sufficient (with the exception of fractionated picosecond lasers in which metal laser eye shields must be worn due to the risk of ocular injury). All individuals in the treatment room should also wear eye protection. When it comes to selection of treatment parameters, a number of factors need to be considered, including clinical indication, anatomic site, and skin phototype of the patients. In general, studies demonstrate that PIH is less common when fractional resurfacing of darker skin is performed using lower density settings, fewer passes, and longer treatment intervals. Treatment of nonfacial sites should be performed with slightly lower density and fluence settings.

PEARL 6

Large treatment areas ($>400\,cm^2$) should be avoided to reduce the risk of lidocaine toxicity.

PEARL 7

In darker-pigmented patients, energy densities should be decreased; also consider lowering the energy and performing fewer passes in an effort to reduce the risk of hyperpigmentation.

GENERAL TECHNIQUE

We find the supine position most comfortable for the patient and practitioner. In this position the practitioner can be seated comfortably with elbows close to 90 degrees to alleviate fatigue and repetitive stress injury. During treatment, patient positioning is crucial to ensure perpendicular application of the laser handpiece. For example, when treating the neck, especially in the submandibular area, it is often helpful to have the chin tilted upward to allow for better exposure.

With the scanning handpiece of the Fraxel systems (Solta Medical, a division of Bausch Medical, Bothell, WA), we deliver eight passes when treating acne scars, rhytides, and photoaging of the face. We use a double-pass, "up-down" 50% overlap technique. One linear pass is delivered, the handpiece is brought to a complete stop, lifted, and then returned along the same path for a second pass. The handpiece is then moved laterally by 50%, and the technique is repeated until the treatment area is completed. As a result, each area is treated with four passes. For the next four passes, we direct the passes perpendicular to the first treatment to ensure complete

CASE STUDY 4　Toxicity

A 45-year-old, petite woman weighing 102 lb presents for nonablative fractional resurfacing of her face, neck, and chest to treat photoaging. She has not had treatment before and has some anxiety over the procedure. After counseling the patient and addressing her concerns, she gives her informed consent and pretreatment photos are taken; 30% lidocaine gel is then applied over the face, neck, and chest.

Prior to her treatment, your schedule begins to run late and you are unable to start her treatment until an hour and a half after the topical anesthesia has been applied. She tolerates the first pass on her cheek but then suddenly becomes agitated and reports significant anxiety. Treatment is immediately stopped, but the woman begins to complain of nausea and perioral paresthesias. You start an infusion of normal saline and closely observe the patient over a couple of hours without further sequelae. Her serum lidocaine levels are elevated at $2\,\mu g/mL$.

To avoid this problem, topical anesthesia application should be limited to no more than 90 minutes. Furthermore, large treatment areas should be avoided at one visit and therefore we typically limit patients to two anatomical locations per treatment sessions (e.g., face and neck or neck and chest but not face, neck and chest).

and even laser coverage. Using this 50% overlap technique the outer most treatment area only receives four passes total with the remainder of the treatment area receiving eight passes; this creates a more elegant transition from treated site to untreated site. Dividing the face into four quadrants also helps to manage the treatment area and reduce the risk of overlap or missing a section.

Our settings are individualized according to patients' needs and tolerability. For 1550 nm facial resurfacing with the Fraxel Dual we often start with energy levels between 40 and 50 mJ and a treatment level of 6–8 (Table 6.2). The settings are often increased during subsequent visits if tolerated. When using the 1927-nm thulium laser component of the Fraxel Dual we often use an energy level of 10 mJ and a treatment level of 5, 4, 3 for the face, neck, and chest, respectively. For patients wanting even less downtime, we sometimes decrease the treatment level to 1 and only perform four passes. With these gentle settings patients typically have less than 1 day of downtime.

TABLE 6.2   Recommended Treatment Parameters

Device	Indication		Energy (mJ)	Pulse Width	Treatment Level[a]	Number of Passes
1550 nm (Fraxel)	Facial resurfacing for wrinkles, acne, and other scarring but not melasma/ dyspigmentation		40–70	—	6–10	8
	Nonfacial resurfacing		20–40	—	6–10	8
	Melasma		10–20	—	3–6	8
1927 nm (Fraxel)	Facial resurfacing		10	—	5	8
	Nonfacial resurfacing		10	—	3	8
	Melasma		5–10	—	2–4	8
1440 nm (StarLux/ Icon)	10-mm tip	Facial resurfacing	25–70	7–10	—	2
	15-mm tip	Facial resurfacing	6–10	7	—	1–3
1540 nm (StarLux/ Icon)	10-mm tip	Facial resurfacing	40–70	10–15	—	3–6
	15-mm tip	Facial resurfacing	10–15	10–15	—	3–4
	15-mm tip	Melasma	5–12	10–15	—	2–5
	14-mm tip	Facial resurfacing	3–4	—	—	2
755 nm (PicoSure Focus Array)	6-mm	Facial resurfacing for wrinkles, scars and dyspigmentation	0.71 J/cm^2	500–750 ps	—	2–6
1,064 + 532 nm (PicoWay Resolve)	6 mm	Facial resurfacing for wrinkles and dyspigmentation	Up to 400mJ	450 ps	—	1–4

[a]Treatment level for darker skin types (IV–VI) should be decreased to reduce the risk of hyperpigmentation.

For stamping handpieces, the fractionated energy is delivered according to the tip size. For example, with the Icon system (Cynosure, Westford, MA) and the 15-mm Lux1540 handpiece, three to four passes are generally delivered with a 50% overlap in both directions. The handpiece should be lifted off the skin between each pulse, and pulse-stacking is not recommended. For facial resurfacing with the Lux1540 15-mm tip, we recommend using 10–15mJ per microbeam with a pulse width of 10–15 milliseconds.

For treatment with fractionated picosecond lasers, 30 minutes of topical anesthesia is usually sufficient. A series of passes is recommended with a total of several thousand pulses delivered per treatment. Patients are treated every 4–6 weeks for up to six treatments or until a satisfactory result has been achieved.

COOLING

A cooling device used in conjunction with the NAFR laser device should be standard for all treatments. A popular forced-air cooling device, the Zimmer Cryo (Zimmer Medizin Systems, Irvine, CA) increases patient comfort significantly. Some laser systems now also come with a built-in cooling device. In a study of 20 patients, 19 noted significant pain reduction with the addition of a cooling device.

POSTTREATMENT

Upon completion of the treatment, patients are advised to ice their skin for at least 10 minutes and then periodically over the next few hours. Not only does this help with patient comfort, but it also reduces postprocedural swelling. Swelling typically lasts 1–3 days, but in the rare individual it can last for a week. Although swelling is hard to predict prior to the first treatment, the pattern usually remains constant during a series of treatments. Patients who do not swell after the first treatment tend not to swell with subsequent treatments. Erythema develops immediately afterwards in all treated patients (Fig. 6.9) and typically resolves in 3 days. Use of noncomedogenic moisturizers is also recommended. Patients are advised to wear sun protection for several weeks after their treatment to reduce the risk of hyperpigmentation. In those with an increased risk of hyperpigmentation, hydroquinone may be started immediately after the procedure. We routinely wait to start lightening agents until we see the first signs of postinflammatory pigmentation, which is usually around day 21 posttreatment. Alster et al. showed that a light-emitting diode device (Gentlewaves, Light BioSciences, Virginia Beach, VA) decreases erythema intensity and duration following treatment, although the precise mechanism of action is unclear.

SAFETY AND COMPLICATIONS

NAFR is a well-tolerated procedure with an excellent safety profile. Fisher and Geronemus studied the immediate and short-term side effects, showing a favorable side effect profile. In their study of 60 patients with skin types I–IV, all patients expectedly developed erythema immediately posttreatment, which in most patients resolved in 3 days. Xerosis occurred in 86.6% of patients, usually presenting 2 days after treatment and resolving by day 5 or 6. This was minimally bothersome and responded well to moisturization. Other frequently reported posttreatment side effects were transient and included facial edema (82%) and flaking (60%). Small, superficial scratches were also reported in 46.6% of patients. These scratches, which all resolve without sequelae, are thought to be related to tangential application of the handpiece or pulse stacking by inexperienced users. Pruritus (37%) and bronzing (26.6%) are also common side effects of treatment. Perhaps the most valuable finding from this short-term study was the impact on the patient's quality of life; 72% reported limiting social activities by an average time of only 2.1 days, which is in stark contrast to the downtime seen with the conventional resurfacing laser. The most commonly attributed reasons were erythema and edema. The treatments were well tolerated, with an average pain score of 4.6 on a scale of 1–10.

Given that NAFR was specifically developed to minimize the extent of complications, long-term

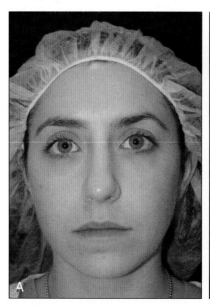 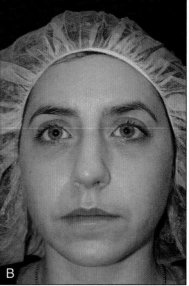

Fig. 6.9 Prior to treatment (A) and immediately after nonablative fractional resurfacing (B) demonstrating erythema.

complications are also extremely rare. Graber et al. performed a large-scale study looking at the complications and long-term side effects of NAFR. Consistent with Fisher and Geronemus' study, they also reported a low short-term complication rate. In their study of 422 patients with a total of 961 treatments, the most common complications were acne eruptions (1.87%), HSV outbreaks (1.77%), and erosions (1.35%), all of which occurred with lower frequency than after ablative procedures. Acne outbreaks were more likely to occur in patients who were acne-prone and thus oral antibiotic prophylaxis may be considered in some patients. Other uncommon complications included prolonged erythema and edema.

When similar treatment parameters were used across different skin phototypes, complications were more likely to occur in those that were more darkly pigmented, especially with regard to PIH. Although an uncommon complication (0.73%), PIH lasted an average of 51 days, significantly longer than any other complication. Studies have shown that, with proper titration of settings, darker-pigmented patients can be treated more safely. Chan et al. provided the first evidence that density of MTZs may specifically increase the risk for PIH. By reducing the density and lengthening the treatment interval, the risk of PIH in darker-skinned patients can be significantly reduced. Although complications, especially long-term ones, are extremely rare, patients should be educated to expect typical side effects, including posttreatment erythema, edema, dry skin, and desquamation (Box 6.4).

FRACTIONAL MICRONEEDLE RADIOFREQUENCY

While lasers remain the gold standard for treatment of rhytides, scars and skin tightening, fractional microneedle radiofrequency (FMRF) devices provide another therapeutic option. These devices have increased in popularity over recent years and new devices continue to come to market. A few commonly used devices include the Profound (Syneron Candela, Wayland, MA), the Genius (Lutronic, San Jose, CA), the Legend (Lumenis, San Jose, CA), and the Secret (Cutera, Brisbane, CA). In contrast to lasers which generate heat through selective photothermolysis, FMRF works by delivering energy in the form of radiofrequency directly to tissues via microneedles in a nonchromophore specific pattern. The energy delivered creates thermal coagulative injury zones which cause contraction and restructuring of collagen. The microneedles have adjustable depth and energy depending on the device and can reach deeper depths than nonablative fractional lasers. The tips of the microneedles can be either insulated or noninsulated, the former being safer in darker skin types given the epidermis is protected from thermal damage.

Some view FMRF as a safer alternative to nonablative fractional lasers in skin of color although data is lacking. Often topical anesthesia is required, and erythema may last from <24 hours to 4 days. A recent study evaluated the biometric changes of the skin after FMRF and found that the density and thickness of the dermis along with collagen content increased after six sessions. Although there are few studies directly comparing nonablative fractional lasers to FMRF, one study showed similar but greater improvement of atrophic acne scarring with 1550-nm fractional laser treatment compared with FMRF.

ADVANCES IN TECHNOLOGY

The field of fractional resurfacing is relatively new, with advances in treatment parameters and new applications for the technology evolving seemingly every month. Since the first fractional resurfacing device was used in 2004, laser systems have continued to be refined and updated. Nonablative laser wavelengths have also been broadened significantly with systems now using picosecond 755- and 1064-nm technology. In addition, Sciton recently released the Halo laser

---

BOX 6.4 **Complications Associated With Nonablative Fractional Resurfacing**	
More Common Complications	**Less Common Complications**
• Acneiform eruptions • HSV outbreaks • Erosions • Postinflammatory hyperpigmentation	• Prolonged erythema • Prolonged edema • Recall erythema • Dermatitis • Impetigo • Scarring • Varicella zoster virus • Lidocaine toxicity

which is the first hybrid fractional laser that delivers both ablative and nonablative wavelengths to the same MTZ.

ADVANCED TOPICS: TREATMENT TIPS FOR EXPERIENCED PRACTITIONERS

Many patients have both the pigmentary changes and rhytides associated with photoaging. A hybrid approach combining two nonablative fractional resurfacing wavelengths optimizes outcomes. Alternating 1927- with 1550-nm treatments addresses both concerns (Case Study 5). An alternative approach uses IPL to address the dyschromia and uneven pigmentation of photoaging, whereas 1550-, 1540-, or 1440-nm NAFR devices address wrinkling. Combining technologies in what are sometimes called "megasessions" produces striking improvement in texture and color. Some combinations include NAFR preceded by Q-switched alexandrite laser, Q-switched Nd:YAG laser, long-pulsed green laser, or IPL. In our own study, the addition of a MaxG IPL (Cynosure, Westford, MA) treatment immediately prior to the Lux1540 nonablative resurfacing device yielded significant improvement in photoaging scores when rated by blinded physicians.

CASE STUDY 5 **Combination Treatment**

A 62-year-old female with numerous lentigines and mild rhytides comes in for cosmetic consultation. She has heard that IPL treatment would improve her brown spots. Although you agree that IPL would significantly improve her dyspigmentation, you recommended the 1550-nm nonablative fractionated device alternating with the 1927-nm device instead. Using this treatment strategy, you realize that you can give her a "bigger bang for her buck" and also improve her rhytides. She does six treatments (three with each laser) over 6 months and has a very dramatic response. She is extremely pleased with the treatment results.

CONCLUSION

The science of NAFR has revolutionized our treatment strategies for a host of dermatologic conditions. Coupled with a very favorable side effect profile and minimal downtime, this relatively new technology will continue to gain in popularity. With new devices and modifications to current systems emerging constantly, its applications will also continue to evolve and broaden. Clinical studies demonstrating efficacy and further scientific scrutiny will help to continue to advance this technology.

Check online video (Video 6.1)

FURTHER READING

Alexiades-Armenakas MR, Dover JS, Arndt KA. The spectrum of laser skin resurfacing: nonablative, fractional, and ablative laser resurfacing. *J Am Acad Dermatol.* 2008;58(5): 719–737.

Amann PM, Marquardt Y, Steiner T, et al. Effects of nonablative fractional erbium glass laser treatment on gene regulation in human three-dimensional skin models. *Lasers Med Sci.* 2016;31(3):397–404. A mechanistic study of the effects of NARFR in scars.

Bogdan Allemann I, Kaufman J. Fractional photothermolysis—an update. *Lasers Med Sci.* 2010;25(1):137–144. This article reviews both ablative and non-ablative fractional photothermolysis. It includes a table of available devices. A little bit cumbersome to read but reviews the literature comprehensively.

Brauer JA, Kazlouskaya V, Alabdulrazzaq H, et al. Use of a picosecond pulse duration laser with specialized optic for treatment of facial acne scarring. *J Am Med Assoc Dermatol.* 2015;151(3):278–284. A study describing the use of a pixilated handpiece affixed to a picosecond alexandrite leaser for treatment of acne scars.

Cohen BE, Brauer JA, Geronemus RG. Acne scarring: a review of available therapeutic lasers. *Lasers Surg Med.* 2016;48(2):95–115. A nice review of all available technologies for the treatment of acne scarring with a large section on NAFR.

Geronemus RG. Fractional photothermolysis: current and future applications. *Lasers Surg Med.* 2006;38(3):169–176. One of the earliest articles discussing the clinical applications of non-ablative fractional photothermolysis through the eyes of one early implementer. Good clinical photos.

Graber EM, Tanzi EL, Alster TS. Side effects and complications of fractional laser photothermolysis: experience with 961 treatments. *Dermatol Surg.* 2008;34(3):301–305. A study with a large population reporting potential complications. The study also documents the safety of non-ablative fractional photothermolysis.

Manstein D, Herron GS, Sink RK, Tanner H, Anderson RR. Fractional photothermolysis: a new concept for cutaneous remodeling using microscopic patterns of thermal injury. *Lasers Surg Med.* 2004;34:426–438. The seminal article on the concept of fractional photothermolysis. It includes an excellent background to the technology, mechanism of action, and clinical data.

Marra DE, Yip D, Fincher EF, Moy RL. Systemic toxicity from topically applied lidocaine in conjunction with fractional photothermolysis. *Arch Dermatol.* 2006;142(8):1024–1026. A case report of systemic toxicity to topical lidocaine during treatment with non-ablative fractional photothermolysis.

Metelitsa AI, Alster TS. Fractionated laser skin resurfacing treatment complications: a review. *Dermatol Surg.* 2010;36(3):299–306. A good review of treatment of complications with non-ablative fractional photothermolysis.

Narurkar VA. Nonablative fractional laser resurfacing. *Dermatol Clin.* 2009;27(4):473–478. A review of non-ablative fractional photothermolysis and its clinical applications with good before and after photos.

Prather H, et al. Laser safety in isotretinoin use: a survey of expert opinion and practice. *Dermatol Surg.* 2017.

Sherling M, Friedman PM, Adrian R, et al. Consensus recommendations on the use of an erbium-doped 1,550-nm fractionated laser and its applications in dermatologic laser surgery. *Dermatol Surg.* 2010;36(4):461–469. In this article, a group of laser experts provide their recommendations of treatment settings on one particular laser, the Fraxel re:store. An excellent resource to obtain guidelines for treatment settings for new practitioners.

Taudorf EH, Danielsen PL, Paulsen IF, et al. Non-ablative fractional laser provides long-term improvement of mature burn scars—a randomized controlled trial with histological assessment. *Lasers Surg Med.* 2015;47(2):141–147.

Tierney EP, Kouba DJ, Hanke CW. Review of fractional photothermolysis: treatment indications and efficacy. *Dermatol Surg.* 2009;35(10):1445–1461.

7

Nonsurgical Skin Tightening

Michael S. Kaminer, Courtney Gwinn, and Karen J. Dover

SUMMARY AND KEY FEATURES

- Nonsurgical skin tightening is a popular concept, with novel devices continually entering the market.
- The main types of nonsurgical skin-tightening technologies include radiofrequency, infrared light, ultrasound, microneedling with radiofrequency, and subdermal minimally-invasive radiofrequency.
- Treatment protocols have evolved over the years to focus on reduced energy settings and multipass techniques, making the procedures safer and more comfortable for patients.
- All skin-tightening devices work by the introduction of energy to create heat within the skin or underlying structures. These devices elicit mechanical and biochemical effects that lead to both immediate contraction of collagen fibers, and delayed remodeling and neocollagenesis via wound healing.
- Patient selection is key for best results and overall patient satisfaction.
- Ideal candidates for nonablative approaches include those patients concerned with risks and recovery of more invasive procedures, and those willing to accept lesser efficacy in exchange for improved side effect and healing time profiles.
- Noninvasive and minimally invasive skin-tightening devices are capable of improving both skin laxity and facial contours. The physician must analyze the patient's three-dimensional facial and neck structures, dynamically and at rest, to determine the regions most amenable to therapy, which typically include the upper face/brow and the lower face/jawline.
- Skin-tightening procedures can be performed along with fillers, neurotoxins, or other laser- or light-based devices to address multiple issues and achieve a more global improvement: synergy amongst these modalities leads to enhanced patient satisfaction.
- Very rarely patients may experience side effects related to overly-aggressive treatment, such as burns, indentations, scars, or changes in pigmentation. The overall incidence of such problems is extremely low with all current devices, owing to updated and improved protocol trends, the use of lower energies, and regular patient feedback as a guide to safe energy delivery.

INTRODUCTION

The appearance of rhytides and skin laxity are near certainties during the aging process. A number of modalities have been used to reduce these phenomena, including laser, mechanical, and surgical techniques. In the mid to late 1990, ablative resurfacing lasers were deemed the gold standard for facial skin tightening. Despite substantial clinical benefits, the technology was beset with significant downtime, and an increased risk of side effects, including erythema, permanent pigmentary changes, infection, and scarring. Patients are now more accustomed to procedures with both reduced downtime and sufficient clinical improvement. This has led to a burgeoning number of nonablative technologies with little to no recovery time and a more favorable risk–reward profile. Unlike ablative

TABLE 7.1 Major Types of Skin-Tightening Technologies

Skin-Tightening Technology	Device
Monopolar radiofrequency	Thermage CPT and FLX (Solta) Pelleve (Cyanosure) NuEra Tight (Lumenis)
Bipolar radiofrequency with light energy	Elos Plus, Galaxy, Aurora, Polaris, ReFirme (Syneron-Candela)
Bipolar radiofrequency with vacuum	Aluma (Lumenis)
Bipolar radiofrequency delivered via a microneedle electrode array	Profound (Syneron-Candela) Infini (Lutronic) Intensif (Endymed) Genius (Lutronic) Legend Pro (Lumenis) Morpheus8 (Inmode)
Broadband infrared light	Titan (Cutera) Icon (Cynosure) SkinTyte (Sciton)
Unipolar and bipolar radiofrequency	Accent (Alma) TruSculpt (Cutera)
Bipolar radiofrequency	Evoke (SpectruMed)
Ultrasound technology	Ulthera (Merz) Sofwave (Sofwave)
Ultrasound with radiofrequency	Exilis (BTL Aesthetics)

BOX 7.1 Mechanism of Skin-Tightening Devices

1. Immediate collagen contraction by direct heating of collagen fibers
2. Delayed remodeling and neocollagenesis via a wound-healing response

lasers, nonablative technologies induce thermal injury to the dermis or subcutaneous tissues, without epidermal vaporization. Epidermal protection is customarily achieved through the use of adjunctive surface cooling.

In terms of skin laxity, specifically, the benchmark remains rhytidectomy or surgical redraping. The goal of this chapter is to review the major types of minimally invasive or nonablative, tissue-tightening techniques, including radiofrequency-, light-, and ultrasound-based devices (Table 7.1). These options are not a replacement for surgical procedures, and appropriate patient selection remains key to overall satisfaction.

THERMAL COLLAGEN REMODELING

All skin-tightening devices work by delivering energy to create heat within the skin or underlying structures.

This elicits mechanical and biochemical effects that lead to both immediate contraction of collagen fibers and delayed remodeling and neocollagenesis via a wound-healing response (Box 7.1).

Collagen fibers are composed of a triple helix of protein chains linked with interchain bonds into a crystalline structure. When collagen fibers are heated to specific temperatures, they contract due to breakage of intramolecular hydrogen bonds. This contraction causes the crystalline triple helix structure to fold, creating thicker and shorter collagen fibers. This is thought to be the mechanism of action of immediate tissue tightening seen after skin-tightening procedures. Studies have also found selective contraction of fibrous septae in the subcutaneous fat, which is thought to be responsible for the inward (Z dimension) tightening (Fig. 7.1). It is also believed that fibroblasts, upon heating, stimulate neocollagenesis. Increased production of type I collagen with reorganization in parallel arrays of compact fibrils then leads to delayed dermal remodeling.

Problems arise if too much heat is delivered, as collagen fibrils denature completely above a critical heat threshold, leading to cell death, and scar formation. If too little heat is delivered, there can be an inadequate tissue response, although it appears mild thermal injury, in the sub-coagulative range, does give rise to new dermal ground substance and tissue remodeling of photodamaged skin over time. The optimal shrinkage temperature of collagen has been cited as 58°C–65°C, with initial onset of fibril shrinkage at 58°C, and the main transition to denaturation occurring at approximately 65°C; however, contraction is, in actuality, determined by a combination of temperature and exposure time. For every 5°C decrease in temperature, a tenfold increase in exposure time is required to achieve an equivalent amount of collagen contraction. Studies demonstrate with exposure times in the millisecond domain, the shrinkage temperature is greater than 85°C, whereas for exposure times over several seconds,

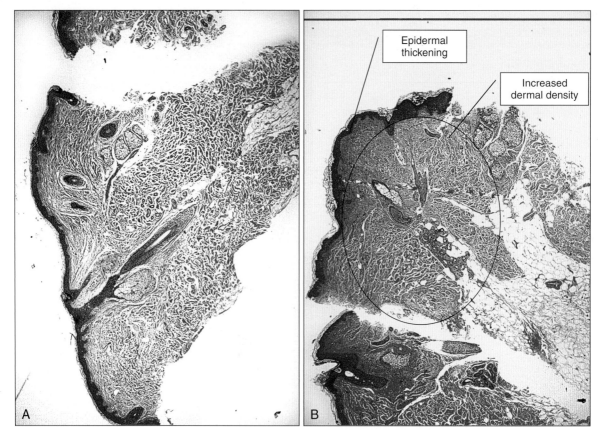

Fig. 7.1 Human skin (A) before and (B) 4 months after treatment with Thermage, showing epidermal thickening and increased dermal density. *(Photographs courtesy Solta.)*

the shrinkage temperature is at the lower range of 60°C–65°C. In conclusion, both temperature and exposure time must be considered.

The other main mechanism in skin rejuvenation is a secondary wound-healing response that produces dermal remodeling over time, which entails activation of fibroblasts to increase deposition of type I collagen and encourages collagen reorganization into parallel arrays of compact fibrils.

RADIOFREQUENCY DEVICES

Radiofrequency (RF) devices are indispensable for hemostasis, electrocoagulation, and endovenous closure in medical dermatology. In the esthetic arena, the technology has been used for skin resurfacing and noninvasive tissue tightening.

Radiofrequency is energy in the electromagnetic spectrum, ranging from 300 MHz to 3 kHz. Unlike most lasers, which target specific absorption bands of chromophores, heat is generated from the natural resistance of tissue to the movement of electrons within the radiofrequency field, as governed by Ohm's law (Box 7.2): of fundamental importance, it is a formula which calculates the relationship between voltage, current and resistance in an electrical circuit (V = IR). This resistance, called impedance, generates heat relative to the amount of current and time by converting electrical current to

---

BOX 7.2   Ohm's Law

Impedance (Z) to the movement of electrons creates heat relative to the amount of current (I) and time (t):

$$\text{Energy(Joules)} = I^2 \times Z \times t$$

thermal energy. Consequently, energy is dispersed to three-dimensional tissue volumes at targeted and controlled depths.

The configuration of electrodes in a noninvasive RF device can be monopolar, unipolar, bipolar, multipolar or fractional. Minimally-invasive platforms include fractional (insulated or noninsulated microneedles) or subcutaneous probes. The main differences are the configuration of electrodes and the type of electromagnetic field that are generated. In a monopolar system, the electrical current passes through a single electrode in the handpiece to a grounding pad (Box 7.3). This type of electrode configuration is common in surgical radiofrequency devices, because there is a high density of power close to the electrode surface, with the potential for deep penetration of tissue heating. In tissue-tightening applications, surface cooling is used to protect the outer layers of the skin and heat only the deeper targets. In a bipolar system, the electrical current passes between two electrodes at a fixed distance (Box 7.4). This type of electrode configuration has a more controlled current distribution; however, the depth of penetration is limited to approximately one-half the distance between the electrodes and will vary with frequency. Unipolar radiofrequency transfers RF energy as electromagnetic radiation rather than as a current, leading to resistive heating requiring no ground. In fractional RF, multiple electrode arrays, or microneedles, are utilized to induce fractional thermal injury. RF microneedling devices can have either insulated or noninsulated needles; insulated needles only heat the area surrounding the sphere at the uninsulated tip whereas noninsulated needles create thermal columns of injury in both the epidermis and dermis relying on the high impedance of the epidermis for epidermal protection. Despite this high impedance, the epidermis is not entirely spared from thermal injury with noninsulated needles. Subdermal, minimally-invasive RF devices utilize a subdermal probe (accessing the dermis through focal skin punctures) to deliver energy in a monopolar or bipolar fashion, heating the dermis to a desired, predictable temperature (55°C–65°C for dermis, 70°C for fat).

With radiofrequency technologies, the depth of energy penetration depends upon the following factors: (1) the configuration of the electrodes (i.e., either monopolar or bipolar), (2) the mode of delivery (i.e., skin surface, needle-based, or probe-based), (3) the type and composition of tissue serving as the conduction medium (i.e., fat, blood, skin), (4) temperature, and (5) the frequency of the electrical current applied (Box 7.5). Tissue is made up of multiple layers, including dermis, fat, muscle, and fibrous tissue, all of which have a different resistance to the movement of radiofrequency energy (Table 7.2). Structures with higher impedance are more susceptible to heating. In general, fat, bone, and dry skin tend to have low conductivities, such that current tends to flow around these structures rather than through them. Wet skin has a higher electrical conductivity, allowing greater penetration of current. For this reason, in certain radiofrequency procedures, improved results can be seen with generous amounts of coupling fluid and increased hydration of the skin. The structure of an individual's tissue (dermal thickness, fat thickness, fibrous septae, number and size of adnexal structures) plays a role in determining impedance, heat perception, and, ultimately, total deposited energy, despite otherwise comparable parameters.

Temperature also influences tissue conductivity and the distribution of electrical current. In general, every 1°C increase in temperature lowers the skin impedance by 2%. Surface cooling will increase resistance

---

BOX 7.3 Monopolar Electrode Devices

- The electrical current passes through a single electrode in the handpiece to a grounding pad
- There is a high density of power close to the electrode's surface, with the potential for deep penetration of tissue heating

---

BOX 7.4 Bipolar Electrode Devices

- The electrical current passes between two electrodes at a fixed distance
- The depth of penetration of the current is limited to approximately one-half the distance between the electrodes

---

BOX 7.5 Factors Influencing the Depth of Penetration of Radiofrequency Technologies

- Frequency of the electrical current
- Electrode configuration (i.e., monopolar or bipolar)
- Type of tissue serving as the conduction medium
- Temperature

TABLE 7.2   Dielectric Properties for Human Tissue at 1 MHz and Room Temperature

Type of Tissue	Electrical Conductivity (siemens/m)
Bone	0.02
Fat	0.03
Dry skin	0.03
Nerve	0.13
Cartilage	0.23
Wet skin	0.22
Muscle	0.50
Thyroid	0.60

to the electrical field near the epidermis, driving the radiofrequency current into the tissue, and increasing the penetration depth. Conversely, target structures that have been prewarmed with optical energy will, in theory, have greater conductivity, less resistance, and greater selective heating by the radiofrequency current. This is the theoretical advantage touted by hybrid, skin-tightening devices, that use a combined approach of light and radiofrequency energy to provide synergistic results.

Noninvasive Monopolar Radiofrequency

The first monopolar tissue-tightening device on the market was Thermage (Solta Medical, Hayward, CA; Valeant Pharmaceuticals, Bridgewater, NJ), introduced in 2001. It remains the apparatus to garner the most scientific studies and publications. The Thermage device uses a capacitive, coupled-electrode, at a single contact point, and a high-frequency current of 6 MHz. A disposable membrane tip is used to deliver the energy into the skin, with an accompanying adhesive grounding pad serving as a low-resistance path for current flow to complete the circuit. The use of capacitive rather than conductive coupling is important, because it allows the energy to be dispersed across a surface to create a zone of tissue heating. With conductive coupling, the energy is concentrated at the tip of the electrode, resulting in increased heating at the contact surface and an increased risk of epidermal injury (Video 7.1). Precooling, parallel-cooling, and postcooling, as delivered through a cryogen spray on the tip of the handpiece, are integral in cooling the epidermis to avoid

injury, increasing skin impedance, and increasing the depth of penetration of the radiofrequency current.

In the early clinical experience, one of the main drawbacks to the Thermage procedure was a high degree of discomfort during the procedure, requiring heavy sedation or frank anesthesia. The protocol at that time was one to two passes at higher energies. The treatments were quite painful, results tended to be inconsistent from patient to patient, and some adverse events, such as fat necrosis and atrophic scarring, were noted. Over the years, treatment protocols have evolved to a paradigm using lower energies, multiple passes, and regular patient feedback on heat sensation as the end-point of therapy. In 2006, Kist et al. noted that twice the amount of collagen denaturation occurred with three passes at lower energy than one pass at higher energy. The multipass technique has all but eliminated the risk of unacceptable side effects, and has greatly reduced the pain involved, such that most procedures can be performed without any anesthesia. Furthermore, the Thermage FLX was recently released, which increased the surface area of the treatment tip from 3 to 4 cm² optimizing the efficiency of treatment, introduced vibration (Comfort Pulse Technology [CPT]) to further enhance patient comfort, and modified the handpiece to be compatible with all tips (eyelid, face, and body) as to avoid need to interchange. Monopolar radiofrequency energy is now commonly used to accomplish skin tightening of the face (Case Study 1), neck, eyelids (Case Study 1), abdomen, and extremities.

Practitioners should focus on delivering multiple passes at modest fluences, titrated to patient comfort, to maximize outcomes. A transferable, temporary ink-grid, supplied by the company, should be applied to the forehead, as well as spanning from the infraorbital rim to the mid-neck inferiorly and from the preauricular line laterally to the nasolabial and mesolabial folds medially, to guide multiple passes. The aim is a minimum of 3 total passes, targeting squares, circles, and lines on the grid, both horizontally and vertically. Various finessed techniques abound, including: (1) zonal approaches, in which the treatment area is divided into blocks for ideal heat accumulation without over-heating, (2) super-passes, (3) vector lines, and (4) superficial muscular aponeurotic system (SMAS)-targeting; the underlying principles and goals remain unchanged, that of comfortable delivery of the optimal amount of energy to

CASE STUDY 1

A 47-year-old woman presents for a consultation regarding skin laxity on the lower face and jawline. She states she has noticed a gradual increase in sagging and jowls over the past several years and she is finding it difficult to camouflage. She has her 30th high school reunion in 4 months and states she wants improvement by then. She tells you she is not trying to look 18 again, but just wants to look as good as she feels. On examination, the patient has mild-to-moderate jowl formation, with a loss of definition to her jawline. She also has a modest amount of submental laxity, absence of platysmal bands, and minimal submental fat. Her skin tone and thickness are average. This patient would be a candidate for either radiofrequency skin tightening or a surgical face-lift. She may be a better candidate for nonsurgical tightening because of her mild-to-moderate skin laxity, without underlying structural deficits. She also has realistic expectations about results and has several months postprocedure for the skin tightening to take effect before her goal event. Most of the skin-tightening technologies can be used over multiple areas of the body; however, there are a few locations that favor some devices over others. The Thermage device is an excellent choice for skin tightening of the lower face because it has a small 0.25 cm^2 tip, a high eye-safety profile, and lack of significant discomfort during treatment.

the desired tissue to heat ideally for best outcomes and greatest patient satisfaction. Sites over which patients often experience some discomfort include over bony prominences, such as the angle of the mandible, lateral to the lateral commissure of the mouth, and inferior to the mid-anterior neck. Techniques for minimizing pain entail generous use of coupling fluid, increased vibration, avoidance of applicator overlap, and reducing fluence (particularly for treatment of the neck). We typically recommend to avoid treating directly over the thyroid. Focus, with additional passes along the jawline and particular attention to mandibular and submental definition, can enhance posttreatment results and patient satisfaction; the same can be said for the forehead to reduce brow ptosis.

Absolute contraindications to treatment with monopolar radiofrequency include treatment on patients with a pacemaker, defibrillator, ICD, or other implantable electronic device. When treating upper or lower eyelids within the orbital rim with a specialized treatment tip, designed specifically for the periorbital region, sterile plastic eye shields are required to avoid scleral thermal injury.

The clinical results of nonablative radiofrequency skin tightening were first reported by Fitzpatrick et al. for the periorbital area in 2003, with at least some degree of clinical improvement reported in 80% of subjects (Figs. 7.2–7.4). Notably, in the 86 patients studied, 61.5% of eyebrows experienced lifting of eyebrows by at least 0.5 mm. Criticism of the objectivity, due to lack of standardization of photos and lack of randomization, as all patients received treatment, has been noted. In a study by Abraham et al., a statistically-significant increase in mean, vertical eyebrow-height of 1.6–2.4 mm was found at 12 weeks after a single session. Alster and Tanzi treated 50 patients with Thermage, with standardization in camera settings, lighting, and patient positioning. Photos were later evaluated independently by three, blinded reviewers. All agreed that change was modest, but the majority of patients experienced improvement, with 28 out of 30 patients experiencing amelioration of the nasolabial and mesolabial folds, and 17 out of 20 appreciated an improvement of neck laxity. The five nonresponders were noted to be over 62 years of age. In 2006, Dover et al. compared the original single-pass, high-energy technique with the updated low-energy, multiple-pass technique, using immediate tissue tightening as a real-time end point. With the original, high-energy treatment algorithm, 26% of patients saw immediate tightening, 54% observed skin tightening at 6 months, and 45% found the procedure overly painful. With the updated protocol, 87% had immediate tissue tightening, 92% had some degree of tightening at 6 months, only 5% found the procedure overly painful, and 94% stated the procedure matched their expectations (Fig. 7.5). The low-energy, multiple-pass protocol has also been reported to be significantly safer, lowering the incidence of adverse events to less than 0.05%. It should be noted, and patient expectations should be established, that results declare themselves gradually over the course of 6 months. After the initial acute enhancement, which often dissipates after 2 weeks, there is typically a lag; there is a very slow, gentle improvement in the first phase, with an exponential change in the later stages. In 2019, Alam et al. put monopolar radiofrequency to the test, enrolling

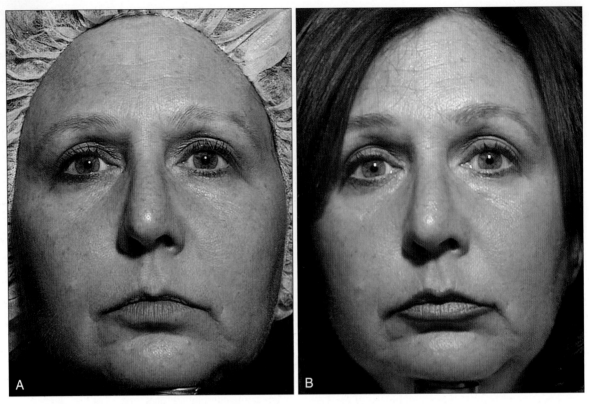

Fig. 7.2 Eyebrow lift following Thermage treatment: (A) baseline and (B) 4 weeks post treatment, with a mean lift of 3.42 mm (right brow) and 3.41 mm (left brow). *(Photographs courtesy Solta.)*

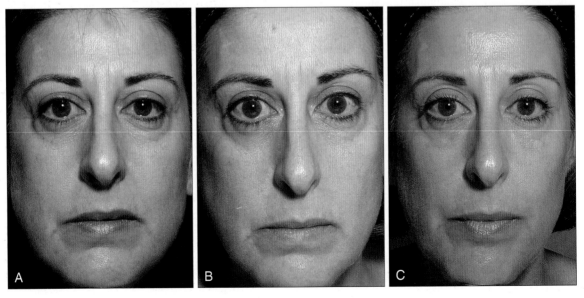

Fig. 7.3 Periorbital rejuvenation following Thermage treatment: (A) baseline, (B) 2 months post-treatment, and (C) 4 months posttreatment. *(Photographs courtesy Solta.)*

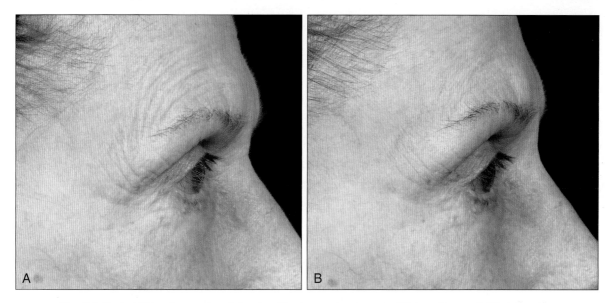

Fig. 7.4 Periorbital rejuvenation following Thermage treatment: (A) baseline and (B) 4 months posttreatment. *(Photographs courtesy Solta Medical Aesthetic Center.)*

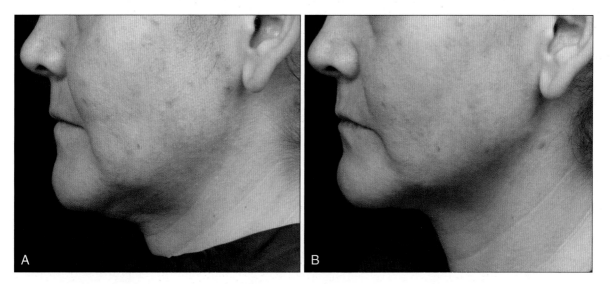

Fig. 7.5 Lower face skin tightening following Thermage treatment: (A) baseline and (B) 3 months posttreatment. *(Photographs courtesy Dr Ivan Rosales.)*

25 female patients with mild- moderate skin laxity of the arms. Micro-tattoos were applied at the treatment sites on the arms, outlining two, 6 × 12 cm rectangles per subject, to provide a fixed, objective landmark for tissue shrinkage assessment. Patients were randomized to two Thermage treatments with multipass or single pass technique. The size of each rectangle was measured with care revealing a statistically-significant skin reduction and shrinkage at 6-week follow up.

The Pelleve (Cynosure, Westford, MA) and Nuera (Lumenis, Israel) devices are both monopolar noninvasive platforms.

Fractional Minimally Invasive Bipolar Radiofrequency

Early radiofrequency devices utilized electrode arrays, which required energy to pass through the epidermis to

---

PEARL 1

Ideal endpoints in Thermage treatments include, but are not limited to, the following: firmer tissue upon palpation; tightening of the brow with elevation of eyebrows and increased eyelid show; smoother, plumper contouring of the cheeks along the zygoma; support of the oral commissure, with gentle upturning of the angle of the mouth; decrease in the appearance of the melomental folds and nasolabial folds; enhanced definition of the mandibular edge; sharpening of sub-mental contouring, with less tissue laxity along the neck; and, an improvement of crepiness in the off-face treatments, such as the abdomen, knees, and arms. These enhancements are evident immediately posttreatment, then often dissipate within 2 weeks, but gradually return over 6 months posttherapy in an exponential manner. Results declare themselves very slowly initially, but the improvements escalate considerably from 4 to 6 months. Recurrent, annual treatments appear to diminish the sagging tendency of the skin.

PEARL 2

Although skin-tightening procedures can cause significant discomfort, they ideally should not do so. For best results, regular, patient-pain feedback should be used as the basis for choosing particular energies in a given treatment area, customized to each individual's comfort. With updated treatment protocols, anesthesia should not be required. The use of nerve blocks and intravenous sedation should not be used, as some degree of pain feedback from the patient is necessary to limit side effects and enhance patient safety and results. Local infiltration anesthesia is also not recommended as it alters the inherent tissue impedance and can increase adverse effects. If a therapeutic plan involves both Thermage and Coolsculpting for the same area, such as submental, arms, or abdominal regions, many clinicians elect to perform Thermage first. The postcryolipolysis alteration in pain perception in the treatment area can lead to erroneously elevated radiofrequency energies and increased risk of to the patient. Prudence pays dividends in this arena, as pain does not lead to gain with this modality; pleasant, comfortable treatments translate to the best outcomes.

---

the dermis. Thermal burns occurred when the epidermis reached 48°C, but the optimal temperature for dermal collagen contraction was established to be 58°C–60°C. Attempts to aggressively cool the skin and the use of multiple treatments of short duration were required, but surface temperatures limited the penetration depth of the RF energy. Microneedling and subcutaneous radiofrequency delivery platforms were developed to circumvent the dermal-epidermal junction and deliver energy directly to the dermis. Bypassing the epidermis also led to increased safety profiles in all skin tones.

The Profound (Candela-Syneron, Wayland, MA) device utilizes a bipolar radiofrequency microneedle electrode array to deliver energy into the reticular dermis, while bypassing the epidermis and papillary dermis. Single-use treatment cartridges are used that contain five independently controlled, 32-gauge, bipolar microneedle pairs. The 250-μm needles are spaced 1.25 mm apart, and each needle pair is independently powered by the generator. The needles are 6-mm long, with the top 3 mm insulated to protect the superficial portion of the skin during treatment, and the bottom 3 mm exposed to allow electrical current flow. The needles are inserted at a 25-degree angle to the epidermal surface plane, so that the tip of the needle is 2 mm from the epidermis. Insertion is affected by spring-loaded injection. Current flows between the two, paired needles, creating a fractionated zone of thermal injury between each of the pairs, situated in the deep dermis, 1–2 mm from the skin surface. Epidermal cooling is achieved via an integrated thermokinetic cooling bar on the applicator. This approach allows for real-time temperature monitoring with sensors in each electrode tip to help to maintain a preselected target temperature, regardless of varying skin conditions: this leads to an improved consistency between patients.

Alexiades-Armenakas et al., compared baseline and 3- to 6-month follow-up photographs of 15 patients who had undergone skin tightening using a microneedle radiofrequency device to those of six patients who had undergone rhytidectomy. The radiofrequency device patients were judged to have a 16% improvement from baseline, while the surgical patients were judged to have a 49% improvement. The authors concluded that the mean laxity improvement from a single microneedle radiofrequency treatment was 37% that of a surgical facelift. In the multicenter clinical trial and multi-arm studies of target dermal temperatures ranging from 52°C to 78°C, it was discovered that the temperature 67°C cohort resulted in maximal neocollagenesis, neoelastogenesis, and hyaluronic acid production and correlated clinically with maximal rhytid and laxity reduction and a 100% response rate. Higher and lower target temperatures demonstrated less efficacy. The findings made possible by needle-delivered radiofrequency support the authors' theory that partially denatured collagen is more effective at triggering a strong wound healing response, and, in fact, sub-coagulative temperatures are more beneficial than coagulative. A clinical example of a subject at baseline and at 6 months, following a single treatment with microneedle radiofrequency (Profound; Syneron Candela, Wayland, MA) is shown in Figs. 7.6–7.8. Relative to other microneedling RF platforms, the Profound is thought to have larger zones of coagulation. Pain is often a limiting factor in treatment.

A number of needle-delivered bipolar radiofrequency devices have emerged, all with unique features:

1. The Infini (Lutronic, Billerica, MA) provides the feature of adjustable needle depths, to 0.5, 1.0, 1.5, 2.0, and 3.5 mm. The device offers a 49-needle tip (10 × 10 mm, 7 × 7 needles) and a 16-needle tip (5 × 5 mm, 4 × 4 needles). The microneedles are made from surgical stainless steel, coated with gold for conductivity and then double-coated with an insulating silicon compound, except for the 300 μm at the tip. The needles have a diameter of 200 μm and a point diameter of 20 μm. The insulation of the needle shaft means that the active area of the microneedle electrodes is restricted to the tip, and there is no electrothermal damage delivered to the epidermis. Clinical trials have demonstrated wrinkle reduction following treatment with this device, with clinician-assessed overall efficacy and patient satisfaction index similar from 80.7% to 88.9% and 81.3% to 85.9%.

2. The Intensif (EndyMed Medical, Caesarea, Israel) uses 25 noninsulated, gold-plated, microneedle electrodes, with a maximum diameter of 300 μm at their base, gradually tapered to a sharp edge. Penetration depth is up to 3.5 mm, with digitally controlled increments of 0.1 mm. Maximal power is 25 W with a maximal pulse duration of 200 milliseconds. When the needles reach the predefined insertion depth, the radiofrequency is emitted selectively, heating the dermis while sparing the epidermis. The difference in the high electrical impedance of the epidermis and the low impedance of the dermis ensures the radiofrequency flows through the dermis. The radiofrequency emission delivered over the whole dermal portion of the needle allows effective coagulation, resulting in minimal or no bleeding combined with deep dermal heating.

3. The Fractora (InMode, Irvine, CA) is the original InMode microneedling with RF handpiece, which uses 24 radiofrequency conducting needles, alternating current, with two long side electrodes. Each needle is 2500 μm long and 200 × 300 μm wide at the base. The coated needles are insulated along 2000 μm, leaving the distal 500 μm uncoated. The handpiece is loaded to the Fractora platform (also applicable to InMode or BodyTite platforms; Invasix Ltd./InMode, Irvine, CA). The device has been reported to result in significant improvement in acne and acne scars. InMode recently modified the Fractora

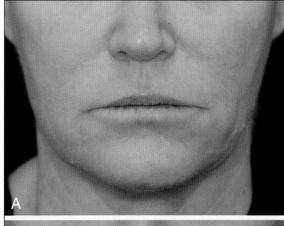
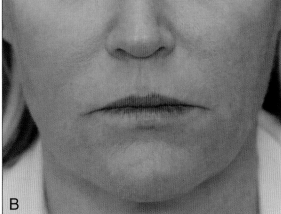

Fig. 7.6 Baseline and after Profound needle-delivered, bipolar radiofrequency.

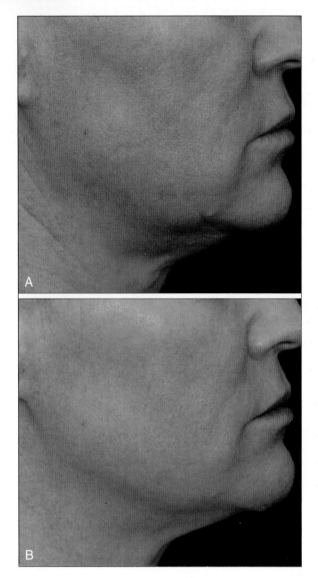

Fig. 7.7 Baseline and after Profound needle-delivered, bipolar radiofrequency.

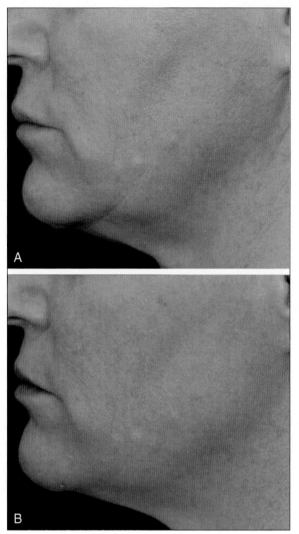

Fig. 7.8 Baselineand after Profound needle-delivered, bipolar radiofrequency.

releasing a new microneedling RF handpiece, called the Morpheus8 (InMode, Irvine, CA); also with 24 coated, insulated needles, it touts multiple programmable pin depths of up to 4 mm, and an additional 1 mm of thermal depth, reaching up to 5 mm. With treatment at multiple depths, this device is intended to allow customizable treatments, not restricted to the face, allowing targeting of fat, as well as deep dermis. Typically, a 2 mm depth of needle penetration

is recommended for bony areas, periorbital skin, forehead, and chin; 3 mm is recommended for soft tissue and neck; and 4 mm is recommended for the body, taking into consideration the thermal zone of treatment reaches an additional 1 mm beyond needle depth. The Morpheus8 device has been studied in combination with subdermal bipolar radiofrequency (FaceTite, InMode, Israel). Prospective evaluation of 247 patients undergoing combination RF therapy for neck laxity and jowling revealed a reduction in average Baker Face Neck Classification from 3.1

(standard deviation +/− 1.4) to 1.4 points (standard deviation +/− 1.1). Ninety-three percent of patients were pleased with the results and would repeat the procedure in the future.

4. The Genius (Lutronic, Billerica, MA) is another bipolar, insulated-needle, microneedling RF device that is unique in precise coagulation zones achieved through real-time impedance monitoring, ensuring consistent energy delivery despite variation in tissue impedance. With the measurement of impedance between needle tips, it is possible to deliver consistent energy throughout the treatment, leading to a predictable zone of coagulation. If impedance rises too quickly, leading to temperatures that could cause desiccation, the power is automatically reduced by the system to a safe level, thus avoiding overheating.

5. The Legend Pro VoluDerm (Lumenis, Yokne'am Illit, Israel) is an additional device that uses delivery of energy by electrodes to thermally ablate the outer surface of skin to reach the dermis, with subsequent delivery of microneedles through the ablative columns, followed by a burst of radiofrequency energy. The formation of fractional ablative columns prior to microneedle insertion minimizes pain relative to other microneedling RF platforms. The electrodes are merely 0.15 mm in diameter. This platform also comes with a Tripollar handpiece for transcutaneous delivery of radiofrequency. Notably, in our practice experience, the Legend Voluderm treatment has been the most well-tolerated by patients with regard to pain, when compared to other platforms.

Not all microneedling with radiofrequency devices are created equally, with variation in depth of penetration, composition and diameter of needles, insulated versus noninsulated needles, and presence or absence of real-time impedance monitoring. Pain is a significant treatment-limiting factor that can lead to early discontinuation, incompletion of treatments, and difficulty reproducing outcomes reported in studies. Even devices such as the Profound with the body tip require tumescent anesthesia for tolerability.

Subdermal Minimally Invasive Radiofrequency

A subdermal, probe-delivered, monopolar radiofrequency device has been developed, Thermi (ThermiAesthetics, Irving, TX), to deliver radiofrequency energy to the subdermal plane. A blunt, 10-cm long, 18-gauge percutaneous treatment probe is inserted, and the distal end administers the radiofrequency. A thermistor is attached to the probe tip, which initiates an automatic feedback loop to maintain subdermal tissue temperatures of 55°C–65°C when treating the dermis, and 70°C when treating fat. The temperature-sensing element detects changes in resistance when exposed to small changes in temperature, with subsequent modulation of RF-current output. Subdermal temperatures of 65°C and 50°C correlate with skin surface temperatures of 41.6°C and 41.1°C, respectively. The Thermistor element has been integrated with a forward looking infrared (FLIR) camera, which continuously monitors epidermal temperatures, with goal temperatures of 42°C–45°C. The ThermiTight system was studied in 35 patients undergoing treatment of submental and jowl skin laxity. Two, blinded reviewers assessed patient photographs at baseline and 30 days after the procedure; grading on a 4-point skin laxity scale revealed 74% of patients demonstrating clinical improvement, with a mean change of -0.78/4.

The BodyTite, FaceTite, and AccuTite (InMode, Irvine, CA) are bipolar radiofrequency devices, utilizing a subcutaneous RF delivery probe to treat septofascial and fasciocutaneous structures of the subdermis, coupled with a superficial electrode that glides along the skin surface, allowing for transepidermal, nonfractionated RF energy delivery to the papillary and reticular dermis. Paul et al. introduced the device in 2009 for RF-assisted liposuction/lipolysis by comparing radiofrequency-assisted liposuction to laser-assisted lipolysis. The BodyTite RF device provided more consistent and uniform RF delivery at sub-necrotic thermal levels with more robust lipolysis, reduced bleeding and bruising, increased tissue contraction, and retraction of the subcutaneous fibrous and dermal matrix in 40 lipoplasty zones of 20 patients treated to a maximal epidermal temperature of 38°C–40°C. Ahn et al. later studied the FaceTite in 42 patients for treatment of skin laxity of the face and neck, targeting maximal skin temperatures of 38°C–40°C, revealing significant tightening and lifting of the brow, lower lid, cheeks, and neck, starting at 3–4 weeks posttreatment and continuing over 6 months.

COMBINED ELECTRICAL AND OPTICAL ENERGY

Another type of skin-tightening device combines radiofrequency energy with optical energy from laser or light sources. The currently-available, combined electrical- and optical-energy devices use bipolar electrodes and include the Galaxy, Aurora, Polaris, and ReFirme systems (Syneron Candela). The hypothetical advantage to these devices is that the two forms of energy may act synergistically to generate heat. Target structures which have been prewarmed with optical energy will, in theory, have greater conductivity, less resistance, and greater selective heating by the radiofrequency current. No grounding pad is required, as the current flows between the electrodes rather than throughout the remainder of the body, as with monopolar systems. One major adverse event noted with these devices is known as tissue arcing, which can result in tissue burns and possible/probable scar formation. Proper technique helps to avoid this issue, as arcing has been associated with the incomplete contact of the handpiece with the skin.

The technology has been used in hair removal, wrinkle reduction, skin tightening, and the treatment of both pigment and vascular disorders (Case Study 2). The premise is that less radiofrequency energy is ultimately needed for proper collagen denaturation and remodeling. The major disadvantage to these devices is that bipolar radiofrequency energy does not penetrate very deeply into the skin. There is also some criticism that bipolar radiofrequency is unable to produce a uniform, volumetric heating response, comparable to monopolar radiofrequency. Furthermore, because the bipolar radiofrequency devices are often combined with other light-based technologies, it is difficult, if not impossible, to accurately assess the role bipolar radiofrequency actually plays in the clinical outcomes of such treatments.

For this type of patient, combined electrical and optical energy may be the best option to treat skin laxity in combination with other signs of photodamage, such as lentigines or telangiectasias. A 2002 study by Bitter evaluating a series of three to five combined intense-pulsed light and radiofrequency energy treatments on photoaged skin revealed a 70% improvement in erythema and telangiectasia, a 78% improvement in lentigines, and a 60% improvement in skin texture, as determined by subject satisfaction levels. Because these devices can also be used for hair removal, caution should be used in treating the lower face and neck in a male patient, so as to not to thin or remove the beard. Prudence should also be used when treating darker skin types, or tanned skin, with devices using an optical component, absorbed by pigment. As a general guideline, optical fluences should be lowered by a minimum of 20% when treating darkly pigmented lesions or dense pigment irregularity, even in light-skinned patients, to avoid side effects such as burns, crusting, or pigmentary alteration.

PEARL 3

Most skin-tightening treatments using radiofrequency, ultrasound, and infrared light are generally safe in all skin types. The exception is technologies that use an optical component absorbed by pigment, such as the intense pulsed light–radiofrequency combination. In these cases, caution should be exercised when treating Fitzpatrick skin types IV–VI, lighter-skin type patients with a tan, darkly pigmented lesions, or areas of dense pigment irregularity.

In 2005, Doshi and Alster conducted one of the first studies using combined diode and radiofrequency

CASE STUDY 2

A 42-year-old woman comes into your office complaining of skin laxity in the upper arm area. She states that she is no longer comfortable wearing sleeveless clothing because she feels like her arms look like what she calls "cottage cheese." She states she has always maintained a relatively normal weight. On examination, she is of a normal weight for her height and build. She has mild-to-moderate skin laxity, predominantly in the posterior portion of her upper arm, and dimpling in the texture of both the anterior and posterior surface of the arms. In this case, the patient has two main options for improvement, which include upper arm liposuction and nonsurgical skin tightening. She may be a better candidate for the latter because the textural abnormality in her upper arms extends around the full circumference. Liposuction would predominantly improve the skin in the "bat wing" area on the posterior portion of the arm. She would not be a candidate for surgical brachioplasty, due to her young age, milder degree of laxity, and desire to wear sleeveless clothing. In this case the hybrid Accent device might be a good choice for tissue tightening, with the added benefit of possible volume reduction.

technology, with a series of three treatments in 20 female subjects (radiofrequency: 50–85 J/cm², optical energy: 32–40 J/cm²). Energy was increased with each session, based on the patient's pain tolerance and a clinical response of immediate erythema and edema. Modest improvement was seen in all patients at 3 months; however, improvement was found to be less so at 6 months. In 2005, Sadick et al. conducted a two-center study using combination intense-pulsed light and radiofrequency (radiofrequency: up to 20 J/cm², optical energy: 30–45 J/cm²) over five treatments for facial rhytides and skin laxity. Modest improvements were reported. Side effects were minimal, but some instances of crusting occurred. In 2007, Yu et al. used combination radiofrequency and infrared energy to study skin tightening in a three-treatment series on 19 female Asian patients (radiofrequency: 70–120 J/cm², optical energy: 10 J/cm²). Objective assessment showed mild-to-moderate improvement in 26%–47% of the areas treated (see Figs. 7.7 and 7.8).

VACUUM-ASSISTED BIPOLAR RADIOFREQUENCY

Bipolar radiofrequency has been combined with an accompanying vacuum apparatus, in an attempt to take advantage of several of the benefits of vacuum technology. The first device to do this was the Aluma (Lumenis, Santa Clara, CA), using what has been termed FACES (functional aspiration controlled electrothermal stimulation) technology. The vacuum apparatus suctions a fold of skin in alignment between two electrodes. Nontarget structures, such as muscle, fascia, and bone are avoided. The theory is that this may help to overcome the depth limitations inherent in bipolar radiofrequency technology by bringing the target tissue closer to the electrodes. Less overall energy may also be required for effective treatment. It has also been hypothesized that increased blood flow and mechanical stress on fibroblasts from the vacuum suction may lead to increased collagen formation. Vacuum technology has the added benefit of helping to reduce procedure discomfort.

In a pilot study of 46 adults, undergoing eight facial treatments with vacuum-assisted bipolar radiofrequency, Gold found significant improvement in skin texture. The mean elastosis score of study participants went from 4.5 pretreatment to 2.5 by 6 months posttreatment, indicating a shift from moderate to mild elastosis. The authors noted a short-term tightening effect, due to collagen

contraction, followed by a gradual, long-term improvement, due to the wound-healing response and neocollagenesis. Although subjects were generally pleased with the treatment outcome, their satisfaction levels declined somewhat during the follow-up period. This can be a common finding in radiofrequency skin treatments owing to delayed neocollagenesis and long-term wound-healing response. Subjects may have difficulty accurately remembering the true condition of their skin before treatment, particularly when 6 or more months have passed.

PEARL 4

It is essential to take standardized photographs before skin-tightening procedures. Care should be taken to use identical positioning and lighting conditions in all photography sessions as subtle differences can distort appearance and alter perceived outcomes. Pretreatment and posttreatment photographs may need to be compared because changes with skin-tightening procedures may be subtle to the patient, especially after several months have passed.

HYBRID MONOPOLAR AND BIPOLAR RADIOFREQUENCY

The first system to combine monopolar and bipolar radiofrequency in one device was the Accent (Alma Lasers, Buffalo Grove, IL). The reason for using both types of radiofrequency was to deliver current to different depths within the skin. The bipolar electrode handpiece allows for more superficial, localized (nonvolumetric) heating based on tissue resistance to the radiofrequency conductive current. The monopolar electrode handpiece targets deeper, volumetric heating via the rotational movement of water molecules in the alternating current of the electromagnetic field. The monopolar handpiece delivers a higher amount of energy because it, theoretically, is heating a greater tissue volume than the bipolar handpiece. The monopolar handpiece is typically used to treat the forehead, cheeks, jawline, and neck. The bipolar handpiece is used to treat the glabella, lateral periorbital area (Fig. 7.9), upper lip, and chin (Fig. 7.10). Despite the use of monopolar radiofrequency, this particular system uses a closed system in which no grounding plate is required (Case Study 3).

In 2007 Friedman treated 16 patients with a hybrid monopolar and bipolar radiofrequency device; 56% of

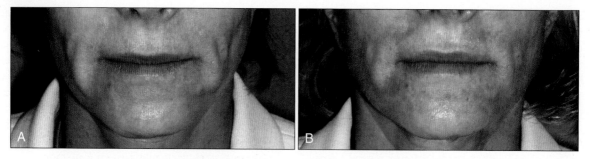

Fig. 7.9 Lower face skin tightening: (A) before and (B) immediately following a single treatment with the Galaxy device.

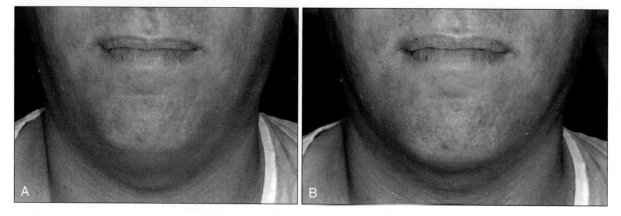

Fig. 7.10 Skin tightening of the neck and jawline region: (A) before and (B) immediately following a single treatment with the Accent treatment. *(Photographs courtesy Dr Alexiades.)*

participants had at least some degree of improvement in the appearance of rhytides and skin laxity. Twelve patients had cheek treatments, with five achieving 51%–75% improvement and two achieving greater than 75% improvement. Nine had jowl treatments, with four achieving 51%–75% improvement and one achieving greater than 75% improvement. Younger patients (25–45 years of age) were found to have a higher satisfaction rate than older patients.

PEARL 5

Studies suggest that younger patients may respond better than older patients. Potentially, this is because heat-labile collagen bonds are progressively replaced by irreducible multivalent crosslinks as the tissue ages, such that the skin of older individuals is less amenable to heat-induced tissue tightening. Skin quality is more important than the absolute age of the patient. Older patients with relatively good skin quality can respond just as well as their younger counterparts.

The Pelleve device (Cynosure Inc., Westford, MA) has modified a dual monopolar and bipolar radiofrequency-based surgical unit, normally used for tissue cutting and coagulation to make it suitable for skin-tightening procedures. The system works with the use of reusable probes that are plugged into the system and applied over the skin in a circular or linear pattern to heat the subdermal tissue. A coupling gel is applied to ensure proper coupling between the electrode and the patient, and to help protect the epidermis. As with other skin-tightening devices, the gentle heating induces collagen denaturation, contraction, and subsequent synthesis. Repeat treatments have been shown to improve the appearance of wrinkles and skin laxity, but results are somewhat limited due to the discrete amount of energy applied. Early protocols recommended 8-weekly treatments for best results, but the treatment paradigm has since been revised to two to four treatments, spaced 1 month apart, with some patients requiring an additional treatment.

CASE STUDY 3

A 78-year-old woman presents for a consultation regarding general photoaging. She has avoided sun exposure her whole life and is a devoted wearer of sunscreen. She tells you she has been going to an esthetician for the past 15 years for light glycolic peels every few months. She has also used a prescription tretinoin cream, given to her by her general dermatologist, for the past 25 years. She is otherwise healthy and would like to improve her appearance, but she would like to get your advice on what she needs. She has never had surgery before and tells you that she would like to avoid having a facelift, if possible. On examination she has remarkably-preserved skin quality, with very few deep lines and no major pigmentary issues, owing to her diligent sun protection and sun avoidance, long-term use of topical rejuvenation therapies. She does have some loss of definition along the jawline, with mild-to-moderate jowling, deepening of the nasolabial folds, descent of the eyebrow, and volume-related changes in the midface region. She also has prominent platysmal banding visible in the neck region. This patient would be an ideal candidate for almost any of the noninvasive skin-tightening approaches, in combination with other therapies, such as neurotoxins and fillers, to augment her results. Although studies have shown that younger patients tend to have better results than older patients after tissue-tightening procedures, this patient has extremely good skin quality and can be expected to have at least some degree of improvement. Because the skin-tightening procedure will not address her underlying changes in facial volume and musculature, performing adjunctive therapies, such as botulinum toxin to the superolateral orbicularis oculi and platysma muscles, would help her to lift the brow, decrease banding on the neck, and achieve a more defined jawline. Filler to her mid-face region, nasolabial folds, prejowl region, and jawline would also be of use to restore underlying structure, increase the lifting effect, and give a more youthful shape to the face. A 2006 study by Shumaker et al. showed monopolar radiofrequency skin tightening to be safe when performed over multiple soft tissue fillers, and indicated it may even have some synergistic effects in terms of long-term collagen growth. The patient has proven she is not averse to maintenance therapies and she will achieve a better overall result with global rejuvenation.

INFRARED LIGHT DEVICES

Broadband, infrared light, in the range of 800–1800 nm, depending on the device, has been used for nonablative tissue-tightening. The infrared rays are selectively filtered to achieve gradual heating of the dermis, with pre-, parallel-, and postcooling, to ensure epidermal protection. The first such light-based system on the market was the Titan (Cutera, Brisbane, CA). It uses light energy in the range of 1100–1800 nm, to target water for absorption, causing collagen-denaturation and, ultimately, collagen-remodeling and tissue-tightening. The Icon (Cynosure) delivers energy through the handpiece of the device at a wavelength range of 850–1350 nm, which also targets water as the principal focus to stimulate neocollagenesis. Multiple treatments are required for optimal results. The SkinTyte device (Sciton, Palo Alto, CA) uses light at a wavelength range of 800–1400 nm.

In 2006, Ruiz-Esparza performed one to three treatments on 25 patients, using broadband infrared light from 1100 to 1800 nm. Most patients showed improvement, ranging from minimal to excellent, with immediate skin tightening visible in 22 of the 25 patients. Three patients showed no improvement. The best results were achieved when using a combination of lower fluences and a high number of pulses. Patients treated at $30 \, J/cm^2$ expressed experiencing no pain during the procedure and had a high degree of satisfaction, immediately postprocedure. The same year, Zelickson et al. looked at ultra-structural changes in cadaver and human skin, post treatment. Collagen-fibril alteration was found to be highest with greater fluences and depths of 1–2 mm. Marginal results were observed at shallower depths and lower fluences, which were possibly due to the effect of contact cooling. Comparison of the two studies emphasizes that clinical skin tightening does not always correlate with immediate positive histologic findings. This supports the fact that full clinical effect usually takes many weeks to months to be demonstrated, due to the secondary wound healing response.

In 2006, a multi-center study reported longer-term, 12- to 18-month results using the 1100- to 1800-nm infrared device at $34–36 \, J/cm^2$. Improvements were seen both immediately posttreatment, and delayed up to 6 months. Clinical outcomes ranged from mild-to-moderate in most patients. The authors concluded that using a lower fluence range of $30–40 \, J/cm^2$, two to three treatments, one to two passes, and extra passes on areas that need immediate contraction or along vector lines, yielded best results.

In 2009, Alexiades-Armenakas demonstrated that mobile delivery of broadband infrared light (1100–1800 nm, Titan; Cutera) allowed for delivery of 30% higher fluences of 44–46 J/cm². Improvement in skin laxity was demonstrated following 2 monthly treatments consisting of 300–450 pulses per treatment. Skin surface temperatures of 41°C–42°C were attained rapidly and maintained throughout the treatment with the mobile technique.

PEARL 6

When treating the face, one approach is to address as distinct regions. Although the entire face can be treated in one session, it is also possible to treat segmental areas alone, such as the forehead, the eyelids, or the cheek/jawline region. Treatment, however, of broader surface areas, and treatment of areas adjacent to the described area of laxity, may improve results.

Complications were limited to minor erythema, but a few blisters were observed in areas that were over-treated. In 2007, Goldberg et al. noted positive results in 11 of 12 patients receiving two treatments with the same device (30–36 J/cm²). The best results were observed in patients who had loose, draping skin, with less significant results in sagging skin, which was more closely associated with the subcutaneous tissue loss. No improvement was noted in the jowl region.

PEARL 7

Nonsurgical skin tightening is best-suited to patients with mild-to-moderate skin laxity, without significant underlying structural ptosis. Patients with underlying structural laxity, including that of the facial musculature or superficial muscular aponeurotic system (SMAS), and patients with an excessive amount of skin laxity are likely to have limited-to-no improvement and should be counseled on other methods of rejuvenation, including surgery.

Other laser wavelengths that have been used for tissue tightening include the 1064- and 1320-nm. The chromophores for the 1064-nm wavelength, in decreasing order, are melanin and hemoglobin, and there is some absorption by water, and the primary target for the 1320-nm wavelength is water. A 2005 study by Taylor and

Prokopenko compared a single treatment using a monopolar radiofrequency system (73.5 J/cm²) with a single treatment using the 1064-nm Nd:YAG laser at 50 J/cm². The 1064-nm laser side was deemed to have better overall results in terms of improvement in wrinkles and skin laxity, although only modest improvements were noted with both modalities. Another study, in 2007 by Key compared a single facial treatment with a monopolar radiofrequency system (40 J/cm²) to the 1064-nm Nd:YAG laser (73–79 J/cm²). The 1064-nm laser resulted in greater improvement on the lower face, whereas improvement on the upper face was equivalent with both modalities. In 2001, Trelles et al. treated 10 patients with a series of eight treatments using a 1320-nm laser system (30–35 J/cm²). Clinical improvement was subtle, with only two patients reporting satisfaction with the procedure. The authors suggested that combining laser treatment with parallel epidermal treatment may yield better results and achieve higher patient satisfaction.

PEARL 8

Combination therapy is a leading theme in cosmetic dermatology. Patients achieve a better overall result when procedures, such as nonsurgical skin tightening, are combined with other therapies, such as botulinum toxin, fillers, and other modalities. For example, patients desiring a brow-lift and a more-defined jawline may achieve benefit from the use of botulinum toxin to the superolateral orbicularis oculi and platysma muscles in addition to skin tightening. Fillers can be used to achieve additional lift in the mid-face, brow/temples, prejowl region, and jawline, as well as to contour and volumize to enhance patient satisfaction.

ULTRASOUND DEVICES (VIDEO 7.2)

High-intensity focused ultrasound (HIFU) has become a foundation in the skin-tightening technology realm. When an intense ultrasound field vibrates tissue, friction is created between molecules, causing them to absorb mechanical energy, leading to secondary generation of heat. Thus, the primary mechanism responsible for tissue necrosis with HIFU treatment is the heating of tissue due to the absorption of acoustic energy. This, ideally, leads to immediate tissue contraction and delayed collagen remodeling, with the coagulative change limited to the focal region of the ultrasound field. In reality, the spectrum of cellular changes depends on the rise in temperature and the exposure duration, and can range from total necrosis to subtler, ultrastructural cell damage with modulation of cellular cytokine expression.

HIFU for skin-tightening applications uses short, millisecond pulses with a frequency in the megahertz domain, rather than kilohertz, as is used in traditional HIFU, to avoid cavitational processes. HIFU for skin applications also uses significantly lower energies than traditional HIFU, 0.5–10 J versus 100 J, which allows thermal tissue changes without gross necrosis. The main advantage to HIFU is the potential for greater depth of skin changes than other technologies, with the added benefit of precisely-controlled, focal tissue injury. Ultrasound energy is able to target deeper structures in a select, focused fashion without secondary scatter and absorption in the dermis and epidermis. Early research on human cadaveric tissue showed HIFU energy was able to target the facial SMAS to produce discrete zones of thermal injury while sparing nontargeted, adjacent structures.

The first HIFU device on the market was the Ulthera system (Merz Aesthetics, Raleigh, NC). The system incorporates ultrasound-imaging capability for visualizing the skin and deep tissue in combination with a therapeutic-ultrasound module; the latter creates small,

approximately 1 mm^3, wedge-shaped zones of thermal coagulation at depths of up to 5 mm within the mid-to-deep reticular dermis and subdermis. The thermally-induced zones result from selective absorption of ultrasound energy in the area of the geometric focus of the beam. The depth and volume of the thermal lesions are determined by the preset focus depth and frequency of the probe, in conjunction with the intrinsic characteristics of the tissue being treated. The source energy is an adjustable parameter. Higher-frequency probes are associated with a more superficial tissue effect, whereas lower-frequency probes are associated with a deeper tissue effect. Typically, higher-frequency probes are used to treat areas of thinner skin, such as that of the neck, whereas the lower-frequency probes are used to treat areas of thicker skin, such as the cheeks.

Current protocols aim for a geometric, focal depth of therapy in the superficial-to-deep dermis. One of the first clinical trials by Alam et al. in 2010 assessed the safety and efficacy of HIFU on skin tightening. Significant improvement was seen in brow-elevation in more than 83% of treated patients, with an average increase in brow elevation of 1.7–1.9 mm (Fig. 7.11). Results developed over the 90-day period following treatment and were still noticeable at the 10-month follow-up. The authors found

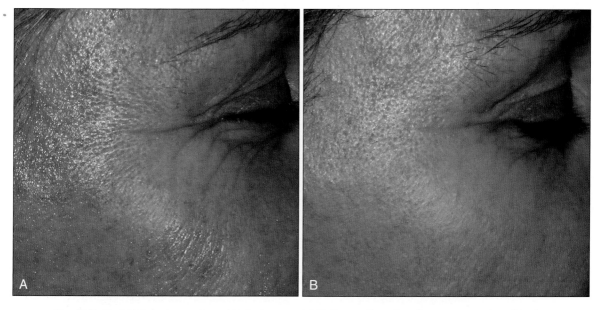

Fig. 7.11 Periorbital rejuvenation: (A) before and (B) 3 months after four treatments with the Accent. *(Photographs courtesy Dr Alexiades.)*

lower face tightening more difficult to assess due to a lack of fixed anatomic landmarks. In 2011, Suh et al. treated 22 Asian patients with facial-skin laxity with HIFU; 77% of patients reported much improvement in the nasolabial folds, and 73% reported much improvement in the jawline. Histologic evaluation of skin samples showed greater dermal collagen, with thickening of the dermis and straightening of elastic fibers in the reticular dermis after treatment (Figs. 7.12–7.15). In 2019, Kapoor et al. treated 50 Indian patients for mid-and lower-face sagging with 3.00 mm probes, targeting the deep dermis and 4.5 mm probes, targeting the superficial dermis. At 6

months, improvement was seen in 93% of patients identified by blinded reviewers, and 85% of patients found the results satisfactory. Results were maintained at the 1 year mark. Currently, limitations of Ultherapy include significant, occasionally unbearable, discomfort for patients during treatment, and lengthy treatment times. Pronox, Toradol, and Demerol have been utilized by practitioners for pain control during HIFU treatments.

The Sofwave device, released in 2019 (Sofwave, Tustin, CA) introduced new Synchronous Ultrasound Parallel Beam Technology (SUPERB) delivering a parallel array of volumetric, cylindrical, thermal zones, separated by undamaged tissue, creating a fractional effect, referred to as Volumetric Directional Thermal Impact (VDTI). The fractional-ultrasound effect leads to a controlled, directional, thermal injury, increasing the temperature of the mid-dermis to 60°C–70°C at a consistent depth of 1.5 mm, avoiding injury to underlying nerves and facial fat. There are seven ultrasound tranducers, along with direct contact-cooling and real-time, epidermal-temperature monitoring in the handpiece to reduce treatment time, while protecting the epidermis from thermal injury. Treatment, typically, only takes about 30–40 minutes, significantly shorter in duration than Ultherapy.

TIPS FOR MAXIMIZING PATIENT SATISFACTION

Patient selection is of utmost importance in ultimate satisfaction with nonsurgical skin-tightening technologies.

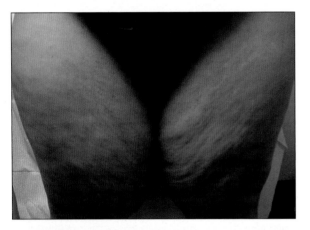

Fig. 7.12 Cellulite treatment on right leg following five treatments with the Accent; left leg serves as an untreated control. *(Photograph courtesy Dr Alexiades.)*

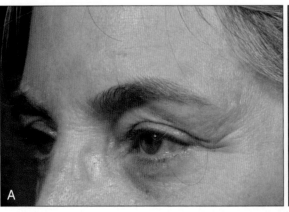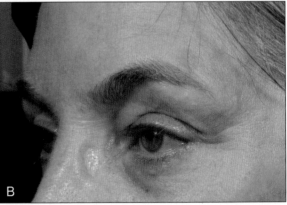

Fig. 7.13 Periorbital rejuvenation and brow lift following Ultherapy treatment: (A) baseline and (B) post single-depth treatment using the 3.0-mm transducer or 4.5-mm transducer depth, based on the periorbital region. *(Photographs courtesy Dr Jeffrey Dover.)*

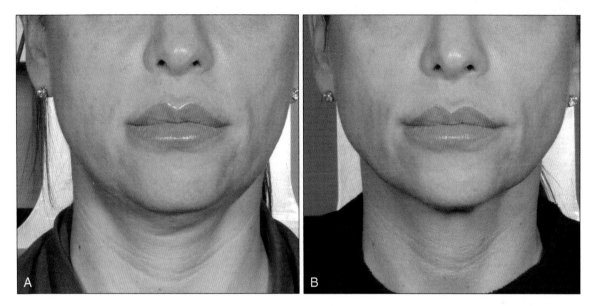

Fig. 7.14 Lower face skin tightening following Ultherapy treatment: (A) baseline and (B) post dual-depth treatment at 3.0- and 4.5-mm depths. *(Photographs courtesy Ulthera Inc.)*

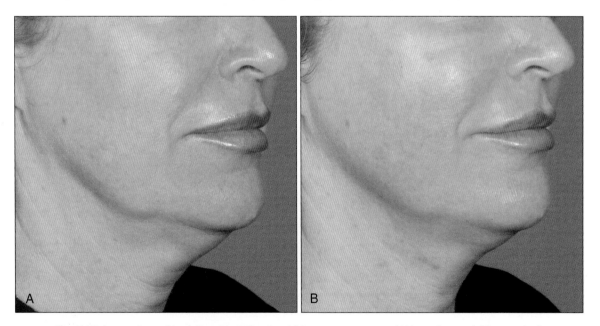

Fig. 7.15 Lower face skin tightening following Ultherapy treatment: (A) baseline and (B) post dual-depth treatment at 3.0- and 4.5-mm depths. *(Photographs courtesy Ulthera Inc.)*

Patients must be counseled that maximum results are slow and gradual, and occur over a period of 3–6 months. In terms of expectations, these technologies should not be thought of as an equivalent to, or a replacement for surgical lifting, but as an alternative option for modest improvement and/or maintenance in a subset of patients. Despite a number of clinical studies reporting significant improvement in the appearance of lax skin, most patients show only mild-to-moderate improvement. It appears that patients who are younger at the first sign of skin descent,

CASE STUDY 4

A 66-year-old woman comes to your office to discuss options regarding skin laxity on her face. She states she has always loved the sun and shares tales of her days lying out on her roof with a foil blanket, covered in baby oil and iodine. She states she does not purposely tan anymore, but her husband loves to play golf and go boating. She normally accompanies him, but she has not been able to since she was diagnosed with an irregular heart rhythm last year when her cardiologist implanted a pacemaker. During the consultation, she pulls her facial skin back tautly with her hands and tells you her wrinkles do not bother her, but she would be happy if she could get rid of her sagging skin. On examination, the patient has a thin body habitus with severe solar elastosis and significant skin laxity.

This patient is not a good candidate for nonsurgical skin tightening for several reasons. The first issue is her pacemaker device, as radiofrequency treatments are contraindicated in patients with pacemakers, internal defibrillators, or metal implants in the face. Although she could undergo nonsurgical skin tightening with ultrasound, or one of the broadband infrared light devices, she has very poor skin quality and a considerable degree of laxity. These issues, combined with her desire for facelift-like results, would most likely lead to disappointment after the procedure. Further discussions would most probably help to tease out an approach suitable for both patient and clinician, a perfect opportunity to practice the true art of cosmetic dermatology.

BOX 7.6 Relative Predictors of Success in Nonablative Skin-Tightening Procedures

- Younger patients, with a lesser degree of skin laxity
- Skin laxity, without significant muscular or osteocutaneous attachments
- Realistic expectations, and willingness to accept a lesser degree of skin tightening in exchange for little to no recovery time and minimal risk

---

with a lesser degree of skin laxity, may yield the most promising clinical outcomes; skin laxity, without significant muscular or osteocutaneous attachments also appears to yield better results (Case Study 4). Very old adults, with severe sagging and wrinkles, are generally sub-optimal candidates for the degree of improvement expected with noninvasive tightening devices. Interestingly, when these elderly patients, who are often not remotely surgical candidates, do choose to proceed with noninvasive skin-tightening procedures, they are often content with the mild improvements. Many patients report that when skin-tightening procedures are performed at regular 1 to 2-year intervals, the progression of sagging and laxity appears to slow significantly over time.

Patients should be told that nonablative skin tightening is not a substitute for a facelift and that results may be modest in comparison (Box 7.6). A small number of patients perceive no improvement at all. Patients should also be counseled that nonablative skin tightening alone is not effective for the textural aspects of photo-aging, including deep wrinkles and pigmentary alterations. Long-term studies to examine the longevity of skin tightening have not been performed, but it appears patients can expect at least a period of a year or more before repeat treatments are required. More research also needs to be done, comparing the devices themselves to determine scientifically the distinct advantages of one over another.

CONCLUSION

The quest for nonsurgical skin tightening has led to a burgeoning number of devices on the market. Although dermal remodeling may occur with radiofrequency-, optical-, and ultrasound-based devices, patients and physicians should not expect results to be similar to those seen after surgical interventions, or possibly even ablative treatments. The techniques appear best-suited for younger patients, with mild-to-moderate skin laxity, without a significant degree of underlying structural ptosis. Physicians must appreciate the indications, complications, benefits, and limitations of each device. The key to success remains rooted in patient selection and management of expectations. It is still uncertain as to how many treatments are ideal for the majority of these medical devices, and how long the effects will be maintained. Future research and clinical trials will continue to refine techniques and delivery systems for optimal results.

Check online videos (Video 7.1 and 7.2).

FURTHER READING

Abraham MT, Chiang SK, Keller GS, Rawnsley JD, Blackwell KE, Elashoff DA. Clinical evaluation of non-ablative radiofrequency facial rejuvenation. *J Cosmet Laser Ther*. 2004; 6(3):136–144.

Ahn DH, Mulholland RS, Duncan Diane, Paul Malcolm. Non-excisional face and neck tightening using a novel subdermal radiofrequency thermo-coaugulative device. *J Cosmet Dermatol Sci Appl*. 2011;1(4):141–146.

Alam M, Pongprutthipan M, Nanda S, et al. Quantitative evaluation of skin shrinkage associated with non-invasive skin tightening: a simple method for reproducible linear measurement using microtattoos. *Lasers Med Sci*. 2019; 34(4):703–709.

Alam M, White LE, Martin N, Witherspoon J, Yoo S, West DP. Ultrasound tightening of facial and neck skin: a rater-blinded prospective cohort study. *J Am Acad Dermatol*. 2010;62(2):262–269.

Alexiades M, Berube D. Randomized, blinded, 3-arm clinical trial assessing optimal temperature and duration for treatment with minimally invasive fractional radiofrequency. *Dermatol Surg*. 2015;41(5):623–632.

Alexiades-Armenakas M, Newman J, Willey A, et al. Prospective multicenter clinical trial of a minimally invasive temperature-controlled bipolar fractional radiofrequency system for rhytid and laxity treatment. *Dermatol Surg*. 2013;39(2):263–273.

Alexiades-Armenakas M, Rosenberg D, Renton B, Dover J, Arndt K. Blinded, randomized, quantitative grading comparison of minimally invasive, fractional radiofrequency and surgical face-lift to treat skin laxity. *Arch Dermatol*. 2010;146(4):396–405.

Alexiades-Armenakas M. Assessment of the mobile delivery of infrared light (1100-1800 nm) for the treatment of facial and neck skin laxity. *J Drugs Dermatol*. 2009;8(3):221–226.

Alster TS, Tanzi E. Improvement of neck and cheek laxity with a nonablative radiofrequency device: a lifting experience. *Dermatol Surg*. 2004;30(4 Pt 1):503–507, discussion 507.

Atiyeh BS, Dibo SA. Nonsurgical nonablative treatment of aging skin: radiofrequency technologies between aggressive marketing and evidence-based efficacy. *Aesthetic Plast Surg*. 2009;33(3):283–294.

Bitter P Jr, Mulholland RS. Report of a new technique for enhanced non-invasive skin rejuvenation using a dual mode pulsed light and radio-frequency energy source: selective radio-thermolysis. *J Cosmet Dermatol*. 2002; 1(3):142–143.

Dayan E, Chia C, Burns AJ, Theodorou S. Adjustable depth fractional radiofrequency combined with bipolar radiofrequency: a minimally invasive combination treatment for skin laxity. *Aesthet Surg J*. 2019;39(3):S112–S119.

Doshi SN, Alster TS. Combination radiofrequency and diode laser for treatment of facial rhytides and skin laxity. *J Cosmet Laser Ther*. 2005;7(1):11–15.

Dover JS, Zelickson B. Physician Multispecialty Consensus P. Results of a survey of 5700 patient monopolar radiofrequency facial skin tightening treatments: assessment of a low-energy multiple-pass technique leading to a clinical end point algorithm. *Dermatol Surg*. 2007;33(8):900–907.

Fitzpatrick R, Geronemus R, Goldberg D, Kaminer M, Kilmer S, Ruiz-Esparza J. Multicenter study of noninvasive radiofrequency for periorbital tissue tightening. *Lasers Surg Med*. 2003;33(4):232–242.

Friedman DJ, Gilead LT. The use of hybrid radiofrequency device for the treatment of rhytides and lax skin. *Dermatol Surg*. 2007;33(5):543–551.

Gold MH, Goldman MP, Rao J, Carcamo AS, Ehrlich M. Treatment of wrinkles and elastosis using vacuum-assisted bipolar radiofrequency heating of the dermis. *Dermatol Surg*. 2007;33(3):300–309.

Goldberg DJ, Hussain M, Fazeli A, Berlin AL. Treatment of skin laxity of the lower face and neck in older individuals with a broad-spectrum infrared light device. *J Cosmet Laser Ther*. 2007;9(1):35–40.

Hellman J. Retrospective study of the use of a fractional radiofrequency ablative device in the treatment of acne vulgaris and related acne scars. *J Cosmet Dermatol Sci Appl*. 2015;5:311–316.

Key DJ. Comprehensive thermoregulation for the purpose of skin tightening using a novel radiofrequency treatment device: A preliminary report. *J Drugs Dermatol*. 2014;13(2):185–189.

Key DJ. Integration of thermal imaging with subsurface radiofrequency thermistor heating for the purpose of skin tightening and contour improvement: a retrospective review of clinical efficacy. *J Drugs Dermatol*. 2014;13(12):1485–1489.

Key DJ. Single-treatment skin tightening by radiofrequency and long-pulsed, 1064-nm nd: Yag laser compared. *Lasers Surg Med*. 2007;39(2):169–175.

Kist D, Burns AJ, Sanner R, Counters J, Zelickson B. Ultrastructural evaluation of multiple pass low energy versus single pass high energy radio-frequency treatment. *Lasers Surg Med*. 2006;38(2):150–154.

Kwon HH, Lee WY, Choi SC, Jung JY, Bae Y, Park GH. Combined treatment for skin laxity of the aging face with monopolar radiofrequency and intense focused ultrasound in korean subjects. *J Cosmet Laser Ther*. 2018;20(7-8):449–453.

Laubach HJ, Makin IR, Barthe PG, Slayton MH, Manstein D. Intense focused ultrasound: evaluation of a new treatment modality for precise microcoagulation within the skin. *Dermatol Surg.* 2008;34(5):727–734.

Locketz GD, Bloom JD. Percutaneous radiofrequency technologies for the lower face and neck. *Facial Plast Surg Clin North Am.* 2019;27(3):305–320.

Mayoral FA. Skin tightening with a combined unipolar and bipolar radiofrequency device. *J Drugs Dermatol.* 2007;6(2):212–215.

Narins RS, Tope WD, Pope K, Ross EV. Overtreatment effects associated with a radiofrequency tissue-tightening device: rare, preventable, and correctable with subcision and autologous fat transfer. *Dermatol Surg.* 2006;32(1):115–124.

Paul M, Mulholland RS. A new approach for adipose tissue treatment and body contouring using radiofrequency-assisted liposuction. *Aesthetic Plast Surg.* 2009;33(5):687–694.

Ruiz-Esparza J. Nonablative radiofrequency for facial and neck rejuvenation. A faster, safer, and less painful procedure based on concentrating the heat in key areas: the thermalift concept. *J Cosmet Dermatol.* 2006;5(1):68–75.

Ruiz-Esparza J, Gomez JB. The medical face lift: a noninvasive, nonsurgical approach to tissue tightening in facial skin using nonablative radiofrequency. *Dermatol Surg.* 2003;29(4):325–332, discussion 332.

Sadick NS, Alexiades-Armenakas M, Bitter P Jr, Hruza G, Mulholland RS. Enhanced full-face skin rejuvenation using synchronous intense pulsed optical and conducted bipolar radiofrequency energy (ELOS): introducing selective radiophotothermolysis. *J Drugs Dermatol.* 2005;4(2):181–186.

Sadick NS, Shaoul J. Hair removal using a combination of conducted radiofrequency and optical energies—an 18-month follow-up. *J Cosmet Laser Ther.* 2004;6(1):21–26.

Shome D, Vadera S, Ram MS, Khare S, Kapoor R. Use of micro-focused ultrasound for skin tightening of mid and lower face. *Plast Reconstr Surg Glob Open.* 2019;7(12):e2498.

Shumaker PR, England LJ, Dover JS, et al. Effect of monopolar radiofrequency treatment over soft-tissue fillers in an animal model: part 2. *Lasers Surg Med.* 2006;38(3):211–217.

Suh DH, Shin MK, Lee SJ, et al. Intense focused ultrasound tightening in asian skin: clinical and pathologic results. *Dermatol Surg.* 2011;37(11):1595–1602.

Taub AF, Battle EF Jr, Nikolaidis G. Multicenter clinical perspectives on a broadband infrared light device for skin tightening. *J Drugs Dermatol.* 2006;5(8):771–778.

Taylor MB, Prokopenko I. Split-face comparison of radiofrequency versus long-pulse Nd-YAG treatment of facial laxity. *J Cosmet Laser Ther.* 2006;8(1):17–22.

Trelles MA, Allones I, Luna R. Facial rejuvenation with a nonablative 1320 nm Nd:YAG laser: a preliminary clinical and histologic evaluation. *Dermatol Surg.* 2001;27(2):111–116.

Yu CS, Yeung CK, Shek SY, Tse RK, Kono T, Chan HH. Combined infrared light and bipolar radiofrequency for skin tightening in asians. *Lasers Surg Med.* 2007;39(6):471–475.

Zelickson B, Ross V, Kist D, Counters J, Davenport S, Spooner G. Ultrastructural effects of an infrared handpiece on forehead and abdominal skin. *Dermatol Surg.* 2006;32(7):897–901.

8

Photodynamic Therapy

Macrene Alexiades

SUMMARY AND KEY FEATURES

- Identify the indications and contraindications PDT.
- Learn the approved PDT protocols for each cutaneous condition.
- Recognize pre and postoperative preparations, side effects and complications.
- Become familiar with off-label PDT applications.

INTRODUCTION

Photodynamic therapy (PDT) involves the application of a photosensitizer, a light-absorbing compound, which accumulates in a subset of cells or tissues, followed by illumination with specified wavelengths, which triggers a reaction that destroys the target. The German professor Hermann von Tappeiner coined the term "photodynamic reaction" circa 1900 to describe an observation made by his student Oscar Raab that acridine orange accumulated in *Paramecia* and resulted in their death upon illumination. The PDT reaction requires photosensitizer, a light source, and oxygen with reactive oxygen species generated that lead to apoptosis and necrosis.

PDT has been conducted using a variety of photosensitizers and light sources. Systemic photosensitizers, such as hematoporphyrin, followed by irradiation with broadband red and blue light were used to treat a variety of cutaneous neoplasms. In 1995, the first US Food and Drug Administration (FDA) approval for PDT was with porfirin sodium for treatment of esophageal carcinoma. Topical 5-aminolevulinic acid (ALA) was introduced in the 1980s for cutaneous applications and eliminated the complication of generalized cutaneous photosensitivity observed with systemic PDT.

PRINCIPLES

The light source used for PDT is determined by the absorption spectrum of the photosensitizer and the wavelength and penetration depth of the light. The porphyrins, the main class of photosensitize rs used in PDT, absorb light maximally in the Soret band ranging from 360 nm to 400 nm, with additional smaller peaks, the Q bands, between 500 nm and 635 nm. ALA is converted within target cells into the protoporphyrin IX (PpIX), with an absorption spectrum large blue peak at 417 nm and small red peak at 650 nm. The penetration depth increases in direct proportion to wavelength across the visible spectrum. The 50% penetration depth is 80 mm for a 355-nm laser and increases to 1200 mm for a 694-nm laser. Noncoherent light sources, while expected to achieve less optical penetration because of scatter, achieve good penetration up to 5 mm for 630-nm light and 1–2 cm for 700-nm to 800-nm light. Broadband light sources in the red and blue range dominate in PDT applications.

Topical ALA has been paired with red and blue light, the latter FDA-approved for the treatment AK in 1999. Various lasers, light sources and incubation protocols have been introduced to treat cutaneous neoplasms and inflammatory disorders. Methyl aminolevulinic acid (MAL) was approved with red light in the European Union (EU) countries starting in 2001 for the treatment of hyperkeratotic AK and basal cell carcinoma (BCC), and in the United States in 2004 for the treatment of hyperkeratotic AK. A nano-emulsion of ALA was introduced and approved for use with red light in the EU in 2011 for the treatment of AK and BCC and FDA-approved in the United States in 2016.

MECHANISM OF ACTION

PDT involves the application of a topical photosensitizing agent over a target area, followed by activation of the agent by light irradiation. The PDT reaction leads to the formation of reactive oxygen species in the presence of oxygen, which exert effects on essential cellular components leading to apoptosis and necrosis due to irreversible oxidization.

PHOTODYNAMIC THERAPY APPLICATIONS

PDT is utilized in dermatology, general oncology, cardiovascular, and ophthalmology. The various indications in dermatology are shown below:

Approved Indications in US and EU

1. Actinic Keratoses (AK):
   - ALA:
     - ALA 20% solution with blue light for the treatment of AK on the face and scalp is FDA-approved in the United States. ALA is applied to AKs only, followed 14–18 hours later by $10 J/cm^2$ of blue light exposure using the BLU-U device.
     - ALA 10% nano-emulsion gel with red light for the treatment of AK on the face and scalp is FDA-approved in the United States and licensed for use in the EU. ALA is applied to AKs for 3 hours followed by $37 J/cm^2$ of red light exposure using the BF-RhodoLED lamp. In the EU it is also approved for use with 2 hours of daylight.
     - ALA $2 mg/cm^2$ patch for the treatment of AK on face and scalp is licensed for use in the EU, applied for 4 hours followed by $37 J/cm^2$ of red light exposure using the BF-RhodoLED lamp.
   - MAL:
     - MAL 16.8% cream is FDA-approved for the treatment of AK on the face and scalp following

curettage with an incubation period of 3 hours under occlusion with $37 J/cm^2$ red light using the Aktilite, two sessions 7 days apart.
     - MAL 16.8% cream is licensed in the EU for AK of face/scalp with curettage and an incubation period of 3 hours under occlusion with $37 J/cm^2$ red light using the Aktilite, two sessions 7 days apart. It may also be combined with 2 hours daylight for AK.
     - Squamous cell carcinoma in situ (SCCis)
     - MAL 16.8% cream is licensed in the EU for SCCis with curettage and an incubation period of 3 hours under occlusion with $37 J/cm^2$ red light using the Aktilite, two sessions 7 days apart.
2. Basal Cell Carcinoma (BCC):
   - MAL:
     - MAL 16.8% cream is licensed in the EU for superficial (s) and nodular (n) BCC with curettage and an incubation period of 3 hours under occlusion with $37 J/cm^2$ red light using the Aktilite, two sessions 7 days apart.
   - ALA
     - ALA 10% nano-emulsion gel is licensed in the EU with red light for the treatment of sBCC and nBCC for 3 hours followed by $37 J/cm^2$ of red light exposure using the BF-RhodoLED lamp.

CONTRAINDICATIONS

Contraindications to PDT include:
- Known hypersensitivity to porphyrins
- Known hypersensitivity to any component of the drug
- Porphyria
- Photodermatoses
- Cutaneous photosensitivity at wavelengths used
- Safety in pregnancy not generally established; pregnancy category C
- Safety in pediatric population 12 years and younger not established

WARNINGS AND PRECAUTIONS

Risk of Eye Injury: Patients and healthcare providers must wear protective eyewear before operating light
Photosensitivity: Protect treated lesions from sunlight exposure for 48 hours posttreatment
Risk of Bleeding: Risk of bleeding may occur during lesion preparation in patients with coagulation disorders.

Ophthalmic Adverse Reactions: Avoid direct contact of photosensitizer drug with the eyes.

Mucous Membranes Irritation: Avoid direct contact with the mucous membranes.

DRUG INTERACTIONS

Concomitant use of certain medications may increase the phototoxic reaction to PDT: St. John's Wort, griseofulvin, thiazide diuretics, sulfonylureas, phenothiazines, sulfonamides, quinolones, and tetracyclines.

TREATMENT PROTOCOLS

This section covers PDT protocols and indications approved for use in the USA and EU.

MATERIALS AND METHODS

Photosensitizers

Currently, two topical photosensitizing drugs are FDA approved for dermatology indications: ALA and MAL.

5-Aminolevulinic Acid

ALA is an unstable molecule with low lipid solubility thereby restricting penetration depth and limitation to use in superficial skin diseases. A nano-encapsulated and patch forms have been developed, which increase penetration and stability.

Levulan: Each applicator device contains an ampule of 354 mg of aminolevulinic acid hydrochloride as a powder and a separate ampule of 1.5 mL of solution vehicle comprised of alcohol USP (ethanol content = 48% vol./vol.), water, laureth-4, isopropyl alcohol, and polyethylene glycol. Upon mixture is a topical solution containing 20% aminolevulinic acid hydrochloride (ALA HCl) by weight.

Ameluz: Each gram of 10% gel contains 100 mg of aminolevulinic acid hydrochloride (equivalent to 78 mg of aminolevulinic acid) in a nanovesicle formulation. One gram (g) gel contains 78 mg of 5-aminolaevulinic acid (as hydrochloride), 2.4 mg sodium benzoate (E211), 3 mg soybean phosphatidylcholine, and 10 mg propylene glycol. Full list of excipients: xanthan gum, soybean phosphatidylcholine, polysorbate 80, triglycerides, medium-chain, isopropyl alcohol, disodium phosphate dihydrate, sodium dihydrogen phosphate dihydrate, propylene glycol, sodium benzoate (E211), purified water.

Also known as BF-200 ALA, Ameluz is an oil-in-water (O/W) dispersion of nano-sized (< 50 nm diameter) vesicles composed of a lipid core surrounded by an emulsifying monolayer of phospholipids for improved delivery. Hydrophilic 5-aminolevulinic acid (ALA) becomes soluble in the aqueous phase of the nanoemulsion, providing chemical stability of the active ingredient ALA, presumably by allowing it to adhere to the external, hydrophilic part of the nano-vesicles' phosphatidylcholine monolayer.

Alacare: Each 4 cm^2 patch contains 8 mg (2 mg/cm^2) ALA with excipient of Poly[(2-ethylhexyl)acrylate-co-methylacrylate-co-acrylicacid-co-glycidylmethacrylate] and a backing film of pigmented polyethylene aluminum vapor coated polyester. Patch application has been shown to increase delivery through fluorescence analysis.

Methyl Aminolevulinic Acid

A more stable molecule with greater lipid solubility MAL is reported to attain deeper penetration as compared to ALA.

Metvix(ia): 16.8% cream is contained in 2 g tubes. Each tube contains 160 mg/g of methyl aminolevulinate (as hydrochloride) equivalent to 16.0% of methyl aminolevulinate (as hydrochloride). Metvix(ia) contains cetostearyl alcohol (40 mg/g), methyl parahydroxybenzoate (E 218; 2 mg/g), propyl parahydroxybenzoate (E 216; 1 mg/g) and arachis oil (30 mg/g). Full list of excipients include: Self-emulsifying glyceryl monostearate, cetostearyl alcohol, poloxyl 40 stearate, methyl parahydroxybenzoate (E 218), propyl parahydroxybenzoate (E 216), disodium edetate, glycerol, white soft paraffin, cholesterol, isopropyl myristate, arachis oil, refined almond oil, oleyl alcohol, purified water.

Light Sources

Three commercial light sources are approved or licensed and in general use currently.

Irradiation

Protective eyewear should be worn by the patient and those in the treatment room.

Blue Light

BLU-U: Blue light source emitting 417 (+/−5) nm and maximum power output of 10 J/cm^2 at 1000 seconds, which corresponds to 16 minutes 40 seconds; dosage requires that the patient's lesions are within 2–4 inches of the device.

Red light

Aktilite: Narrow output spectrum red light with a peak at 630 nm and a spectral half-width of approximately 20 nm at a light dose of 37 J/cm^2 in 7–10 minutes session. Illumination surface is $18 \times 8\,cm = 144\,cm^2$.

BF-RhodoLED lamp: Red light source with a narrow spectrum with peak at 635 nm that delivers a light dose of approximately 37 J/cm^2 within 10 minutes session.

US Food and Drug Administration-Approved Procedures

Levulan Kerastick and BLU-U

▶ Check online video (Videos 8.1–8.4 and 8.9–8.13)

Step 1. Skin Preparation: AKs targeted for treatment should be clean and dry prior to applying the Levulan Kerastick topical solution.

Step 2. Levulan Application: The applicator consists of an applicator tube containing two sealed glass ampules. One ampule contains 1.5 mL of solvent vehicle, the other ALA HCl as a dry solid. Holding the applicator with tip up, crush the bottom ampule containing the solution vehicle by applying finger pressure to Position A on the cardboard sleeve. Then, crush the top ampule containing the ALA HCl powder by applying finger pressure to Position B on the cardboard sleeve and continue crushing the applicator downward to Position A. Shake in an up and down motion for at least 30 seconds to completely dissolve the drug powder in the solution vehicle. Remove the cap and dab applicator on a gauze pad until uniformly wet with solution. Apply the solution directly to the target lesions to uniformly wet the lesion surface, including the edges without excess running or dripping. Once the initial application has dried, repeat application second time. Avoid periorbital area and do not allow contact with ocular or mucosal surfaces.

Step 3. Incubation

1. Face and Scalp: FDA label incubation time for Levulan Kerastick is 14–18 hours. The actinic keratoses should not be washed during this time. The patient should be advised to wear a wide-brimmed hat or other protective apparel to shade the treated actinic keratoses from sunlight or other bright light sources until BLU-U illumination. The patient should be advised to reduce light exposure if the sensations of stinging and/or burning are experienced.

2. Upper Extremities: Occlude the upper extremity with low density polyethylene plastic wrap and hold in place with an elastic net dressing for 3 hours. Remove the occlusive dressing prior to light treatment and gently rinse the treated area(s) with water and pat dry before light illumination.

Step 4: Illumination

BLU-U Blue Light Photodynamic Therapy Illuminator: A 1000 second (16 minutes 40 seconds) exposure is required to provide a 10 J/cm^2 light dose. During light treatment, both patients and medical personnel should be provided with blue blocking protective eyewear.

The light is positioned so the entire surface area to be treated lies between 2 and 4 inches from the BLU-U surface:

Ameluz and BF-RhodoLED

Check online video (Videos 8.5–8.8) ▶

Step 1. Degreasing the Skin:

Before applying AMELUZ, wipe lesions with an ethanol or isopropanol-soaked cotton pad to ensure degreasing of the skin.

Step 2. Ameluz Application:

Use glove protected fingertips or a spatula to apply gel approximately 1 mm thick to lesion and to approximately 5 mm of surrounding skin. Application area should not exceed 20 cm^2 and no more than 2 grams (one tube) at one time. Avoid mucous membranes such as the eyes, nostrils, mouth, and ears (keep a 1 cm distance from these areas). Allow the gel to dry for approximately 10 minutes before applying occlusive dressing.

Step 3. 3 Hour Incubation Under Occlusion

Cover the area where the gel has been applied with a light-blocking, occlusive dressing. Following 3 hours of occlusion, remove the dressing and wipe off any remaining gel.

Step 4. Illumination With Red Light

During illumination, patient and medical personnel must wear red light protective eyewear. Immediately after removing occlusion and any remaining gel, illuminate the treatment area with BF-RhodoLED, red light source with a narrow spectrum around 635 nm that delivers a light dose of approximately 37 J/cm^2 within 10 minutes. Position the lamp 5–8 cm from the skin surface. When an area of $8 \times 18\,cm$ is illuminated, the effective treatment area is 6 × 16 cm. Larger areas may be illuminated in several steps.

Metvixia and Aktilite

Step 1. Curettage: The lesion surface is prepared with a dermal curette to remove scales and crusts and roughen the surface of the lesion. Only nitrile gloves should be worn as vinyl and latex do not provide adequate protection.

Step 2. Metvixia Application: Apply a layer approximately 1 mm thick to the lesion and the surrounding 5 mm of normal skin. Multiple lesions may be treated but do not apply more than one gram (half tube) per treatment session.

Step 3. Occlusion: Cover area with an occlusive, non-absorbent dressing.

Step 4. Incubation: Incubate occluded for 3 hours. Patients should avoid exposure of the photosensitive treatment sites to sunlight or bright indoor light during incubation.

Step 5. Illumination: Remove the occlusive dressing, clean the area with saline and gauze. Position the lamp over the area to be illuminated so the distance between the LED panel and the lesion surface should be 50–80 mm (2–3.2 in). The patient and operator should wear appropriate eye protection during illumination. The required illumination time (7–10 minutes) is calculated automatically, and remaining time displayed at the control panel. Each treatment field is limited to an area of 80 × 180 mm.

Step 6. Repeat Treatment: Two treatment sessions should be administered one week apart.

Ameluz/Metvix(ia) and Daylight

Daylight is approved in the EU for AK with Metvix and additionally for field cancerization with Ameluz. In these protocols, first sunscreen is applied and then lesion preparation and drug application are performed as aforementioned. Within 30 minutes of drug application, patients are exposed to daylight for 2 hours. Daylight is not FDA-approved in the United States.

Step 1. Sunscreen application: Sunscreen is applied to the entire area to be treated. Wait for adsorption approximately 15 minutes.

Step 2. Skin preparation: As above for Ameluz or Metvix

Step 3. Drug application: As above for Ameluz or Metvix. Alert: No occlusion.

Step 4. Incubation: None or limited to maximum of 30 minutes.

Step 5. Illumination: Within 30 minutes of drug application, patients are exposed to daylight for 2 hours.

Peri-operative Side Effects: Patients should be advised that transient pain, burning or stinging at the target lesion sites may occur during the period of light exposure. The illumination may be paused and restarted.

Post-treatment Instructions:

After light treatment, patients should wear a broad-brimmed hat and not expose themselves to sunlight or intense light for at least 48 hours. Noncompliance can result in a severe phototoxic reaction.

Treated lesions that have not completely resolved after 8 weeks may be treated a second time with ALA PDT. Regular patient follow-up is recommended.

TREATMENT SITE ADVERSE REACTIONS

Levulan BLU-U: The most common local adverse reactions (AE) (incidence ≥ 10%) to Levulan and BLU-U are erythema, edema, stinging/burning, scaling/crusting, itching, erosion, hypo/hyperpigmentation, oozing/vesiculation/crusting, scaling and dryness.

Ameluz and RhodoLED: Most common AEs include application site erythema, pain/burning, irritation, edema, pruritus, exfoliation, scab, induration, vesicles.

Metvixia and Aktilite: The most common AEs (>1%) include skin burning/pain, erythema, scabbing/crusting/blistering/erosions, pruritus, edema, exfoliation, discharge, skin hemorrhage, skin tightness, hyperpigmentation.

Complications: Complications of PDT include:

1. Short-term localized AEs include pain, erythema, edema, pruritus, urticaria, contact dermatitis, erosive pustular dermatosis of the scalp, decreased delayed-type hypersensitivity responses
2. Systemic AEs: Extensive ALA application could lead to systemic absorption and systemic phototoxicity
3. Long-term AEs: Pigmentary changes and scarring including hyper/hypopigmentation and rare incidences of bullous pemphigoid.
4. Immunomodulation: Studies have shown both immunostimulatory and immunosuppressive effects following PDT, which warrant further study.
5. Carcinogenicity: Keratoacanthomas, BCC, invasive squamous cell carcinoma, melanomas have been reported posttreatment with PDT. The author reported a prevalence of biopsy-proven skin carcinoma in

as high as 45% of non-responding lesions post-PDT, emphasizing the need to follow up and perform evaluations on non-responding lesions. The role of PDT in causing tumor has not been clearly defined and requires further elucidation.

CLINICAL CLEARANCE RATES

ACTINIC KERATOSES

Multiple retrospective analyses have concurred that the typical clearance rates for AKs of face and scalp using topical ALA or MAL PDT approved protocols of blue or red light range between 89% and 92% with quality of evidence I and strength of recommendation A. Efficacy rates are lower for trunk and extremities and when using daylight PDT. A photographic example of outcome for AK following ALA PDT is shown (Fig. 8.1).

BASAL CELL CARCINOMA

The initial clearance rates for sBCC after MAL PDT are 92%–97%, 91% at 1 year, and 78% at 5 years follow up. For nBCC, 91% primary lesions were clear at 3 months

and 76% at 5 years. Histological clearance rates are lower with overall 73% clearance for nBCC and 82% for BCC reported.

SQUAMOUS CELL CARCINOMA IN SITU

MAL and red light treatment of SCCis is associated with 86%–89% clearance rate of lesions to 17–50 month follow up.

OFF-LABEL PROTOCOL VARIATIONS

This section covers unapproved protocol variations, including off-label skin preparation, photosensitizer incubation times, illumination methods, and clinical applications.

5-AMINOLEVULINIC ACID BLUE LIGHT ACTINIC KERATOSIS APPLICATIONS

Off-label protocol variations of ALA PDT for the treatment of AK are presented including unapproved skin preparation methods, incubation durations, and light sources.

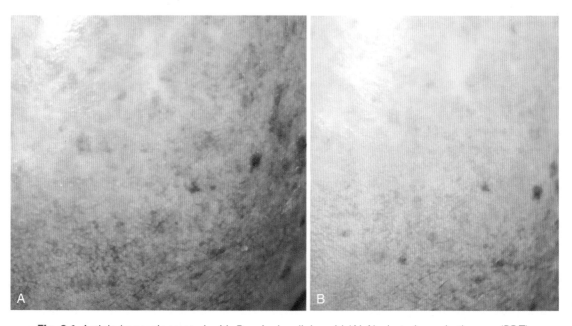

Fig. 8.1 Actinic keratosis treated with 5-aminolevulinic acid (ALA) photodynamic therapy (PDT). Patient prior to (A) and following (B) one session of PDT with Levulan and BLU-U. (Macrene Alexiades.)

SKIN PREPARATION VARIATIONS

Skin may be prepared or degreased using a variety of methods to increase drug penetration or PDT efficacy. Acetone wipe, gentle curettage, pre-treatment with urea, topical retinoids or 5-fluorouracil have been tested and studied. Another common variation is eliminating the wash off step of the drug prior to illumination; while increasing background, it boosts the PDT reaction.

5-AMINOLEVULINIC ACID INCUBATION VARIATIONS

1. Levulan Kerastick: While the product labeling specifies a 14 to 18-hour ALA incubation of ALA, this results in a greater incidence of unwanted AEs. Short incubation ALA was introduced by the author in 2003 and since then ALA incubations varying between 15 minutes to 3 hours have been reported. Short incubation has eliminated intense phototoxic reactions while maintaining satisfactory albeit lower AK clearance rates.

2. Ameluz: While the approved incubation time for this photosensitizer is 3 hours, short incubation times of 1 hour have been reported with satisfactory efficacy.

ILLUMINATION VARIATIONS

The greatest variation in protocol has been in the application of alternative light sources to ignite the PDT reaction. Lasers, intense pulsed light, broadbrand light sources, light emitting diodes (LED), lamps, and fiberoptic illumination systems have all been studied. The most pertinent for the laser community include the following:

Intense pulsed light: IPL devices have been extensively utilized as a PDT light source with most significant results in patients with diffuse actinic damage. When IPL is applied to PDT, short incubation of 1–3 hours followed by long pulse duration and reduced fluence are recommended with improvements in AK clearance as well as photoaging, including telangiectasiae and lentigines [35–37]. Caution is recommended as posttreatment erythema and exfoliation is proportionate to the degree of actinic damage.

Pulsed dye laser: PDL has been reported in the treatment of AK and AC, but with most significance in the PDT treatment of acne and acne scars, lichen sclerosus, and vascular malformations. When PDL is applied to

PDT, long-pulsed PDL (595 nm) is recommended at 10 milliseconds pulse durations and moderate fluences of 5–7 J/cm^2 in two passes for actinic damage and acne/acne scars (Fig. 8.2). When using 585 nm PDL, similar parameters but shorter pulse durations of 1.5 ms have been used (with purpura expected in these instances) for the treatment of vascular malformations such as port wine stains.

Fractionated Illumination: Discontinuous light exposure periods have been proposed to improve PDT efficacy by theoretically allowing for re-oxygenation between exposures. Published reports indicate superiority of fractionated illumination ALA PDT for AK (94% vs. 85% at 1 year follow up) and sBCC (88% vs. 75% at 5-year follow-up). Interestingly, no difference in efficacy has been observed for MAL PDT with fractionation, purportedly due to the differential localization of the drug.

ALTERNATIVE CLINICAL APPLICATIONS

BCC: Ameluz and Metvix are licensed for treatment of sBCC and nBCC in the EU in combination with red light in the aforementioned protocol. These are off label protocols in the Unites States.

Actinic Cheilitis: Extensively published for the treatment of AC, the approved protocols have been employed with demonstrated efficacy, as have variations with other devices such as PDL and with the Alacare patch which is available in the EU. Long-term follow-up studies have shown a complete remission rate of 62% (3–30 months) and a histological cure of 47% (1.5–18 months) following PDT of AC.

Keratoacanthoma (KA): While case reports of KA treated with PDT exist, post-PDT incidence of KA have also been reported; therefore, this is not a recommended off-label use at this time.

Bowen's Disease (SCCis): Metvix and red light is licensed for treatment of SCCis in the EU with the aforementioned protocol with 86%–89% clearance rate of lesions.

Erythroplasia of Querat: Studies reported 62.5% of patients treated with MAL PDT and 58.3% of patients treated with ALAP DT achieved complete remission.

Acne: The application of PDT protocols involving all aforementioned photosensitizers and all illumination options to the treatment of acne has been widely studied with numerous reports of safety and efficacy

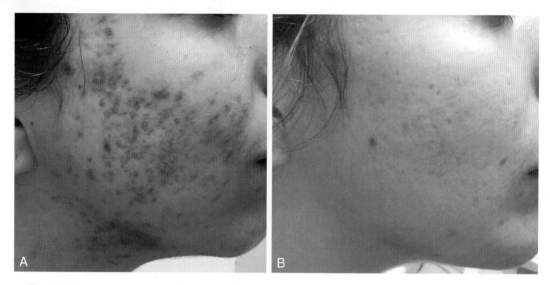

Fig. 8.2 Acne and acne scarring treated 5-aminolevulinic acid (with ALA) photodynamic therapy (PDT). Patient prior to (A) and following (B) treatment with ALA and long-pulsed PDL at 7 J/cm², 10 milliseconds, 10 mm, 30 milliseconds cryo/20 milliseconds delay. (Macrene Alexiades.)

in the literature. While PDL is effective, red light is the most widely used due to its penetration depth, adequate sebaceous uptake and reduced cost. A representative example of acne treated with ALA PDL PDT is shown (see Fig. 8.2).

Vascular Malformations: Port wine stains and other vascular malformations have been successfully treated mainly with systemic PDT protocols.

Lichen Sclerosus: A systematic review revealed efficacy in the treatment of lichen sclerosus with PDT; however, further clinical trials are required to ascertain clearance rates.

Sebaceous Hyperplasia: While some improvement in sebaceous hyperplasia has been reported following PDT, long-term follow up studies are lacking; given incomplete clearance, recurrence is expected.

CONCLUSION

Topical PDT is a well-established and highly effective treatment modality for AK in the United States, and additionally for BCC and SCCis in the EU. Approved photosensitizers include ALA and MAL, while illumination options include blue light and red light in the United States and additionally daylight in the EU. The advantage of PDT is that it provides a well-tolerated

option for field cancerization. Alternative off label uses include variant skin preparation and incubation methods, including short incubation; alternative illumination methods, including lasers, IPL, and fractionated exposures; and a number of additional applications including skin neoplasia, acne, and inflammatory disorders.

FURTHER READING

Alam M, Dover JS. Treatment of photoaging with topical aminolevulinic acid and light. Skin Therapy Lett. 2004;9(10):7–9.

Alexiades M. Randomized, controlled trial of fractional carbon dioxide laser resurfacing followed by ultrashort incubation aminolevulinic acid blue light photodynamic therapy for actinic keratosis. Dermatol Surg. 2017; 43(8):1053–1064.

Alexiades-Armenakas MR, Geronemus G. Laser-mediated photodynamic therapy of actinic keratoses. Arch Dermatol. 2003;139(10):1313–1320.

Alexiades-Armenakas MR. Laser-mediated photodynamic therapy. Clin Dermatol. 2006;24(1):16–25.

Alexiades-Armenakas MR. Aminolevulinic acid photodynamic therapy for actinic keratoses/actinic cheilitis/acne: vascular lasers. Dermatol Clin. 2007;25:25–33.

Basset-Seguin N, Ibbotson SH, Emtestam L, et al. Topical methyl aminolaevulinate photodynamic therapy versus cryotherapy for superficial basal cell carcinoma: a 5-year randomized trial E. *J Dermatol.* 2008;18:547–553.

Boen M, Brownell J, Patel P, Tsoukas MM. The role of photodynamic therapy in acne: an evidence-based review. *Am J Clin Dermatol.* 2017;18(3):311–321.

Borgia F, Giuffrida R, Caradonna E, Vaccaro M, Guarneri F, Cannavò SP. Early and late onset side effects of photodynamic therapy. *Biomedicines.* 2018;6(1):12.

Calzavara-Pinton PG, Venturini M, Sala R, et al. Methyl aminolaevulinate-based photodynamic therapy of Bowen's disease and squamous cell carcinoma. *Br J Dermatol.* 2008;159:137–144.

Cavicchini S, Serini SM, Fiorani R, et al. Long-term follow-up of methyl aminolevulinate (MAL)-PDT in difficult-to-treat cutaneous Bowen's disease. *Int J Dermatol.* 2011;50:1002–1005.

Channual J, Choi B, Osann K, Pattanachinda D, Lotfi J, Kelly KM. Vascular effects of photodynamic and pulsed dye laser therapy protocols. *Lasers Surg Med.* 2008;40(9):644–650.

De Haas ERM, Kruijt B, Sterenborg HJCM, Neumann HAM, Robinson DJ. Fractionated illumination significantly improves the response of superficial basal cell carcinoma to aminolevulinic acid photodynamic therapy. *J Invest Dermat.* 2006;126:2679–2686.

De Vijlder HC, Sterenborg HJCM, Neumann HAM, Robinson DJ, de Haas ERM. Light fractionation significantly improves the response of superficial basal cell carcinoma to ALA-PDT: five-year follow-up of a randomized, prospective trial. *Acta Dermatol Venereol.* 2012;92:641–647.

Fantini F, Greco A, Del Giovane C, et al. Photodynamic therapy for basal cell carcinoma: clinical and pathological determinants of response. *J Eur Acad Dermatol Venereol.* 2011;25:896–901.

Foley P, Freeman M, Menter A, et al. Photodynamic therapy with methyl aminolevulinate for primary nodular basal cell carcinoma: results of two randomized studies. *Int J Dermatol.* 2009;48:1236–1245.

Gold MH, Bradshaw VL, Boring MM, Bridges TM, Biron JA, Lewis TL. Treatment of sebaceous gland hyperplasia by photodynamic therapy with 5-aminolevulinic acid and a blue light source or intense pulsed light source. *J Drugs Dermatol.* 2004;3(6 suppl):S6–S9.

Kennedy JC, Pottier RH, Pross DC. Photodynamic therapy with endogenous protoporphyrin IX: basic principles and present clinical experience. *J Photo- chem Photobiol B.* 1990;14:275–292.

Kim MM, Darafsheh A. Light sources and dosimetry techniques for photodynamic therapy. *Photochem Photobiol.* 2020;96:280–294.

Lehmann P. Methyl aminolaevulinate-photodynamic therapy: a review of clinical trials in the treatment of actinic keratoses and nonmelanoma skin cancer. *Br J Dermatol.* 2007;156:793–801.

Maranda EL, Nguyen AH, Lim VM, Shah VV, Jimenez JJ. Erythroplasia of Queyrat treated by laser and light modalities: a systematic review. *Lasers Med Sci.* 2016;31:1971–1976.

Meyer-Betz F. [Investigation of biological (photodynamic) actions of hematoporphyrins and other de-rivatives of blood and bilirubin]. *Dtsch Arch Klin Med.* 1913;112:476 [in German].

Morton C, Szeimies RM, Basset-Seguin N, Calzavara-Pinton P, et al. European Dermatology Forum guidelines on topical photodynamic therapy 2019 Part 1: treatment delivery and established indications—actinic keratoses, Bowen's disease and basal cell carcinomas. *J Eur Acad Dermatol Venereol.* 2019;33(12):2225–2238.

Nestor MS, Berman B, Patel J, Lawson A. Safety and efficacy of aminolevulinic acid 10% topical gel versus aminolevulinic acid 20% topical solution followed by blue-light photodynamic therapy for the treatment of actinic keratosis on the face and scalp: a randomized, double-blind study. *J Clin Aesthet Dermatol.* 2019;12(3):32–38.

Passeron T, Lacour JP, Ortonne JP. Comparative treatment of extragenital lichen sclerosus with methylaminolevulinic acid pulsed dye laser-mediated photodynamic therapy or pulsed dye laser alone. *Dermatol Surg.* 2009;35(5):878–880.

Piccolo D, Kostaki D. Photodynamic therapy activated by intense pulsed light in the treatment of nonmelanoma skin cancer. *Biomedicines.* 2018;6(1):18.

Prodromidou A, Chatziioannou E, Daskalakis G, Stergios K, Pergialiotis V. Photodynamic therapy for vulvar lichen sclerosus—a systematic review. *J Low Genit Tract Dis.* 2018;22(1):58–65.

Raab O. Uber die Wirkung, fluorescirender Stoffe auf Infusorien. *Infusaria Z Biol.* 1900;39(524):9.

Radakovic S, Dangl M, Tanew A. 5-Aminolevulinic acid patch (Alacare) photodynamic therapy for actinic cheilitis: data from a prospective 12-month follow-up study on 21 patients. *J Eur Acad Dermatol Venereol.* 2020;34(9):2011–2015.

Rhodes LE, de Rie MA, Leifsdottir R, et al. Five year follow up of a randomized prospective trial of topical methyl aminolevulinate-photodynamic therapy versus surgery for nodular basal cell carcinoma. *Arch Dermatol.* 2007;143:1131–1136.

Szeimies Rolf-Markus, Dräger Julia, Abels Christoph, Landthaler Michael. History of photodynamic therapy in dermatology. In: Calzavara-Pinton Piergiacomo, Szeimies Rolf-Markus, Ortel Bernhard, eds. *Comprehensive Series in Photosciences.* Volume 2. Elsevier; 2001:3–15.

Szeimies R, Ibbotson S, Murrell D, et al. A clinical study comparing methyl aminolevulinate photodynamic therapy and surgery in small superficial basal cell carcinoma (8–20 mm), with a 12-month follow-up. *J Eur Acad Dermatol Venereol.* 2008;22:1302–1311.

Tampa M, Sarbu M, Matei C, et al. Photodynamic therapy: a hot topic in dermato-oncology (review). *Oncol Lett.* 2019; 17:4085–4093.

Tappeiner HV, Jodlbauer A. Uber die Wirkung der photody-namischen (fluoreszierenden) Stoffe auf Infusorien. *Dtsch Arch Klin Med.* 1904;1904(80):427–487.

Touma D, Yaar M, Whitehead S, Konnikov N, Gilchrest BA. A trial of short incubation, broad-area photodynamic therapy for facial actinic keratoses and diffuse photodam-age. *Arch Dermatol.* 2004;140(1):33–40.

Truchuelo M, Fernandez-Guarino M, Fleta B, et al. Effectiveness of pho- todynamic therapy in Bowen's disease: an observa-tional and descriptive study in 51 lesions. *J Eur Acad Derma-tol Venereol.* 2012;26:868–874.

Yazdani Abyaneh MA, Falto-Aizpurua L, Griffith RD, Nouri K. Photodynamic therapy for actinic cheilitis: a systematic review. *Dermatol Surg.* 2015;41:189–198.

Yuan KH, Li Q, Yu WL, Zeng D, Zhang C, Huang Z. Com-parison of photodynamic therapy and pulsed dye laser in patients with port wine stain birthmarks: a retrospective analysis. *Photodiagnosis Photodyn Ther.* 2008;5(1):50–57.

Zhang B, Zhang TH, Huang Z, Li Q, Yuan KH, Hu ZQ. Comparison of pulsed dye laser (PDL) and photodynamic therapy (PDT) for treatment of facial port-wine stain (PWS) birthmarks in pediatric patients. *Photodiagnosis Photodyn Ther.* 2014;11(4):491–497.

9

Ablative Laser Skin Resurfacing

Jacob J. Inda and Joel L. Cohen

SUMMARY AND KEY FEATURES

- Ablative laser resurfacing has long been a very popular cosmetic procedure.
- A variety of carbon dioxide, erbium:yttrium-aluminum-garnet, and yttrium-scandium-gallium-garnet lasers are included in the category of ablative lasers.
- "Full-field" means 100% of the treated area is removed to the selected depth.
- Fractional means discontinuous portions of the treated area are removed in columns.
- Hybrid fractional lasers are a combination of ablative and nonablative fractional resurfacing.

- Recovery time is linked to depth of treatment and percentage of surface damaged.
- Fractional treatments have less downtime than full-field treatments.
- Experience with these lasers is important to achieving optimal results.
- Posttreatment care is very important, especially infection precautions.
- Complications can arise with these laser modalities.

INTRODUCTION

Ablative laser resurfacing encompasses a group of popular procedures in the United States and worldwide. These treatments can be broadly divided into two categories: "full-field" ablative resurfacing and "fractional" ablative resurfacing. Full-field ablative resurfacing is defined by confluent vaporization of treated epidermis and superficial dermis, allowing for impressive outcomes but significant associated downtime following treatment. In contrast, ablative fractional resurfacing results in vertical columns of vaporized tissue called microscopic thermal zones, but leaves the skin adjacent to these zones intact. These areas of intact skin expedite wound healing and reduce the associated downtime relative to full-field ablative resurfacing.

In the mid-1990s, full-field ablative procedures with (CO_2) lasers were extremely popular. Cases of postoperative infections, delayed hypopigmentation and of scarring led to a rapid decline in the use of CO_2 lasers in the early 2000s. The introduction of nonablative technology at the turn of the 20th century then caused full-field ablative resurfacing to largely fall out of favor. Ablative resurfacing resurged after 2004 with the introduction of fractional ablative lasers, which for many patients allowed a more acceptable compromise between downtime, the risk of complications, and clinical improvement with the skin only being treated in microthermal zones.

Recent trends in the number of resurfacing procedures performed reflect growing public interest in these treatments. From 1997–2016, the American Society for Aesthetic Plastic Surgery reported cosmetic procedure data from core specialties including dermatology, plastic surgery, and otorhinolaryngology. Overall, ablative resurfacing was the eighth most common nonsurgical procedure performed in 2016, with over 525,000 procedures performed (Table 9.1).

TABLE 9.1   American Society for Aesthetic Plastic Surgery Top 10 Procedures for 2016
1. Toxins—Botox, etc.
2. Hyaluronic acid
3. Laser hair removal
4. Photorejuvenation (IPL)
5. Chemical peel
6. Microdermabrasion
7. Nonsurgical skin tightening
8. Laser resurfacing—full-field and fractional
9. Sclerotherapy
10. Nonsurgical fat reduction

IPL, Intense-pulsed light.

HISTORY

Continuous wave lasers were first introduced into the dermatology and plastic surgery world in the 1970s for the treatment of vascular lesions and for treatment of a variety of benign cutaneous lesions. The introduction of the pulsed CO_2 laser for skin resurfacing in the mid-1990s rapidly became popular, and largely replaced chemical peels and dermabrasion in many practices. The CO_2 laser has a wavelength of 10,600 nm, has an absorbing chromophore of water, and is used to vaporize tissue. Continuous wave lasers were initially used but often resulted in excessive depths of ablation and unwanted collateral thermal damage. To limit both, competing technologies were developed to either deliver short pulses, each of which contained enough energy to cause tissue ablation (Ultrapulse laser, Lumenis lasers, Yokneam, Israel) or an optomechanical flash scanner used to scan a continuous laser beam in a spiral pattern (Silk-touch and Feather-touch lasers, (ESC) Lumenis lasers, Yokneam, Israel). Both methods created a tissue exposure time of less than 1 millisecond, which allowed tissue ablation with limited residual thermal damage of approximately 75–100 µm. Short-term results of eradicating wrinkles and tightening lax tissue were excellent, but hypopigmentation was seen at longer-term follow-up in some cases. These pigmentary complications and the considerable downtime created for the patient led to the demise of "full-field" CO_2 laser resurfacing around the turn of the last millennium.

Erbium:yttrium-aluminum-garnet (Er:YAG) lasers (2940 nm) were introduced around 2000 and marketed for superficial resurfacing. Erbium lasers have a higher water absorption coefficient than CO_2 lasers (approximately 10–15 times) and ablate tissue with much less residual thermal damage (5–10 µm). Initial machines were low-powered, lacked pattern generators, and needed a considerable number of passes and treatment time to achieve deeper depths of ablation. Subsequent systems had more significant power and thus could be used for efficient deeper resurfacing. There is a linear relationship between the energy delivered and depth of ablation, with approximately 3–4 µm ablated per joule of Er:YAG laser fluence delivered. Complications were fewer, yet the healing and downtime appeared to be similar to that of CO_2 systems. Conclusions of comparative studies were that the combined depth of ablation and coagulation was the determining factor in length of recovery. Combination systems of CO_2 and Er:YAG lasers were popular for a short time (Derma-K, Lumenis lasers, Yokneam, Israel) with the beams being delivered either sequentially or at the same time.

Variable or long-pulse Er:YAG lasers (Sciton Inc., Palo Alto, CA) allow control over the amount of residual thermal injury produced for a given amount of tissue removal. These variable pulse Er:YAG systems seem to produce etched-wrinkle reduction and some skin tightening similar to CO_2 lasers, with a much shorter period of erythema and much lower risk of hypopigmentation. These devices have remained very popular since their introduction in 1998.

Other wavelengths for skin resurfacing have been introduced (2780 and 2790 nm) (Cutera Lasers, Palomar Lasers), which allow variable degrees of thermal damage and ablation settings, but have not had significant commercial success. Plasma skin resurfacing uses nitrogen plasma energy to coagulate a very controlled depth of skin. Healing times and results appear to be similar to Er:YAG lasers. These devices were popular for some time but were removed from the marketplace due to financial problems of the manufacturer. They were recently reintroduced into the market.

In 2004, Manstein and Anderson introduced the concept of fractional photothermolysis. Full-field or traditional laser resurfacing as described previously removes the entire skin surface in the area being treated, with depth of injury depending upon energy level. Fractional laser resurfacing, on the other hand, treats a small "fraction" of the skin at each session, leaving skip

Traditional Ablative Laser Resurfacing

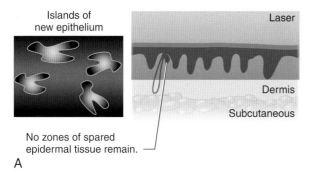

A

Nonablative Fractional Laser Treatment

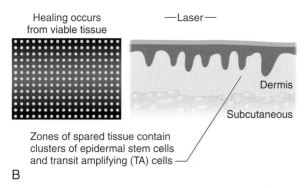

B

Ablative Fractional Laser

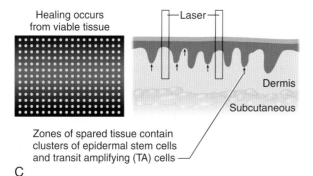

C

Fig. 9.1 (A) Traditional ablative laser resurfacing (full-field). (B) Fractional treatment. (C) Ablative fractional laser treatment.

areas between each exposed area (Fig. 9.1). This was first performed commercially using nonablative fluences at 1550 nm ([Reliant] Solta Medical, Mountain View, CA). These nonablative fractional lasers created a column of

thermal damage with intact epidermis. Healing occurred from deeper structures, as well as from adjacent structures. This differs from full-field resurfacing in which healing occurred from only deeper structures. Deeper treatments (i.e., to the reticular dermis) can safely be performed using this approach than would be tolerated using a full-field treatment. Advantages of this approach include avoidance of an open wound and very low risk of pigment disturbance or scarring. Disadvantages have included the need for multiple treatments and somewhat less clinical response than with full-field ablative resurfacing. Since the introduction of the original system, there have been many manufacturers that have introduced similar nonablative fractional devices with wavelengths of 1440, 1540, and 1550 nm. These devices differ in power output, spot size, density, etc., and comparisons of clinical efficacy are difficult, yet similar degrees of tissue injury should produce similar clinical results.

> **PEARL 1**
>
> Full-field ablative resurfacing means the entire top layer of the skin (to whatever depth is specified) is removed.

> **PEARL 2**
>
> Fractional ablative resurfacing means a "fraction" or percentage of the skin is removed (to whatever depth is specified).

Fractional ablative resurfacing with CO_2, Er:YAG, and yttrium-scandium-gallium-garnet (YSGG) systems was introduced with the intent of providing more significant results than nonablative fractional systems, while achieving shorter healing times and complications when compared with full-field ablative systems. During fractional ablative resurfacing, vertical columns of vaporized tissue termed microscopic thermal zones are created. Importantly, the epidermis between the microscopic thermal zones remains intact, allowing for more rapid healing relative to full-field ablative treatments (see Fig. 9.1).

These devices differ not only in wavelength but in system power, spot size, and amount of thermal damage created adjacent to and deep to the ablated hole. One popular Er:YAG system, the Sciton ProFractional, allows one to vary the amount of thermal damage similarly to their full-field system. Other newer CO_2 fractional lasers allow variation of the thermal damage zones (Deka Medical), whereas others allow superficial and deeper penetration with a single scan (Syneron, Yokneam, Israel). As with the nonablative fractional systems, direct comparison between devices is difficult because devices differ in power output, spot size, density, and degree of thermal damage, but conceptually similar degrees of injury should produce similar clinical results.

The newest wavelength to be introduced into the fractional arena is the Thulium (1927 nm) by Solta Medical. This nonablative fractional device is especially effective in removing superficial pigment and treating actinic keratosis. Given the nonablative, minimal downtime and minimal discomfort aspects of thulium 1927 nm, other companies have now entered this space including Lutronic (Ultra) and Sciton (MOXI).

The newest fractional laser on the market is a hybrid fractional laser made by Sciton called the Halo. This is a very interesting device because it allows coincident delivery of first their Er:YAG fractional laser then a nonablative 1470-nm pulse in the same hole. This device is very efficacious and creates minimal healing times.

PATIENT SELECTION

Patient selection and a clear understanding of potential complications are important to achieving consistent results. The most common indications for both full-field and fractional laser resurfacing are superficial dyschromias, dermatoheliosis, textural anomalies, superficial to deep rhytides, acne scars, and surgical scars. Other conditions that may respond favorably to ablative lasers (either full-field or fractional) include rhinophyma, sebaceous hyperplasia, xanthelasma, syringomas, actinic cheilitis, and diffuse actinic keratoses. Dyschromias, such as melasma, have been successfully treated with fractional resurfacing, but results are not consistent. It seems that the thulium wavelength lasers do better with melasma over a series of treatment sessions. The most commonly treated area is the face, but body and neck skin may be resurfaced with variations of the technique. Non-facial areas lack the appendages necessary for skin rejuvenation, and treatment must be performed non-aggressively to avoid complications. These devices are generally used with patients with Fitzpatrick skin types I to

IV but can be used in skin types V and VI, with modification of technique.

Patient assessment starts at the consultation with observation of the patient's Fitzpatrick skin type, ethnicity, and pathology to be treated. For example, deep acne scarring will not be successfully treated with a single treatment of nonablative fractional treatment, but mild textural issues may respond to superficial treatment. The next assessment is of the patient's tolerance of healing period "downtime." A busy executive with no urgency for end point of clinical results may be able to be treated only with a series of no-downtime nonablative fractional therapy, whereas the bride's mother looking for maximum improvement in a short time to look her best for her daughter's wedding may need a single session with more aggressive treatment. The last parameter is one not usually discussed in medical journals or book chapters: patient finances. A deep full-field resurfacing performed under general anesthesia will be more expensive for the patient than a superficial treatment performed with topical anesthesia. However, in patients with deep rhytides a more aggressive procedure under general anesthesia may be more cost-effective than multiple more superficial treatments. Another consideration is same-session laser resurfacing while patients are undergoing other procedures, such as facelift, abdominoplasty, or esthetic breast surgery. These patients often have built-in downtime from other procedures and have the recovery time available for deep resurfacing.

PEARL 3

Patient assessment starts at the consultation with observation of the patient's Fitzpatrick skin type, ethnicity, and pathology to be treated.

PEARL 4

Assessment of patients' ability to subject themselves to "downtime" of a healing period is important. Full-field erbium can take 10–14 days to reepithelialize, but then postinflammatory erythema often takes 6–10 weeks to subside.

Many of us with various devices in our offices can offer patients a plethora of treatment options, and this can be very confusing to the patient. An effective consultation will encompass a thorough evaluation of the pathology and provide options to the patients in terms of downtime, efficacy, risks, and cost.

EXPECTED BENEFITS AND ALTERNATIVES

The potential for improvement depends upon the device used, as well as the depth and degree of injury produced. There are many options for superficial treatment of texture issues, dyschromias, and superficial rhytides, including nonaggressive full-field resurfacing with Er:YAG, CO_2, YSGG, or plasma devices or with nonablative or ablative fractional treatment. Many practitioners are using combination therapy with superficial full-field treatment combined with fractional treatment, whereas others are combining fractional ablative and nonablative therapy and others again are using intense-pulsed light (IPL) therapy combined with resurfacing. Other treatments that may yield similar results for superficial lines and photodamage include light chemical peels, such as 15%–30% trichloroacetic acid, IPL devices, and Q-switched lasers (532 nm for dyschromias). We prefer lasers to chemical peels, owing to the uniformity and predictability of treatment because the device produces consistent tissue effects with minimal variability from pulse to pulse or patient to patient. The learning curve with lasers is less than with chemical peels, due to the predictability of the treatment. Expert chemical peelers may get similar results to laser treatment at a fraction of the laser cost, but years of experience are necessary to achieve consistency of results. IPL devices may be used to treat dyschromias and superficial vasculature—but these are rather non-specific devices with "filters" to target chromophores and require multiple sessions and do not address textural issues or rhytides. Q-switched lasers (532, 694, 755, 1064 nm) are excellent at removing dyschromias in one session but have resultant erythema that lasts for up to 10 days.

PEARL 5

The potential for improvement depends upon the device used and depth and degree of injury produced.

More significant pathology requires deep treatment to achieve results in a single session. Full-field resurfacing can produce impressive outcomes in a single treatment session, with a low rate of complications when appropriate treatment guidelines are followed. There is still a question of whether repeated superficial therapies with ablative fractional devices will achieve similar results to one more aggressive full-field session, although in the authors' opinion this is not the case. Deep ablative full-field resurfacing may be performed with either Er:YAG or CO_2 systems. YSGG in full-field mode and plasma devices do not ablate deep enough to treat more significant pathology. Acne scars appear to respond better to fractional therapy than to full-field therapy, although these treatments are not mutually exclusive and may be complementary. For instance, full-field single shot erbium may be applied to the shoulders surrounding acne scars prior to fractional therapy during the same treatment session. Alternative treatments may be deeper chemical peels, such as phenol, or dermabrasion. The authors think that lasers provide more consistent and reproducible results than chemical peels or dermabrasion.

LASERS AND TECHNICAL OVERVIEW

As discussed previously, current devices used for ablative laser resurfacing include CO_2, Er:YAG, and YSGG lasers, in both full-field and fractional modes, and nonablative devices in a variety of wavelengths, including 1440, 1540, 1550, and 1927 nm (Table 9.2). Some machines offer upgradeable expandable platforms in which full-field devices and fractional devices are available in one machine, whereas other companies offer only isolated full-field or fractional devices.

Carbon Dioxide Full-Field

Pulsed or scanned full-field CO_2 lasers were very popular from 1995 to approximately 2000. These devices were powerful, with a typical single pass ablating

TABLE 9.2	**Types of Ablative Systems**			
Type of Laser	**Wavelength**			
Full-field	10,600 CO_2	2940 Erbium	2910 EDFGF	2780 YSGG
Ablative fractional	10,600 CO_2	2940 Erbium	2910 EDFGF	2780 YSGG

CO_2, Carbon dioxide; *EDFGF*, erbium-doped fluoride glass fiber; *YSGG*, yttrium-scandium-gallium-garnet.

approximately 75 μm and creating thermal damage of approximately 75–100 μm. This residual area of desiccated tissue reduced the amount of absorbing chromophore (water) and made subsequent passes less efficient, and in fact excessive stacked passes acted as a heat sink and created excessive thermal damage and the potential for scarring. Up to three passes were usually performed with the original CO_2 resurfacing lasers, owing to diminishing efficiency of tissue removal and rapidly increasing risk of complications. The ablated tissue and underlying thermal damage led to long-term collagen changes and tissue remodeling. Healing time with deep full-field CO_2 laser resurfacing took approximately 10–14 days, and caused erythema that typically lasted a few months. Complications of prolonged erythema and then many cases of delayed hypopigmentation occurred—leading to diminished use of these devices. Further complications will be addressed in the complications section.

Erbium:Yttrium-Aluminum-Garnet Full-Field

The Er:YAG laser (2940 nm) has an absorption coefficient 10–16 times greater than the CO_2 laser and ablates tissue more efficiently and leaves less residual thermal damage (5–10 μm). There is a linear relationship between energy density (fluence) delivered and tissue ablated with 3–4 μm of tissue removed per J/cm², and multiple passes can be used to produce deeper tissue removal without additive residual thermal injury. This leads to recovery time of deep full-field Er:YAG laser resurfacing of 7–14 days to full epithelialization followed by 4–8 weeks of erythema. Superficial and deep resurfacing can be performed with these devices with increasing results and increasing recovery times with deeper treatments (Figs. 9.2 and 9.3). Complications, including hypopigmentation, are much less than with CO_2 laser full-field resurfacing. In the opinion of one author (JLC) this is related to the fact that full-field erbium treatment is done to a recognized endpoint of pinpoint dermal bleeding.

Variable pulse Er:YAG systems allow a shorter ablative pulse followed by longer sub-ablative pulses to create increasing thermal damage. These devices are typically used to achieve CO_2 laser-like results, but without the long healing times and complications, such as hypopigmentation.

Yttrium-Scandium-Gallium-Garnet Full-Field

The 2790-nm YSGG (Pearl, Cutera, Brisbane, CA) provides half the affinity for water as the Er:YAG laser at

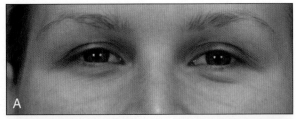

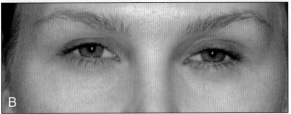

Fig. 9.2 Periocular treatment—a 38-year-old female (A) before and (B) 3 years after full-field variable pulse width Er:YAG laser treatment of the lower lids.

2940 nm. This device in full-field mode produces ablation of approximately 20–30 μm and residual thermal damage of approximately 20 μm per pass. Healing times and downtime are a few days. Deeper resurfacing is not performed with this device.

Plasma Resurfacing

Plasma resurfacing systems create tissue ablation and thermal damage but also a coagulated eschar that remains in place as a biologic bandage until underlying skin is reconstituted. Complications and recovery are reported to be less than for aggressive laser skin resurfacing, but certainly cases of scarring have been reported. This device was recently reintroduced to the marketplace (Energist NA Inc., Nyack, New York).

Nonablative Fractional Resurfacing

Nonablative fractional resurfacing involves the simultaneous or sequential placement of multiple small spots of laser light onto the surface of the skin with intervening skip areas of unexposed skin. The chromophore used is water, and the wavelengths used are 1440, 1470, 1550, and 1540 nm. The lasers create a column of tissue coagulation from 300 to 1200 μm and are called microthermal zones (MTZs). This subject is covered in Chapter 6, and readers are referred there for a more extensive discussion.

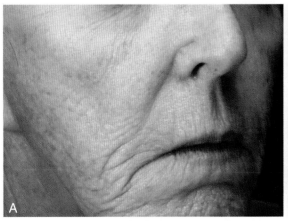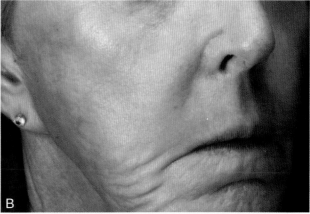

Fig. 9.3 Perioral treatment—a 71-year-old woman (A) before and (B) 2 months after BBL, full-field 2940 Erbium, and also fractional ablative Erbium. (Courtesy of Joel L. Cohen, MD. Denver, Colorado).

Fractional Ablative Technology

Ablative fractional resurfacing can be performed with CO_2, Er:YAG, and YSGG devices. There are many devices available from many well-known laser manufacturers. Differences in devices are the mode of spot placement—scanning versus stamping, size of holes (width and depth) created, and power output of devices. Differences between fractional CO_2 systems, fractional Er:YAG systems, and YSGG systems are similar to their full-field counterparts in that the CO_2 systems cause more residual thermal damage. Newer Er:YAG systems have variable pulse widths, which cause CO_2-like thermal damage. Reepithelialization is quicker than with full-field ablation, and recovery time varies from hours to a few days, depending upon depth and density of treatment.

Both ablative fractional and nonablative fractional devices are used to treat acne and other scars (Fig. 9.4). Multiple treatments are needed, and there is no current consensus as to the best technology for this at present. It was very common in our offices to perform combination treatment with superficial full-field Er:YAG resurfacing followed by Er:YAG fractional treatment. The superficial Er:YAG treatment improves skin texture and minor irregularities, whereas the fractional treatment is useful for collagen remodeling. This treatment regimen was replaced by treatment with a hybrid fractional laser with or without simultaneous IPL treatment.

As fractional CO_2 laser treatments have been pushed to higher and higher coverages in an attempt to maximize efficacy, healing times predictably have increased. More importantly, complications, such as scarring and hypopigmentation, have been observed at coverages in excess of 45%. CO_2 resurfacing histology consistently shows a significant component of tissue ablation and coagulation. Efficacious resurfacing is believed to require a significant component of both. One strategy that has been explored to increase coverage percentage and maximize efficacy involves a combination treatment with ablative Er:YAG fractional and nonablative fractional exposures in a single treatment session. This provides a component of largely ablative exposure with the fractional Er:YAG treatment and a component of coagulation with the nonablative fractional treatment. Rather than being spatially overlapped as in a fractional CO_2 MTZ, the coagulation and ablation are separated. Coverages up to 65% are routinely applied with only a modest increase in healing time and erythema compared with fractional Er:YAG treatment alone and somewhat less than that reported for fractional CO_2. Advantages of this approach include preservation of the short recovery and low incidence of complications seen with

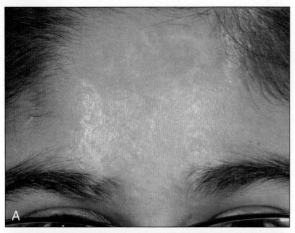

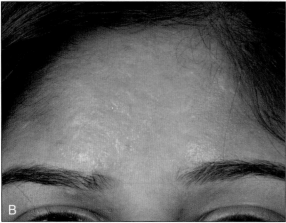

Fig. 9.4 (A and B) This patient had scars of the forehead treated with ablative fractional resurfacing.

fractional Er:YAG treatments and the potential for significant improvement even in perioral rhytides. Disadvantages include the need for two lasers or a single laser platform that offers both options and the time-consuming nature of the treatments (Fig. 9.5).

This combined treatment regimen led to the introduction of the Sciton Halo hybrid laser. This device allows either nonablative fractional resurfacing with a 1470-nm laser or coincident treatment with both a fractional ablative wavelength (2940 nm) and a fractional nonablative wavelength 1470 nm. Treatment with this device has very little downtime, and the results of coincident ablative/nonablative resurfacing on pigment, texture, and pores appear to surpass that achieved with

either nonablative or ablative fractional resurfacing alone (Fig. 9.6). Fewer treatments are needed then with other fractional devices to achieve similar results. Newer protocols with this device are for combined treatment with an IPL device (Broad Band Light) and initial results we have seen appear to be better than non-combined treatments.

OVERVIEW OF TREATMENT STRATEGY

Laser Safety

Laser safety is critical to both practitioner and patient. There are excellent published guidelines on laser safety and courses available on the subject. Specifically relevant to ablative and nonablative resurfacing is the risk of fire and that of eye safety. Fire is an extremely rare occurrence, but one must be cognizant not to fire an ablative laser on paper products or gauze. In the operating room, one must be especially careful in the presence of exposed oxygen sources, such as nasal cannulas. Some recommend the use of wet towels around the patient's face to prevent a fire hazard.

PEARL 6

Laser safety is critical to both practitioner and patient. Room signage on the door and appropriate glasses should always be worn.

Eye protection is critical for all personnel and the patient. Laser-specific eyewear is used for the treating practitioner and all people in the treatment room. External or internal metal contact lens-type eye shields must be used on the patient.

Treatment Approach

Patient selection, as described previously, is important to achieve desired results. In summary, patient selection depends upon the following factors:
- skin type
- ethnicity
- pathology—rhytides, acne scars, etc.
- recovery time
- finances
- patient expectations.

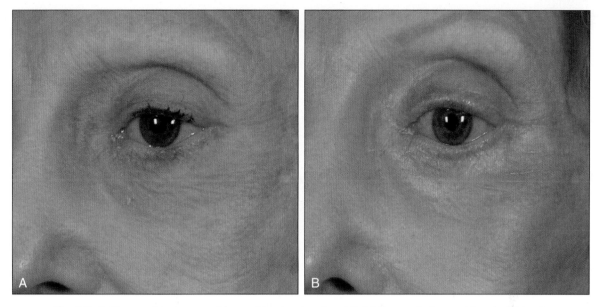

Fig. 9.5 A 68-year-old woman with combination fractional Er:YAG resurfacing and fractional 1540-nm nonablative resurfacing with total coverage of 55%. Time to epithelialization was 4 days. Duration of erythema was 11 days. (A) Before and (B) 6 months after treatment.

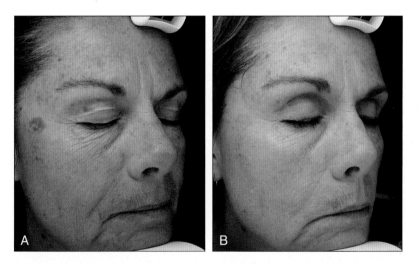

Fig. 9.6 (A) Before and (B) 30 days after treatment with a hybrid fractional laser.

There are a few absolute contraindications for laser treatment and some areas of caution.

Absolute Contraindications
Active Infection
This surgical and elective esthetic procedure should not be performed in the face of active infection. This is true for bacterial, viral, and fungal infections.

Appendageal Abnormality
Laser wounds heal in full-field resurfacing from the deep tissues toward the surface from precursor cells in the hair follicles and sebaceous glands, and in fractional resurfacing from those areas and adjacent normal tissue. Patients with abnormalities of the hair follicles and sebaceous glands may have problems with wound healing. Concurrent or recent oral retinoid treatment used to be considered an absolute contraindication to laser resurfacing but at present time is considered less controversial. The data are confusing as to whether fractional resurfacing is safe with oral retinoid use. Most newer consensus statements agree that nonablative and fractional ablative resurfacing procedures can be performed during systemic retinoid therapy, but that full-field ablative procedures are best delayed until several months after completing treatment. Most experts agree that with return of sebaceous function at 6 months to 2 years post cessation of oral retinoids it is safe to perform deep full-field resurfacing. Previously X-ray irradiated skin lacks appendageal structures and, as such, should not undergo ablative resurfacing procedures.

Extensive electrolysis may also be an absolute contraindication for deep full-field resurfacing, but fractional or superficial full-field resurfacing should be safe.

Relative Contraindications
Unrealistic expectations are a problem we deal with regularly in plastic surgery and esthetic dermatology. Laser resurfacing in all its variations can produce some remarkable results but should not be overstated and oversold. Acne scarring especially can be improved dramatically but may require multiple treatments.

Keloid or Scarring History
Patients with a history of abnormal scarring, particularly keloidal scarring, are at higher risk for this complication. They should be counseled on this risk and approached with caution, and in many cases a test treatment area (test spot) may be helpful.

Regional Resurfacing in Darker-Skinned Individuals
Deep full-field resurfacing in darker-skinned patients may create color differences in adjacent areas. Superficial or fractional regional resurfacing is generally considered safe.

Previous Deep Chemical Peel or Deep Dermabrasion
Caution needs to be taken in patients with previous deep laser or phenol peels or deep dermabrasion because appendages may be damaged and skin may not heal normally.

Previous Deep Laser Resurfacing
Caution also needs to be taken in patients who have had deep full-field resurfacing as appendages may have been damaged. We routinely resurface patients who have had previous deep CO_2 or Er:YAG treatments, but we adjust settings appropriately.

History of Cold Sores/Herpes Simplex 1
Patients with a strong history of cold sores need a modified prophylaxis regimen compared with patients with no history of cold sores. This should start earlier, by 2–3 days, and extend longer after healing. Even after being fully epithelialized, recently resurfaced skin seems to have increased susceptibility to viral infection, unlike bacterial infection risk, which seems largely eliminated by full epithelialization.

Pretreatment and Posttreatment Regimens

Pretreatment with topical retinoids and bleaching creams is another controversial subject, with proponents on either side of this debate and with data from chemical peel and laser literature being mixed. Our feeling is that, in full-field resurfacing greater than 100 μm in depth, the treated melanocytes are ablated so no benefit to pretreatment is seen. In superficial full-field and fractional resurfacing, pretreatment may be beneficial in preventing hyperpigmentation. Most recommend cessation of these products a few days prior to treatment.

The use of antiviral prophylaxis is important with ablative resurfacing. There is debate in the literature as to when to start antiviral therapy, with some proposing 3 days prior to treatment, whereas others recommend starting on the day of treatment. Most agree that therapy should continue until complete reepithelialization occurs. This time is laser-, patient-, and treatment parameter-dependent. The use of antiviral therapy with fractional treatments is controversial. We recommend its use because the risk of these medications is low.

Prophylactic oral antibiotic use is controversial. We know of no controlled studies of their use, and we don't all routinely recommend this. Bacterial infection is extremely rare and is covered in the next section.

After laser treatment, there are a myriad of ways to care for the treated skin. For full-field procedures, most recommend an occlusive ointment (such as white petrolatum) or dressing until epithelialization is complete. Once epithelialization occurs, the patient can be transitioned to a nonocclusive moisturizer such as Cetaphil lotion (Galderma Laboratories). One author (JLC) routinely uses Lasercyn HOCL Post Procedure Gel (Sonoma Pharmaceuticals) as well as Sente Dermal Repair Ultra Nourish (Sente, Inc.). Occlusive dressings, such as Flexzan (Flagship Medical), work well for CO_2 full-field resurfacing but are difficult to keep on Er:YAG patients, owing to the transudate that occurs following this procedure. Deep ablative fractional treatments are usually treated with a similar occlusive regimen for 24–48 hours, although some may prefer a nonocclusive dressing, owing to the incomplete epidermal removal.

Use of sunblock is mandatory for all laser-resurfacing patients after epithelialization is complete. We also recommend institution of a skin care regimen after epithelialization is complete and the skin has had a chance to "calm down." This may mean a few days

for fractional treatments to a few weeks for full-field treatments. There are many good skin care regimens appropriate after laser resurfacing. The combination of 4% hydroquinone and low-strength Retin-A (tretinoin) is still used, although newer regimens with added growth factors are favored by some. The key is to start these regimens slowly to avoid irritation of the skin (see later—dermatitis).

Complications and Their Treatment

Infection

Infection after laser resurfacing can be viral, bacterial, or fungal. The most well-known complication is due to herpes simplex virus (HSV). Many patients have been infected previously and so are carriers. The current recommendation, as outlined previously, is for all patients to be prophylaxed against herpes viral infections (Fig. 9.7). The treatment of an active HSV infection is early recognition and treatment with oral antiviral agents. For very severe infections with herpes simplex or zoster, intravenous antiviral medication may be needed.

PEARL 10

Infection after laser resurfacing can be viral, bacterial, or fungal.

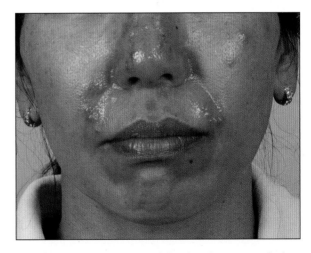

Fig. 9.7 Herpes infection following laser resurfacing. Patient failed to take prescribed antiviral medication and noticed these lesions. Patient was treated with valacyclovir 1000 mg three times a day and responded without scarring.

Bacterial infection after laser resurfacing using open treatment is uncommon, but with increasing methicillin-resistant *Staphylococcus aureus* there have been patients who have had infection after laser resurfacing. The treatment is administration of broad-spectrum antibiotics with culture of the skin and targeted antibiotic treatment after culture results are obtained.

True fungal infections are rare, but infection with yeast (*Candida albicans*) is slightly more common (Fig. 9.8). The patient usually presents with an extremely red face, with a history of having improvement in the healing and suddenly appearing much redder. Culture is essential to confirm the diagnosis and guide therapy. Treatment is topical antifungal therapy with or without an oral antifungal medication, such as fluconazole.

Erythema

Erythema after laser resurfacing is a normal part of the inflammatory healing process. It is directly related to the depth of laser resurfacing and to the amount of thermal damage created. Some patients will experience an amount of erythema disproportionate to the treatment. They may be left untreated for the erythema to resolve spontaneously (which it will), or else they may be treated with mild topical corticosteroids, light emitting diode treatments, IPL treatments, or with a vascular laser such as a pulsed dye laser or nonablative fractional lasers that offer some degree of coagulation.

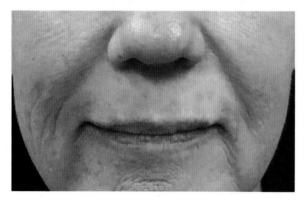

Fig. 9.8 64 year old woman with porcelain-like hypopigmentation several years after full-field CO_2 resurfacing (Photo courtesy of Joel L. Cohen, MD. Denver, Colorado).

Skin Eruptions

Skin eruptions due to acne or milia are common following laser resurfacing. They may be due to occlusion with topical products or to activation of gland function. Acne may be treated with discontinuation of occlusive agents. If this fails, oral antibiotics and/or acne laser treatment with mid-infrared lasers may be used. Milia are treated by nicking the overlying skin with a small-gauge needle and expressing them with a comedone extractor.

> ### PEARL 11
> Acneiform eruptions and milia are common following laser resurfacing.

Dermatitis

Two types of dermatitis are seen following laser resurfacing: irritant and allergic. This is very likely related to the "barrier" of the skin not being completely intact following the treatment, and thus higher chance for irritation or even allergic contact dermatitis. Irritant dermatitis, as mentioned previously, may be due to the start of topical skin care treatments, such as retinoids, too early or too aggressively. Allergic contact dermatitis is due to true allergy, usually to one of the topical agents, but may also be due to one of the oral antibiotics. Treatment for both conditions is discontinuation of the offending agent and application of a mild topical corticosteroid.

Hypopigmentation

This is a dreaded complication of deep laser resurfacing and has been reported both with CO_2 and Er:YAG treatments and with full-field and fractional treatments. It is not uncommon with deep CO_2 resurfacing, with some series reporting up to 70% of patients getting hypopigmentation. It is rare with deep Er:YAG full-field resurfacing (again believed to be due to the pinpoint bleeding endpoint as something that is visualized versus CO_2), and very rare with all fractional treatments. Options for treatment include fractional nonablative 1927 resurfacing with the addition of bimatoprost applied to the affected area twice daily and treatment with fractional CO_2 laser resurfacing. Blending of the noticeable line of demarcation is often helpful.

Hyperpigmentation

Postinflammatory hyperpigmentation (PIH) is a very common problem following laser resurfacing. It is more common in darker skin types and in patients who have had early sun exposure (Fig. 9.9). Prevention as outlined above is key. Treatment is with topical bleaching creams, often combined with retinoids. Failures of this regimen are usually treated with IPL.

> **PEARL 12**
>
> PIH is commonly seen following laser resurfacing.

Scarring

Scarring after laser resurfacing may occur, owing to overly aggressive full-field or fractional treatment, infection, or even scratching by the patient. Full-field resurfacing is a controlled first- or second-degree burn and anything, such as infection, may convert that controlled second-degree burn into a third-degree burn with resultant scarring. Overly aggressive fractional resurfacing may be due to too deep a treatment or too much density, creating a full-field defect when a fractional treatment was intended. We prefer early treatment of thickened areas that appear to be heading toward scarring with potent topical corticosteroids,

such as a pulsed regimen with clobetasol. Intralesional corticosteroids, intralesional 5-fluorouracil, vascular lasers or IPL treatment, and fractional lasers have all been used to improve hypertrophic scars after laser resurfacing (Fig. 9.10).

Slow Healing

Slow healing has been reported in some cases, with reepithelialization of many months and up to a year. This has led to hypertrophic scarring. This scenario of slow healing may represent an indolent infection. Patients with this scenario should be cultured and potentially biopsied to determine and underlying cause.

Ectropion

Ectropion is caused by laser resurfacing by tightening of the lower eyelid skin in the face of weak lower eyelid canthal support. A snap test or other measurement of lower eyelid laxity is recommended prior to laser resurfacing. Patients with significant laxity are offered either canthal support surgery (rare) or canthal temporary support (temporary tarsorrhaphy—common).

Synechia

This is caused by healing of two epidermal surfaces and appears as a line (usually in the lower eyelid). If

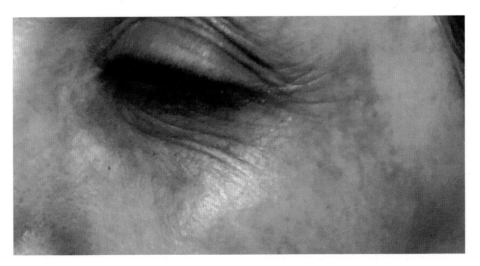

Fig. 9.9 Hyperpigmentation 5 weeks post-ablative fractional resurfacing in 43 year old hispanic patient who was cavalier about sun-protection. (Photo courtesy of Joel L. Cohen, MD. Denver. Colorado).

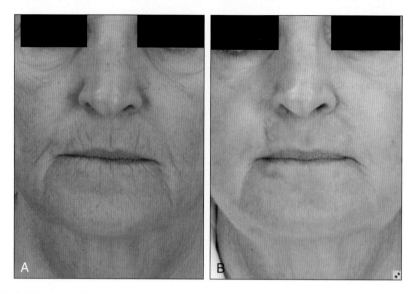

Fig. 9.10 A 64-year-old woman who developed a hypertrophic scar after laser resurfacing: (A) before and (B) after treatment with intralesional corticosteroids and IPL.

untreated this may lead to cyst formation. Treatment is to manually stretch the edges of the synechia until the line opens.

Check online videos (Video 9.1).

CONCLUSION

Ablative laser resurfacing is a popular cosmetic procedure that is best performed by an experienced operator following evidence-based guidelines. A variety of CO_2, Er:YAG, and YSGG lasers are available. During fractional treatments, discontinuous vertical columns of tissue are removed and skin adjacent to those columns remains intact. In full-field treatments, the entire surface of treated skin is removed to the selected depth. Over the past several years, fractional ablative treatments have increased in popularity as they require less downtime relative to full-field ablative resurfacing. However, fractional ablative resurfacing typically requires more treatment sessions than full-field ablative resurfacing, so treatment selection should be informed by the specific goals and preferences of each patient. Appropriate patient selection and postprocedural care are both critically important for optimizing outcomes.

FURTHER READING

Bass LS. Erbium:YAG laser skin resurfacing: preliminary clinical evaluation. *Ann Plast Surg.* 1998;40:328–334.

Bass LS, DelGuzzo M, Doherty S, Seckel B. Combined ablative and non ablative fractional treatment for facial skin rejuvenation. *Lasers Surg Med.* 2009;15(suppl):29.

Bogle MA, Arndt KA, Dover JS. Evaluation of plasma skin regeneration technology in low fluence full-facial rejuvenation. *Arch Dermatol.* 2007;143:168–174.

Chan H. Effective and safe use of lasers, light sources, and radiofrequency devices in the clinical management of Asian patients with selected dermatoses. *Lasers Surg Med.* 2005;37:179–185.

Clementoni MT, Gilardino P, Muti GF, Beretta D, Schianchi R. Non-sequential fractional ultrapulsed CO_2 resurfacing of photoaged facial skin: preliminary clinical report. *J Cosmet Laser Ther.* 2007;9:218–225.

Cohen JL, Ross EV. Combined fractional ablative and nonablative laser resurfacing treatment: a split-face comparative study. *J Drugs Dermatol.* 2013;12:175–178.

Fisher GH, Geronemus RG. Short-term side effects of fractional photothermolysis. *Dermatol Surg.* 2005;31:1245–1249.

Fitzpatrick RE, Rostan EF, Marchell N. Collagen tightening induced by carbon dioxide laser versus erbium:YAG laser. *Lasers Surg Med.* 2000;27:395–403.

Geronemus RG. Fractional photothermolysis: current and future applications. *Lasers Surg Med.* 2006;38:169–176.

Kilmer S, Fitzpatrick R, Bernstein E, Brown D. Long term follow-up on the use of plasma skin regeneration (PSR) in full facial rejuvenation procedures. *Lasers Surg Med.* 2005;36:22.

Kim KH, Fisher GH, Bernstein LJ, et al. Treatment of acneiform scars with fractional photothermolysis. *Lasers Surg Med.* 2005;36:31.

Langlois JH, Kalakanis L, Rubenstein AT, et al. Maxims or myths of beauty? A meta-analytic and theoretical review. *Psychol Bull.* 2000;126:390–423.

Laubach H, Tannous Z, Anderson RR, Manstein D. A histological evaluation of the dermal effects after fractional photothermolysis treatment. *Lasers Surg Med.* 2005;26:86.

Manstein D, Herron GS, Sink RK, Tanner H, Anderson RR. Fractional photothermolysis: a new concept for cutaneous remodeling using microscopic patterns of thermal injury. *Lasers Surg Med.* 2004;34:426–438.

Morrow PC, McElroy JC, Stamper BG, Wilson MA. The effects of physical attractiveness and other demographic characteristics on promotion decisions. *J Manag.* 1990;16:723–736.

Onwudiwe OC, Marmur ES, Cohen JL. Are we too cavalier about antiviral prophylaxis? *J Drugs Dermatol.* 2013;12(2):199–205.

Pozner JN, Goldberg DJ. Histologic effect of a variable pulsed Er:YAG laser. *Dermatol Surg.* 2000;26:733–776.

Pozner JN, Goldberg DJ. Superficial erbium:YAG laser resurfacing of photodamaged skin. *J Cosmet Laser Ther.* 2006;8(2):89–91.

Pozner JN, Roberts TL 3rd. Variable-pulse width Er:YAG laser resurfacing. *Clin Plast Surg.* 2000;27(2):263–271.

Rahman Z, Alam M, Dover JS. Fractional laser treatment for pigmentation and texture improvement. *Skin Therapy Lett.* 2006;11:7–11.

Rahman Z, Rokhsar CK, Tse Y, Lee S, Fitzpatrick R. The treatment of photodamage and facial rhytides with fractional photothermolysis. *Lasers Surg Med.* 2005;36:32.

Sanniec K, Afrooz PN, Burns AJ. Long-term assessment of perioral rhytide correction with erbium:YAG laser resurfacing. *Plast Reconstr Surg.* 2019;143:64–74.

Tannous ZS, Astner S. Utilizing fractional resurfacing in the treatment of therapy-resistant melasma. *J Cosmet Laser Ther.* 2005;7:39–43.

Tannous Z, Laubach HJ, Anderson RR, Manstein D. Changes of epidermal pigment distribution after fractional resurfacing: a clinicopathologic correlation. *Lasers Surg Med.* 2005;36:32.

Tanzi EL, Alster TS. Fractional photothermolysis: treatment of non-facial photodamage with a 1550 nm erbium-doped fiber laser. *Lasers Surg Med.* 2005;36:31.

Weinstein C, Ramirez OM, Pozner JN. Postoperative care following CO_2 laser resurfacing: avoiding pitfalls. *Plast Reconstr Surg.* 1997;100:1855–1866.

Weinstein CW, Ramirez OM, Pozner JN. Carbon dioxide laser resurfacing complications and their prevention. *Aesthet Surg J.* 1997;17:216–225.

Weiss RA, Gold M, Bene N, et al. Prospective clinical evaluation of 1440-nm laser delivered by microarray for the treatment of photoaging and scars. *J Drugs Dermatol.* 2006;5:740–744.

10

Nonsurgical Body Contouring of Fat

Lauren Meshkov Bonati and Omer Ibrahim

SUMMARY AND KEY FEATURES

- Given the dramatic rise of obesity and the obsession with losing weight and improving appearance, the treatment of fat and cellulite is a common cosmetic issue.
- Excess fat and cellulite are distinct entities. Cellulite is best considered a hormonally based structural phenomenon of adipocytes and fibrous septae, whereas excess fat is an overabundance of normal adipocytes.
- The treatment options for excess fat and cellulite are different—a treatment that improves one may have no discernible impact on the other.
- Noninvasive body contouring is a rapidly expanding cosmetic field, with many new technologies recently developed and promising new technologies expected in the near future.
- Topical agents, such as retinoids and methylxanthines, have theoretical benefits on the appearance of fat and cellulite, although objective clinical improvements are limited.
- Injectable therapies, including collagenase, mesotherapy, and injection lipolysis, are also options.

- Physical massage of the affected areas may improve the appearance of fat and cellulite by modulating blood and lymphatic flow.
- Radiofrequency devices use alternating current to generate ionic flow and localized heat in adipocytes, moderately improving the appearance of fat and cellulite.
- Focused ultrasound also specifically targets adipocytes by using pressure waves to damage the cellular membrane, ultimately improving the appearance and thickness of the fat layer.
- Several laser devices using near-infrared wavelengths in combination with physical manipulation have been developed to improve the appearance of fat and cellulite by stimulating dermal collagen formation.
- An adipocyte targeting laser has been developed which selectively heats the adipocytes, thereby leading to apoptosis and clinical reduction in fat volume.
- Cryolipolysis is a therapy by which controlled cold exposure (heat extraction) is used to selectively damage adipocytes, cause apoptosis, gradually and permanently improving the appearance and thickness of the fat layer over several months following the treatment.

INTRODUCTION

Obesity is reaching epidemic proportions in the United States, and weight loss remains a challenging goal for many people. Not only does excess fat present cosmetic challenges to our patients, but it is increasingly obvious that there are also associated significant and dangerous medical effects.

In this chapter, we will focus on noninvasive techniques to improve the appearance of fat and cellulite, the benefits of these technologies, and their limitations. The devices and techniques reviewed herein should be thought of not as ways to achieve weight loss, but rather modest body contouring.

These body-contouring treatments are one of the most rapidly expanding areas in medicine and our general culture. According to the American Society for Dermatologic Surgery (ASDS), approximately 1 million body sculpting procedures were performed in 2019, an increase of 60% from 2018.

Although liposuction remains the true gold standard for treating excess fat, it is an invasive procedure with associated discomfort, bruising, and downtime. The last decade has witnessed the advent of many new technologies that have been developed to treat excess adipose tissue through noninvasive techniques. These noninvasive devices use a multitude of techniques to improve the appearance of excess adipose tissue, including a reduction in the overall volume of fat and improvement in the appearance of cellulite.

FAT VERSUS CELLULITE

Prior to discussing therapeutic options, it is necessary to first differentiate fat and cellulite. Excess fat and obesity are an epidemic, mainly resulting from poor dietary and exercise habits. Fat represents a deposition of excess, but structurally normal, adipose tissue. In contrast, cellulite is best considered a hormonally based structural phenomenon of adipose tissue. It is seen almost ubiquitously in post-pubescent women and rarely in men. As a result of these differences, the techniques and technology that effectively treat excess fat may not have any effect on the appearance of cellulite, and vice versa.

PEARL 1

Excess fat is due to accumulation of normal adipocytes, whereas cellulite is best thought of as a hormonally based structural phenomenon of adipocytes and fat septae. As a result, the evaluation and treatment of these conditions are often divergent.

It is thought that hormones likely play a significant role in the formation of cellulite. Estrogens stimulate lipogenesis and inhibit lipolysis, resulting in adipocyte hypertrophy. Cellulite is typically rare in pre-pubertal women and men of any age but is extremely common in post-pubertal women. In fact, it has been suggested that cellulite is best considered a secondary sexual characteristic of females. It has also been proposed that cellulite develops in at-risk

areas, due to less effective lymphatic and vascular circulation. Exactly how these differences ultimately cause the structural abnormalities of adipose tissue that result in the appearance of cellulite has not been fully elucidated.

Ultrasound and magnetic resonance imaging (MRI) studies have demonstrated the significant structural alterations between male adipose tissue and female cellulite structure. In male adipose tissue the fibrous septae of the adipose tissue are arranged in an overlapping crisscross pattern. This theoretically provides greater strength to the overall scaffolding of the adipose tissue and prevents herniation of fat cells. In contrast, cellulite has fibrous septae that are arranged parallel to each other and perpendicular to the skin surface (Fig. 10.1). This structure is weaker and allows for the focal herniation of adipose tissue. It is this focal herniation that is thought to cause the classic undulating, lumpy, "cottage cheese" appearance of cellulite. MRI has demonstrated that women with cellulite do indeed have fibrous septae that are oriented in parallel to each other, although these septae may actually be more similar to pillar-like columns (Figs. 10.2 and 10.3). In addition to this structural difference, MRI, ultrasound, and biopsies have also demonstrated that women with cellulite typically have an undulating, lumpy interface between the adipose tissue and the dermis, known as *papillae adipose*. This interface also likely contributes to the appearance of cellulite. Notably, MRI images showed no correlation between cellulite severity and the thickness of the adipose layer. Therefore, we believe that excess fatty tissue and cellulite should be considered as two distinct entities and that they should be evaluated and treated as such.

Evaluation of Fatty Tissue and Cellulite

Body mass index (BMI), a person's weight in kilograms divided by the square of their height in meters, remains the classic method for determining obesity. However, this may be an oversimplification because it does not necessarily take into account the patient's mixture of muscle and adipose tissue or their overall body type. Furthermore, many patients presenting for noninvasive body sculpting may be in very good shape overall with only a few small problem areas, such as the thighs or flanks (Case Study 1). Although BMI may be a useful tool for defining obesity in large populations, we do not find it particularly useful in our practice. More commonly, we use such measurements as thigh circumference, waist circumference, skinfold thickness, visual assessment, and photographic comparisons pre- and

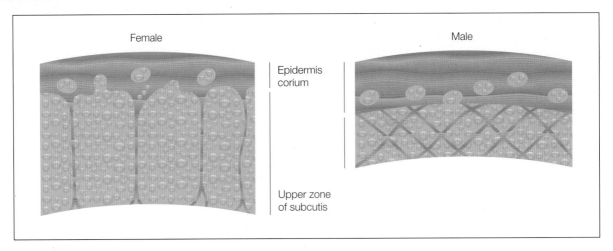

Fig. 10.1 Orientation of subcutaneous fibers extending from dermis to fascia in males and females. (Reprinted from Nurnberger F, Muller G. So-called cellulite: an invented disease. *J Dermatol Surg Oncol.* 1978;4:221.)

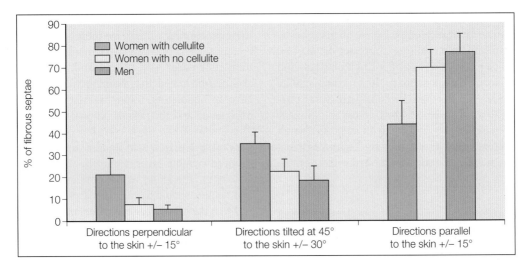

Fig. 10.2 Structured patterns of the fibrous septae network according to gender and presence of cellulite. Our quantitative findings give more evidence about the heterogeneity in the directions of the septae and highly suggest that modeling the three-dimensional (3D) architecture of fibrous septae as a perpendicular pattern in women but tilted at 45 degrees in men would be an oversimplification. (Reprinted from Querleux B, Cornillon C, Jolivet O, Bittoun J. Anatomy and physiology of subcutaneous adipose tissue by in vivo magnetic resonance imaging and spectroscopy: relationships with sex and presence of cellulite. *Skin Res Technol.* 2002;8:118–124.)

post-procedure in our practice because these more typically reflect the patient's ultimate clinical presentation and outcome. It is important to note that there can be a great deal of variability in these measurements if not performed properly. For example, if the waist circumference is not measured at precisely the same location or in the exact same manner, measurements will be inconsistent and the treatment effect will be difficult to determine. Lighting of before and after photographs can also greatly impact the appearance of the images, leading to over exaggeration

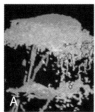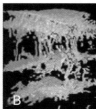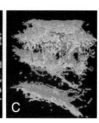

Fig. 10.3 Visualization of the three-dimensional (3D) architecture of fibrous septae in subcutaneous adipose tissue: (A) woman with cellulite, (B) normal woman, and (C) man. (Reprinted from Querleux B, Cornillon C, Jolivet O, Bittoun J. Anatomy and physiology of subcutaneous adipose tissue by in vivo magnetic resonance imaging and spectroscopy: relationships with sex and presence of cellulite. *Skin Res Technol.* 2002;8:118–124.)

CASE STUDY 1

A female patient presents to discuss noninvasive fat treatment options. She is 35 years old, weighs 185 pounds (84 kg) and is 5′4″ (1.63 m) tall. She has also developed early-onset type II diabetes. She has previously tried to lose weight with diet and exercise but has been unsuccessful. She was recently evaluated by her PCP, who encouraged her to lose weight to improve her diabetes and overall health. She presents to your office because she would like a procedure to treat her excess adipose tissue.

This patient has a common misconception that noninvasive fat treatment can substitute for large-scale weight loss. This patient's BMI is 31.8, which defines her as obese. Furthermore, she already has a medical comorbidity, diabetes, associated with her obesity. This patient absolutely needs help losing weight and improving her medical health, particularly because she has tried and failed previous weight loss strategies. She should be referred to a bariatric weight loss program to help her to achieve her goals of weight loss.

If she is interested in a procedure to help to improve her chances of successfully losing weight, this patient may be a good candidate for laparoscopic banding, partial gastrectomy, or gastric bypass. After the patient has lost weight and is closer to her ideal weight, if she continues to have focal trouble spots of excess fat, she may benefit from a noninvasive body-sculpting procedure at that time.

---

or under appreciation of a treatment effect. It is therefore essential that staff be properly trained to perform these measurements and photographs reliably and consistently.

PEARL 2

BMI is a simple tool to assess overall body habitus. However, BMI is often not the best method to assess localized areas of fat excess and is not often used in our clinical assessments. Furthermore, obese patients (BMI > 30) are often not good candidates for noninvasive body contouring and may require diet, bariatric, or other surgical interventions.

Cellulite can similarly be assessed with various measurements and scales, each of which comes with specific pros and cons. Typically, direct observation with side lighting is the simplest and most effective assessment. Based upon these observations, a relatively simple scoring system for the appearance of cellulite has been described (Table 10.1).

More recently, technologies such as ultrasound, MRI, and electrical conductivity have been used to assess adipose tissue and cellulite. These technologies are often used in clinical trials to assess the potential efficacy of a novel therapeutic option. However, they are typically not necessary in the evaluation and management of patients in general practice.

THERAPEUTIC OPTIONS

There are many different technologies and techniques for noninvasive body sculpting. Options include topical creams, injectable agents, physical manipulation, lasers

TABLE 10.1	Cellulite Classification
Grade I	No or minimal skin irregularity upon standing, pinch test, or muscle contraction
Grade II	No or minimal skin irregularity upon standing. Dimpling becomes apparent by pinching or muscle contraction
Grade III	Classic skin dimpling at rest with palpable, small subcutaneous nodularities
Grade IV	More severe puckering and nodularity

and light sources, and cryolipolysis. The best option for your patient is dependent on their clinical presentation, treatment goal, and most importantly, their preferences. It is important to emphasize that none of these treatments provides more than a modest, local contouring benefit in most instances, and that these procedures are not intended for actual decreases in body weight.

Topical Creams

A simple trip to any cosmetic aisle or beauty store demonstrates that there are numerous topical creams that purport to melt away fat and cellulite. Generally speaking, the active ingredients in these products are thought to stimulate improved circulation, improve lymphatic drainage, or cause lipolysis to improve the appearance of fat and cellulite. The most commonly used ingredients include caffeine, aminophylline, and retinoids. Although there are a few limited studies on these creams, many agents have little or no hard evidence to support their claims and the ability of the active ingredients to penetrate to the necessary depth is a matter of significant debate.

PEARL 3

Many topical creams are advertised to improve the appearance of fat and cellulite. In our view, these claims should be regarded skeptically. There is little scientific evidence to support claims.

Topical vitamin A derivatives compounds have long been a mainstay in cosmetic regimens, owing to their ability to stimulate neocollagenesis. Topical retinoids could theoretically improve the appearance of cellulite by increasing collagen deposition and promoting glycosaminoglycan synthesis, thereby resulting in stronger and denser fibrous septae. In clinical studies the results have been modest. Kligman et al. conducted a double-blind study of 20 patients who applied topical retinol twice daily for 6 months and demonstrated a clinical improvement. A further study of 15 patients by Pierard-Franchimont et al. demonstrated a phenotypic shift of connective tissue cells but no visible improvement in overt cellulite appearance following 6 months of application of topical retinol. Thus, although topical retinoids may be of benefit in improving the appearance of fat and cellulite, this benefit is likely modest at best.

Methylxanthines (e.g., caffeine) have also been reported to be effective in treating cellulite. These agents act as phosphodiesterase inhibitors, which, when applied, result in an increase in cyclic adenosine monophosphate (cAMP) levels. This increase in cAMP could theoretically activate hormone-sensitive lipase and thereby stimulate lipolysis in the treated areas. Studies have shown conflicting results in their effectiveness to reduce fat and cellulite. Most recently micronized phospholipid carriers have been developed to increase the penetration of methylxanthines.

Numerous herbal therapies have also been reported to be effective in treating fat and cellulite (Table 10.2). Many of these herbal supplements have not undergone rigorous testing to determine their efficacy, and there is therefore little or no scientific evidence to support their use. Of note, one study demonstrated that even when topical therapies resulted in appreciable improvements in cellulite, results were short term (< 2 weeks).

Injectable Agents

Many different agents have been injected with the goal of dissolving excess adipose tissue and cellulite. Mesotherapy, or intradermotherapy, is performed by the direct injection of pharmacologic agents into the dermal–subcutaneous junction of the skin. This procedure is purported to work by acting directly on the adipocyte to promote lipolysis or adipolysis and thereby improve the appearance of fat and cellulite.

A closely related but separate technique is known as injectable lipolysis, in which detergents, such as bile salts, are injected into the subcutis to chemically ablate adipose tissue. In 2015 Kybella (deoxycholic acid, Allergan (AbbVie), Irvine, California) became the first US Food and Drug Administration (FDA)-approved injectable fat-reduction agent. It is indicated for the treatment of adults with moderate-to-severe fat in the submental neck. The product is injected into the pre-platysmal fat in 0.2-mL aliquots spaced 1 cm apart in a grid-like pattern. In clinical trials the average dose was 4–6 mL per treatment session. In these trials 28%, 43%, and 55% of treated patients had a ≥1-grade composite improvement after two, three, and four treatment sessions, respectively. In addition to submental fat, deoxycholic acid has demonstrated efficacy in the reduction of fat in other off-label areas of the body such as the jowls, abdomen, and pre-axillary area.

TABLE 10.2 Herbal Treatments for Cellulite

Herbal Name	Concentration (%)	Parts of the Plant	Main Constituents	Mechanism of Action
Bladderwrack	1	Whole dried thallus	—	Stimulates vascular flow
Butcher's broom	1–3	Rhizome and flowering tops	Saponins, ruscogenin, and neororuscogenin	Improves microcirculation
Ginkgo biloba	1–3	—	—	Improves microcirculation
Cynara scolymus or artichoke	—	Leaves, flower heads, and roots	Enzymes, cynarin, ascorbic acid, caffeoylquinine acid derivatives, and flavonoids	Reduces edema and promotes diuresis
Common ivy	2	Dried leaves, stems	Saponins (especially hederin)	Improves venous and lymphatic drainage and reduces edema
Ground ivy	2	—	Flavonoids, triterpenoids, and phenolic acids	Increases microvascular flow
Indian or horse chestnut	1–3	Seeds, shells	Triterpenoid saponins and flavones, coumarins and tannins	Reduces lysosomic enzyme activity and capillary permeability
Sweet clover	2–5	Flowers and leaves	Coumarin	Reduces lymphatic edema and capillary permeability
Centella asiatica	2–5	Leaves and roots	Asiaticoside, madecassic acid, asiatic acid	Antiinflammatory and potent healing effects
Red grapes	2–7	—	Tannins, procyanidins	Contains antioxidants that decrease lipid peroxidation and increase permeability of lymphatic and microarterial vessels
Corynanthe yohimbe, *Pausinystalia yohimbe*, and *Rauwolfia serpentina*	—	Leaves, shells, roots	Yohimbe	Stimulates metabolism of fat cells
Papaya	2–5	Fruits, leaves	Papain and bromelain (proteolytic enzymes)	Antiinflammatory effects, decreases edema

In 2020, injectable collagenase *Clostridium histolyticum* (CCH) was approved by the US FDA for the treatment of moderate-to-severe cellulite. Women treated with a series of CCH injections demonstrated appreciable improvement in cellulite as measured by investigator-performed global esthetic improvement scores (GAIS), and 10.6% and 44.6% of subjects were 2-level and 1-level composite responders, respectively.

Physical Manipulation

Endermologie (LPG Systems, Valence, France) is an FDA-cleared device that massages and kneads the skin to improve the appearance of cellulite. The device uses two rollers, as well as positive and negative pressure, to manipulate the patient's skin. The technique is thought to stimulate blood and lymphatic flow, thereby altering the architecture of the fat and improving the appearance of cellulite. In clinical studies, modest clinical improvements have been observed. A study by Gulec of 33 women who were treated with Endermologie for 15 sessions demonstrated a statistically significant improvement in the appearance of cellulite, as assessed by a visual scale; however, few of the patients (5 of the 33) actually demonstrated clinical improvement. A study by Collis et al. compared twice-weekly treatment with Endermologie with a combination treatment of aminophylline cream and Endermologie. The authors concluded that Endermologie is not an effective treatment of cellulite, although 10 out of 35 patients with Endermologie-treated legs reported that their cellulite appearance improved. In summary, Endermologie may result in modest improvements in the appearance of fat and cellulite in some patients, although it likely requires continuing treatments to maintain any improvement. Home therapy units, such as Well Box, are available to facilitate ongoing convenient treatment and may be of benefit to patients.

PEARL 4

Physical manipulation, such as Endermologie, may result in very modest, temporary improvement in the appearance of cellulite, but the results are transient and often require ongoing treatments. At-home units may be a convenient option for patients.

Subcision

Subcision is a relatively simple technique to attempt to improve the appearance of cellulite. A special notched catheter needle is placed into the subcutis of the affected area. The catheter is then physically manipulated by pushing and pulling to break up the fibrous stranding and tethers that are thought to be responsible for the appearance of cellulite. By destroying these fascial tethers, the appearance of cellulite is thought to improve. Side effects, such as ecchymosis and edema, are common. The clinical utility of this method likely varies depending on the skill of the surgeon, and its clinical utility remains to be fully determined.

In 2015, Cellfina (Merz, Frankfurt, Germany) became FDA cleared for long-term (>2 years) improvement in the appearance of cellulite on the buttocks and thighs. The device uses a vacuum-assisted approach to lyse the fibrous bands underlying cellulite. Using a motorized module, a small blade is inserted into individual dimples under local anesthesia to subcise the connective tissue band and release the dimple associated with the cellulite. In the Cellfina Registry Under Investigation for Safety and Efficacy (CRUISE) study, a total of 53 female patients underwent a single Cellfina treatment. Eighty-one percent of patients self-reported improvement in the appearance of cellulite on buttocks and thighs, with 44.4% of patients reporting improvement and 30.5% reporting much improvement. The average Clinician Global Aesthetic Improvement Score was 2.05, corresponding to much improved. The most common side effects were bleeding, blanching, fluid accumulation, ecchymosis, and induration.

Extracorporeal Shock Wave Therapy

Extracorporeal shock wave therapy (ESWT) uses electrical energy to create mechanical disruption of targeted tissues, without cytolysis. This results in tissue remodeling, neocollagenesis, and angiogenesis. ESWT on the thighs has been shown to decrease the thickness of the adipose layer, disrupt fibrous septae, and improve the appearance of cellulite. The intensity and frequency of the shockwaves in ESWT is device-dependent, and these factors may affect the clinical outcomes. Larger randomized trials are necessary to further elucidate the safety and efficacy of ESWT in adipolysis and the treatment of cellulite.

Radiofrequency Devices

Radiofrequency (RF) devices pass sinusoidal, alternating current (AC) through tissue to generate heat. The AC causes ionic flow in the treatment tissue, thereby creating heat from molecular friction. In essence, the tissue itself is the source of the heat, rather than the actual device. As a result, RF is thought to cause localized heating of a targeted tissue mass, while limiting the potential for collateral spread of energy, neuromuscular reaction, or electrolysis. Adipose tissue has high tissue resistance and a relatively low heat transfer coefficient; as a result, adipose tissue can be readily heated and the heat will be predominantly confined to the adipocytes.

Many RF devices have been advertised to improve the appearance of fat and cellulite.

The VelaSmooth and VelaShape (Syneron Candela, Irvine, California) devices combine physical manipulation (massage and suction), with bipolar RF energy and infrared light (700 to 2000 nm) to treat excess fat and cellulite. It has been proposed that these devices improve fat and cellulite by heating the subcutaneous tissue and fat, thereby causing increased localized blood flow and lipolysis. In a randomized clinical study by Nootheti et al. comparing the VelaSmooth device with another laser device for cellulite (TriActive, Cynosure Inc., Westford, Massachusetts), patients were treated twice weekly for 6 weeks. Following the treatments, patients were observed to have a reduction in the upper and lower thigh circumference, as well as in the appearance of cellulite (Figs. 10.4 and 10.5). Seventy-five percent of patients were observed to have an improvement, when comparing pre- and post treatment photographs, but the results were modest. There were no statistically significant differences in the efficacies of the two devices. Bruising can occur following treatment with the VelaSmooth device and was more common with this device than the Triactive device (Fig. 10.6).

The BodyFX (InMode, Inc., Yokneam, Israel) is an FDA-cleared device that uses a suction-coupled, bipolar RF configuration, with a built-in infrared skin surface temperature sensor to heat deep dermis and adipocytes. In addition, the device also uses trains of high-amplitude, high-voltage, ultra-short (nanosecond) pulse duration RF pulses into the preheated adipose tissue, causing irreversible electroporation (IRE) of the adipocyte cell membrane. This starts the cascade of apoptosis, ultimately resulting in permanent, programmed cell death of the adipocytes. In a clinical study of 21 patients by Boisnic et al., significant reductions in abdominal circumference (113.4 to 110.7 cm), reduction of subcutaneous adipose tissue thickness (40.5 to 38.5 mm), and reduction in adipose tissue weight were observed following a series of six treatments with the BodyFX. Importantly, histologic changes were observed, including adipocytes with decreased size and withered shape, increased levels of adipocyte apoptosis, increased collagen synthesis, and compaction and reorganization of the dermis.

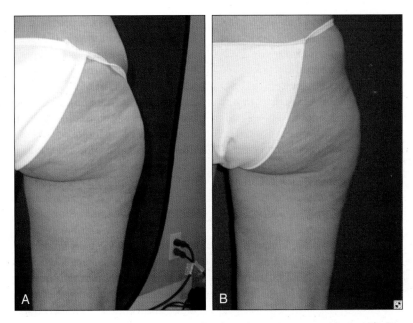

Fig. 10.4 A 47-year-old woman (A) before and (B) after six treatments with the VelaShape device. Photos courtesy of Neil S. Sadick, MD. Reprinted from Sadick NS. VelaSmooth and VelaShape. In Goldman MP, Hexsel D, eds. Cellulite: Pathophysiology and Treatment. 2nd ed. New York, NY: Informa Healthcare; 2010: 108–114.

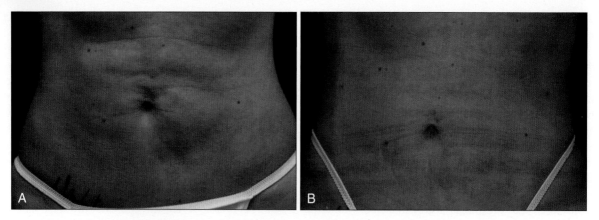

Fig. 10.5 A 37-year-old woman (A) before and (B) after seven treatments with the VelaShape device. Photographs courtesy of Neil S. Sadick, MD. Reprinted from Sadick NS. VelaSmooth and VelaShape. In Goldman MP, Hexsel D, eds. Cellulite: Pathophysiology and Treatment. 2nd ed. New York, NY: Informa Healthcare; 2010: 108–114.

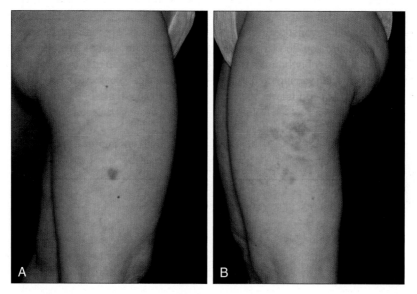

Fig. 10.6 Purpura after treatment with (A) Triactive and (B) Velasmooth. Reproduced from: Nootheti PK, Magpantay A, Yosowitz G, Calderon S, Goldman MP. A single center, randomized, comparative, prospective clinical study to determine the efficacy of the Velasmooth system versus the Triactive system for the treatment of cellulite. *Lasers Surg Med.* 2006;38:908–912.

PEARL 5

Bruising is a common side effect of laser and light source and nonsurgical device treatments for fat. Most commonly, the bruising is related to the vacuum pressure and physical manipulation of the device rather than the actual laser, light source or device

Unipolar, volumetric RF devices with more diffuse, deep heating have also been advocated for the treatment of fat and cellulite. Goldberg et al. treated 30 patients with a unipolar RF device (Accent, Alma Lasers, Buffalo Grove, Illinois) every other week for a total of six treatment sessions. A decrease in mean leg circumference of 2.45 cm was observed, although the study was limited due to a lack of comparative controls. In general, circumference is not a good end point to assess cellulite improvement. Histologic specimens did demonstrate dermal fibrosis that could explain the clinical improvement, although the results were limited.

The TruSculpt ID device (Cutera, Brisbane, CA) uses monopolar RF to selectively heat the adipose layer, resulting in an average fat reduction of 24%. With multiple stationary or gliding hand pieces, specific body areas including the abdomen, flanks, arms, extremities and submentum can be individually targeted (Video 10.1). The device allows for continuous real-time temperature monitoring, automatically adjusting the temperature to keep the fat layer at >45 deg C, while maintaining a skin temperature of 2–3 degrees cooler. A pivotal study demonstrated a mean fat thickness reduction of 1.9 cm at 3 months after a single treatment of the abdomen and flanks. Side effects include mild and self-limited discomfort, erythema, edema, and transient palpable subcutaneous nodules. Recently, RF devices have been combined with other modalities such as infrared light and ultrasound to yield even more promising results. Further clinical studies are necessary to establish the potential role for these RF devices.

Ultrasound Devices

Patients are typically accustomed to the diagnostic utility of ultrasound imaging devices. Focused ultrasound devices have also been developed to treat the subcutis and adipocytes. The Liposonix device (Solta Medical, Bausch, Bothell, WA) is FDA cleared for noninvasive waist circumference reduction. A study by Jewell et al. of the Liposonix device documented significant improvement following a single treatment session. One hundred and eighty patients were randomized to either a sham treatment or one of two doses of high-intensity focused ultrasound. Twelve weeks after the ultrasound treatment, the patients treated with the higher dose had achieved a statistically significant improvement in waist circumference compared with the sham group (−2.44 cm vs −1.43 cm). Patients were observed to have "improved" or "much improved" outcomes as assessed by physicians, and patients were satisfied with their treatments. The procedure is often painful, and bruising and edema develop after treatments. However, no significant laboratory abnormalities were observed following treatment, including lipid profiles, markers of inflammation, coagulation, liver or renal function, hematologic assessments, or blood chemistry.

The nonthermal pulsed ultrasound Ultrashape System (Syneron Candela, Marlborough, MA) received FDA approval in 2014 for the treatment of excess adipose tissue. A prospective, nonrandomized, controlled trial of 164 patients was conducted by Teitelbaum et al. to determine the efficacy of the device; 137 patients underwent one ultrasound treatment to the abdomen, thighs, or flanks; 12 weeks later, mean circumference reductions of 2.3 cm (abdomen), 1.8 cm (thighs), and 1.6 cm (flanks) were observed. The majority (77%) of the improvement in circumference was noted to occur within the first 14 days following the treatment. A later study demonstrated similarly significant improvements in abdominal fat following treatment with nonthermal pulsed ultrasound system.

Ultrasound technologies represent an evolving area within the field of noninvasive fat treatment. Initially, many of the ultrasound technologies were incorporated into liposuction treatments, known as ultrasound-assisted liposuction (UAL). However, more recently, high-intensity focused ultrasound is being developed as a stand-alone, noninvasive treatment for improving the appearance of fat and cellulite. These devices require further clinical study to determine their long-term efficacy and safety profile. Nevertheless, they represent an exciting and promising opportunity within this field.

Lasers and Light Sources

Many different light sources and lasers have been advocated as therapeutic options for fat and cellulite. Many are incorporated into liposuction procedures, known as laser-assisted liposuction (LAL); however, these devices still require invasive liposuction. Other devices have been marketed as being effective, noninvasive therapies for fat and cellulite, although definitive objective evidence of their efficacy may be lacking. Several devices that are advertised to improve fat and cellulite do not actually affect the adipocytes themselves but rather target the dermis in an attempt to stimulate collagen formation/remodeling. Devices with wavelengths in the near-infrared region, as well as intense pulsed-light (IPL) sources, fall into this category.

The TriActive device combines deep tissue massage and suction (similar to Endermologie), with contact cooling and a low-intensity diode laser (808 nm). The device purports to increase lymphatic drainage, improve blood flow, and simultaneously tighten skin in the treated areas, which is thought to improve the appearance of cellulite. Patients typically are treated with the device twice weekly, with a progressive improvement following the treatments. In clinical studies, patients were noted to achieve improvement in the appearance of cellulite, as well as objective improvement in hip and thigh circumferences. Subjective improvement included reduction in the appearance of skin dimpling, improvement in the overall contour of the limb, and improvement in overall skin texture (Fig. 10.7). The treatments were well tolerated, although many patients (approximately 20%) developed mild bruising.

The SmoothShapes device (Eleme Medical, Merrimack, New Hampshire) combines two different wavelengths with a massage system similar to Endermologie. The 915-nm diode wavelength is reported to cause liquefaction of the fat, and the 650-nm wavelength is thought to improve fat membrane permeability, thereby allowing the adipocytes to be mobilized to the interstitium. Multiple passes with the device are typically performed during a treatment session, with two to three sessions being performed each week for best results. In clinical studies by Lach and Kulick the SmoothShapes device resulted in reduction of the thickness of the subcutaneous fat pad, as assessed by MRI. The device was well tolerated with no significant associated adverse events.

The VelaSmooth and VelaShape devices combine physical manipulation with RF energy, as well as infrared energy, to facilitate a multimodality approach to fat and cellulite treatment. The efficacy of these devices was previously discussed in the above section on RF. In addition to combining different types of modalities, recent studies have investigated the use of combining lasers of different wavelengths to achieve reductions in the adipose layer and induce skin tightening. One study investigating the combination of 1064 nm Nd:YAG and 2940 nm Er:YAG wavelengths in the treatment of abdominal fat demonstrated significant reductions in waist circumference, diminution of the fatty layer, and improvement of skin laxity.

Fat-specific Laser

SculpSure (Cynosure Inc., Westford, Massachusetts) is an FDA-cleared laser-based device for noninvasive lipolysis (Video 10.2). In comparison with the laser devices discussed previously, SculpSure uses a 1060-nm diode laser to specifically target adipocytes. This wavelength of light effectively heats the adipocytes with minimal heating of the dermis and surrounding tissue. The device cycles through heating and cooling phases during the 25 minutes of treatment to heat and maintain the adipocytes to a temperature between 42°C and 47°C. This heating of the adipocytes causes them to undergo heat-stimulated apoptosis, and the adipocytes

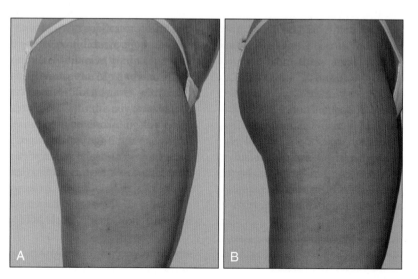

Fig. 10.7 Cellulite treatment with Triactive: subject (A) before and (B) following 10 treatments. (Reproduced from Boyce S, Pabby A, Chuchaltkaren P, Brazzini B, Goldman MP. Clinical evaluation of a device for the treatment of cellulite: Triactive. *Am J Cosmet Surg.* 2005;22:233–237.)

are then cleared by the body's lymphatic system over the 6–12 weeks. Fat volume (as measured by MRI) may be reduced by an average of 24% following a single treatment with SculpSure.

Cryolipolysis

CoolSculpting (Allergan (AbbVie), Pleasanton, California) is an FDA-cleared device for noninvasive fat reduction; it uses cryolipolysis technology to selectively cool fat, extracting energy, and ultimately causing apoptosis. The treatment consists of applying a treatment applicator to the patient's desired treatment area. Areas that can be effectively and safely treated with cryolipolysis include the abdomen, flanks, upper arms, pre-axillary fat, inner and outer thighs, and the sub-mentum (Videos 10.3 and 10.4). A moderate vacuum is then created by the device, drawing the tissue between the treatment plates and clamping down on local cutaneous blood flow to increase the efficiency of cooling. The treatment cycle ranges from 35 to 75 minutes, at the conclusion of which the skin appears cool, firm, and red. The tissue is typically molded into the shape of the treatment applicator. At the conclusion of the treatment, the clinician massages the area manually or with the help of an acoustic wave device to break up any crystallized adipocytes. Over the next several weeks to months, the adipocytes are mobilized and eliminated by the body (Case Study 2).

In a clinical study a significant reduction in the thickness of the fat in the treatment area was observed following a single CoolSculpting treatment (mean fat pad thickness reduction of 22.4%, as measured on high-resolution ultrasound). Of the 32 patients in the study, all had achieved a significant visible contour improvement following a single treatment. The best results were in patients with localized, discrete fat bulges. Another study demonstrated that 79% of patients reported clinical improvement in the appearance of their abdominal fat 2–4 months following a single CoolSculpting treatment. A study of 42 patients treated on the inner thighs showed a 0.9-cm circumferential reduction and 2.8-mm reduction in fat thickness, as measured by ultrasound. In these studies, the treatment was well tolerated, and may even lead to some degree of skin tightening.

Patients may bruise following the procedure, likely due to the vacuum effect of the device. With the newer applicators suction has been modified which has reduced

> ## CASE STUDY 2
>
> A 53-year-old female, who is 5'6" (1.68 m) tall and weighs 145 pounds (66 kg), presents for treatment of small pockets of excess fat around her abdomen. She would like to discuss noninvasive treatment options because she is concerned about the risks of invasive surgery.
>
> This patient's BMI is 23.4, which is within the normal range. She does have localized pockets of excess adipose tissue below the umbilicus, without substantial skin redundancy. This patient could be a good candidate for localized, tumescent liposuction, if she desired. However, she states she does not want an invasive procedure. After discussing options, she elects to have the area treated with CoolSculpting. The proposed treatment area is marked (a separate, but representative patient is shown in Fig. 10.8A). Due to the size, two applications in the same treatment session will be necessary to treat the complete area, each marked with an X (see Fig. 10.8B). A pinch test is performed to ensure that the area can be effectively elevated in the device (see Fig. 10.8C). The patient undergoes treatment with no adverse effects.
>
> It is important to remind the patient that the full effect of the treatment will not be visible for 2–3 months. In the post-procedure photo, taken 16 weeks after the patient's single cryolipolysis treatment session, a noticeable reduction in the volume and appearance of the abdominal fat "muffin top" is clearly observable (see Figs. 10.8D and 10.8E).

the frequency of bruising. Many patients develop transient altered sensation, numbness, or even sharp pain in the treatment area, lasting up to 2 weeks. In rare instances the pain is sufficient to warrant treatment with medications such as pregabalin or gabapentin. No significant changes in lipid profiles or liver function tests following cryolipolysis have been demonstrated in either the initial animal studies or human clinical studies. There is a cost for each treatment cycle for the treating physician (i.e., disposable). No cases of scarring or ulceration of the skin have been reported to date. However, there have been reports of paradoxical adipose hyperplasia (PAH), where the treated area develops increased fat following the CoolSculpting; fortunately, this event is rare, occurring in 0.02%–0.39% of patients. If PAH occurs, we recommend avoidance of any other noninvasive fat reduction procedures and treatment with traditional liposuction.

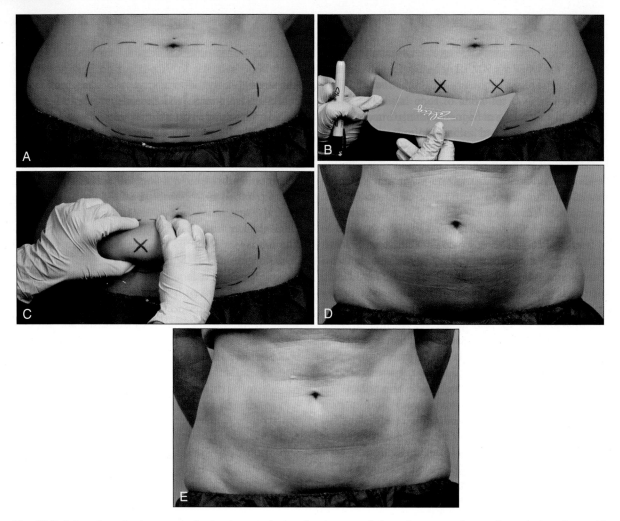

Fig. 10.8 A female patient presents for treatment of a localized accumulation of excess adipose tissue below the umbilicus. (A) The treatment area is outlined by the treating physician. (B) The treating physician then compares the size of the treatment applicator with the planned treatment area. In this case, given the size of the planned treatment area, two treatment applications will be necessary to treat the entire area. The center of each treatment area is marked with an X. (C) A pinch test is performed on the area prior to the treatment to ensure that the area can be effectively elevated in the device. (D) A baseline photograph of the treatment area is taken prior to the patient's cryolipolysis treatment. (E) The patient is shown 16 weeks after a single cryolipolysis treatment to the abdomen. Note the significant improvement in the appearance of the thickness of the fat pad. (Photos (A to C) courtesy of Zeltiq Inc., Pleasanton, CA. Photos (D) and (E) courtesy of Dr Flor Mayoral, Coral Gables, FL and Zeltiq Inc., Pleasanton, CA, USA.)

Since its introduction to the market, the CoolSculpting device has evolved over the years with the addition of multiple applicators for use on different body areas. Furthermore, the applicators have developed similarly, affording the patient quicker, more effective, and more comfortable treatments. The latest CoolSculpting Elite handpieces allow for more tissue contact, more suction, more even cooling, and faster treatments, as now each device can deliver two simultaneous treatments through two separate Elite handpieces. As such, practices with two devices can treat 4 body areas at once.

PEARL 6

Following a CoolSculpting treatment, gentle massage of the treated area should be performed to break up crystallized adipocytes and improve the efficacy of the treatment.

In sum, cryolipolysis is a safe, effective, and simple procedure, which will gradually reduce the appearance of unwanted fat over 2–4 months post treatment. It should be noted that the device works best for localized, discrete fat bulges and is not intended for the treatment of obesity or as a substitute for large-volume liposuction.

CONCLUSION

The field of noninvasive body contouring has evolved rapidly in the last several years. Although liposuction and surgical procedures remain the gold standard for patients seeking large-volume fat removal, these noninvasive options represent simple procedures with limited or no downtime to improve the appearance of fat and cellulite. Topical creams, injectable agents, and physical manipulation all represent options for patients seeking noninvasive treatments.

Within the realm of lasers, light sources, and devices, there are numerous options for patients, including RF, focused ultrasound, lasers, and cryolipolysis. These technologies are relatively new within the last decade, and the ultimate treatment efficacy will continue to be established through controlled clinical trials. Head-to-head studies comparing the devices are currently limited, and as a result it is difficult to definitively compare the efficacy of the devices. The best option for your patient ultimately depends on their treatment goals and expectations.

FURTHER READING

ASDS Survey on Dermatologic Procedures. ASDS. American Society for Dermatologic Surgery. 2021. https://www.asds.net/medical-professionals/practice-resources/asds-survey-on-dermatologic-procedures.

Bass LS, Kaminer MS. Insights into the pathophysiology of cellulite: a review. *Dermatol Surg*. 2020;46(suppl 1):S77–S85.

Bhatia A, Hu E, Kothare A. Abdominal circumference reduction using a non-invasive monopolar radiofrequency device—a pivotal study with 70 subjects. Paper presented at 2017 Annual ASLMS Meeting; San Diego, CA.

Boisnic S, Divaris M, Nelson AA, Gharavi NM, Lask GP. A clinical and biological evaluation of a novel, noninvasive radiofrequency device for the long-term reduction of adipose tissue. *Lasers Surg Med*. 2014;46(2):94–103.

Byun SY, Kwon SH, Heo SH, Shim JS, Du MH, Na JI. Efficacy of slimming cream containing 3.5% water-soluble caffeine and xanthenes for the treatment of cellulite: clinical study and literature review. *Ann Dermatol*. 2015;27(3):243–249.

Carruthers J, Stevens WG, Carruthers A, Humphrey S. Cryolipolysis and skin tightening. *Dermatol Surg*. 2014;40(suppl 12):S184–S189.

Collis N, Elliot LA, Sharpe C, Sharpe DT. Cellulite treatment: a myth or reality: a prospective randomized, controlled trial of two therapies, endermologie and aminophylline cream. *Plast Reconstr Surg*. 1999;104(4):1110–1114.

Derrick C, Shridharani S, Broyles J. The safety and efficacy of cryolipolysis: A systemic review of available literature. *Aesthet Surg J*. 2015;35(7):830–836.

Dierickx CC, Mazar JM, Sand M, Koenig S, Arigon V. Safety, tolerance, and patient satisfaction with noninvasive cryolipolysis. *Dermatol Surg*. 2013;39(8):1209–1216.

Dover JS, Kenkel JM, Carruthers A, Lizzul PF, Gross TM, Subramanian M, et al. Management of patient experience with ATX-101 (deoxycholic acid injection) for reduction of submental fat. *Dermatol Surg*. 2016;42(suppl 1):S288–S299.

Dover JS, Shridharani SM, Bloom JD, Somogyi C, Gallagher CJ. Reduction of submental fat continues beyond 28 days after ATX-101 treatment: results from a post hoc analysis. *Dermatol Surg*. 2018;44(11):1477–1479.

Glogau RG, Glaser DA, Callender VD, Yoelin S, Dover JS, Green JB, et al. A double-blind, placebo-controlled, phase 3b study of atx-101 for reduction of mild or extreme submental fat. *Dermatol Surg*. 2019;45(12):1531–1541.

Goldberg DJ, Fazeli A, Berlin AL. Clinical, laboratory and MRI analysis of cellulite treatment with a unipolar radiofrequency device. *Dermatol Surg*. 2008;34(2):204–209.

Goldman MP, Sadick NS, Young L. Phase 2a, randomized, double-blind, placebo-controlled dose-ranging study of repeat doses of collagenase *Clostridium histolyticum* for the treatment of edematous fibrosclerotic panniculopathy (cellulite). *J Am Acad Dermatol*. 2015;72:AB19.

Gulec AT. Treatment of cellulite with LPG endermologie. *Int J Dermatol*. 2009;48(3):265–270.

Hexsel D, Siega C, Schilling-Souza J, Porto MD, Rodrigues TC. A comparative study of the anatomy of adipose tissue in areas with and without raised lesions of cellulite using magnetic resonance imaging. *Dermatol Surg*. 2013;39(12):1877–1886.

Hugul H, Oba MC, Kutlubay Z. Efficacy of focused radiofrequency with ultrasound in body contouring: A study of 64 patients. *J Cosmet Dermatol.* 2021;20(8):2507–2511.

Humphrey S, Sykes J, Kantor J, Bertucci V, Walker P, Lee DR, et al. ATX-101 for reduction of submental fat: a phase III randomized controlled trial. *J Am Acad Dermatol.* 2016;75(4):788–797.e7.

Jewell ML, Baxter RA, Cox SE, et al. Randomized sham-controlled trial to evaluate the safety and effectiveness of a high-intensity focused ultrasound device for noninvasive body sculpting. *Plast Reconstr Surg.* 2011;128(1):253–262.

Jones DH, Carruthers J, Joseph JH, Callender VD, Walker P, Lee DR, et al. REFINE-1, a multicenter, randomized, double-blind, placebo-controlled, phase 3 trial with ATX-101, an injectable drug for submental fat reduction. *Dermatol Surg.* 2016;42(1):38–49.

Kaminer MS, Coleman 3rd WP, Weiss RA, Robinson DM. Coleman WP, 4th, Hornfeldt C. Multicenter pivotal study of vacuum-assisted precise tissue release for the treatment of cellulite. *Dermatol Surg.* 2015;41(3):336–347.

Kesty K, Goldberg DJ. Combination treatment with 150 W bipolar radiofrequency, infrared light, and ultrasound-induced lipolysis for thigh circumference reduction. *J Cosmet Dermatol.* 2020;19(9):2301–2305.

Klein KB, Zelickson B, Riopelle JG, et al. Non-invasive cryolipolysis for subcutaneous fat reduction does not affect serum lipid levels or liver function tests. *Lasers Surg Med.* 2009;41(10):785–790.

Kligman AM, Pagnoni A, Stoudemayer T. Topical retinol improves cellulite. *J Dermatolog Treat.* 1999;10:119–125.

Kulick MI. Evaluation of a noninvasive, dual-wavelength laser-suction and massage device for the regional treatment of cellulite. *Plast Reconstr Surg.* 2010;125(6): 1788–1796.

Lach R. Reduction of subcutaneous fat and improvement in cellulite appearance by dual-wavelength, low-level laser energy combined with vacuum and massage. *J Cosmet Laser Ther.* 2008;10(4):202–209.

Manstein D, Laubach H, Watanabe K, et al. Selective cryolysis: a novel method of non-invasive fat removal. *Lasers Surg Med.* 2008;40(9):595–604.

Ngamdokmai N, Waranuch N, Chootip K, Jampachaisri K, Scholfield CN, Ingkaninan K. Cellulite reduction by modified thai herbal compresses; a randomized double-blind trial. *J Evid Based Integr Med.* 2018;23: 2515690X18794158.

Nikolis A, Enright KM. A multicenter evaluation of paradoxical adipose hyperplasia following cryolipolysis for fat reduction and body contouring: a review of 8, 658 cycles in 2, 114 patients. *Aesthet Surg J.* 2021;41(8):932–941.

Nootheti PK, Magpantay A, Yosowitz G, Calderon S, Goldman MP. A single center, randomized, comparative, prospective clinical study to determine the efficacy of the Velasmooth system versus the Triactive system for the treatment of cellulite. *Lasers Surg Med.* 2006;38(10):908–912.

Pierard-Franchiemont C, Pierand GE, Henry F, Vroome V, Cauwenbergh G. A randomized, placebo controlled trial of topical retinal in the treatment of cellulite. *Am J Clin Dermatol.* 2000;1(6):369–374.

Rudolph C, Hladik C, Hamade H, Frank K, Kaminer MS, Hexsel D, et al. Structural gender dimorphism and the biomechanics of the gluteal subcutaneous tissue: implications for the pathophysiology of cellulite. *Plast Reconstr Surg.* 2019;143(4):1077–1086.

Sadick NS, Goldman MP, Liu G, Shusterman NH, McLane MP, Hurley D, et al. Collagenase *Clostridium histolyticum* for the treatment of edematous fibrosclerotic panniculopathy (cellulite): a randomized trial. *Dermatol Surg.* 2019;45(8):1047–1056.

Schilling L, Saedi N, Weiss R. 1060 nm diode hyperthermic laser lipolysis:the latest in non-invasive body contouring. *J Drugs Dermatol.* 2017;16(1):48–52.

Shridharani SM. Injection of an adipocytolytic agent for reduction of excess periaxillary fat. *Aesthet Surg J.* 2019;39(12):NP495–NP503. 13.

Shridharani SM. Improvement in jowl fat following ATX-101 treatment: results from a single-site study. *Plast Reconstr Surg.* 2020;145(4):929–935.

Vas K, Besenyi Z, Urban S, Badawi A, Pavics L, Eros G, et al. Efficacy and safety of long pulse 1064 and 2940 nm lasers in noninvasive lipolysis and skin tightening. *J Biophotonics.* 2019;12(9):e201900083.

Weinstein Velez M, Ibrahim O, Petrell K, Dover JS. Nonthermal pulsed ultrasound treatment for the reduction in abdominal fat: a pilot study. *J Clin Aesthet Dermatol.* 2018;11(9):32–36.

Young VL, DiBernardo BE. Comparison of cellulite severity scales and imaging. *Methods. Aesthet Surg J.* 2021;41(6):NP521–NP537.

Zelickson BD, Burns AJ, Kilmer SL. Cryolipolysis for safe and effective inner thigh fat reduction. *Lasers Surg Med.* 2015;47(2):120–127.

11

Muscle Toning and Contouring

Leah Spring and John Peters

SUMMARY AND KEY FEATURES

- Enhancement of muscular tone is a new frontier in noninvasive body contouring, with both cosmetic and functional implications.
- Treatment of the muscle must be always considered in context with the overlying adipose layer—an excess amount of adipose will reduce or obscure the cosmetic effect of treatment.
- Electromagnetic muscle stimulation (EMMS) utilizes electromagnetic muscle induction to stimulate motor nerves and induce repetitive and maximal muscular contraction
- Neuromuscular electrical stimulation (NMES) utilizes applied electrical current via surface electrodes on the skin to directly stimulate motor nerves, resulting in maximal contraction of skeletal muscle fibers.
- Muscle toning and contouring devices can be combined with other technologies such as cryolipolysis for a synergistic effect.

INTRODUCTION

A "toned and tight" physique has traditionally been the hard-won outcome of a long-term healthy diet, consistent strength training regimen, and a little bit of genetic luck. Attrition rates for those attempting a disciplined diet and exercise program can be high due to waning motivation and lack of time, and the goal of "chiseled abs" is frequently replaced by other pursuits. Alternatively, those who either approximate or achieve their body goals are frequently interested in gaining an esthetic edge.

Until recently, the field of noninvasive body contouring has focused on the reduction of subcutaneous fat by inducing adipocyte apoptosis. As interest has grown to further enhance body contouring by inducing muscle hypertrophy and improving tone, established technologies with historically functional applications have been repurposed for novel esthetic applications.

With a maturing body of supporting literature and growing practitioner experience, two technologies, electromagnetic muscle stimulation (EMMS) and neuromuscular electrical stimulation (NMES), have emerged as options for patients interested in toning the underlying muscle layer as an alternative or supplement to traditional resistance training programs. Available EMMS (EmSculpt® and CoolTone®) and NMES (truSculpt flex®) devices provide patients with a more firm and toned appearance with favorable risk-reward profiles. The goal of this chapter is to review these emerging technologies with emphasis on their mechanisms, clinical results, side effect profiles, and patient selection so as they may be best applied in the clinical setting to further improve esthetic body contouring.

PEARL 1

Photographs, weight, and circumference measurements (thigh, abdomen, and arm as applicable) should be included in each patient's baseline evaluation and posttreatment assessment.

PEARL 2

Patients should be instructed to maintain a healthy diet and regular exercise program to enhance and prolong the durability of their results.

ELECTROMAGNETIC MUSCLE STIMULATION

EMMS utilizes the concept of electromagnetic muscle induction, first described by Faraday in 1831, to stimulate motor nerves. A rapidly alternating magnetic field produced by a wire coil applied near the treatment area secondarily generates an electrical current within the tissue. The current depolarizes motor neurons which leads to muscle contractions. The application of magnetic stimulation is generally painless as it preferentially depolarizes larger diameter, lower-resistance motor nerves and leaves smaller diameter, higher-resistance nerves unaffected, such as cutaneous nociceptors.

EMMS-induced motor nerve stimulation bypasses central and peripheral neural pathways. Thus, full activation of the skeletal muscle can be achieved, as contraction is not limited (as during voluntary muscle contraction) by firing rates and conductivity of these pathways. Additionally, by delivering pulses in a high frequency, EMMS prevents full relaxation of the muscle. The result is a supramaximal or tetanic contraction, a phenomenon not achieved by voluntary muscle contraction. This highly stressful condition triggers changes in the muscles as an adaptive response to these conditions which is felt to be beneficial for hypertrophy and hyperplasia.

EMMS has been used historically for the treatment of musculoskeletal and urogynecological disorders. A growing body of literature now supports the application of EMMS technology in the field of esthetic medicine, specifically noninvasive body contouring.

Currently, there are two commercially available, esthetically marketed, FDA approved EMMS devices: EmSculpt® (BTL Industries, Marlborough, MA) and CoolTone® (Zeltiq Aesthetics Inc, Pleasanton, CA). EmSculpt® received approval in 2016 for strengthening, firming, and toning the abdomen, buttocks, thighs, arms, and calves. Of note, studies investigating EmSculpt® often refer to "HIFEM" (high intensity focused electromagnetic) therapy, a proprietary term specific to this device. CoolTone® was approved in 2019 for strengthening,

toning, and firming of abdomen, buttocks, and thighs. Treatment protocols for both devices generally consist of four 30-minute treatment sessions over the course of 2 weeks, at 2- to 3-day intervals.

When applied to the abdomen of subjects, four treatments using EMMS resulted in an average waist circumference reduction of $4.37 +/- 2.63$ cm ($P < .01$) and improved esthetic appearance of the abdomen. Katz et al. observed a 19% and 23% reduction in subcutaneous abdominal fat thickness using ultrasound assessment at 1 and 3 months respectively. MRI assessment after four EMMS treatments showed simultaneous muscle growth (15.4% increase in rectus abdominis muscle thickness), fat reduction (18.6% reduction in adipose tissue thickness), and improvement in diastasis recti (10.4% reduction in rectus abdominis separation). The result was an average reduction in abdominal waist circumference by 3.8 cm, and these changes were sustained at 6 months. Similar findings were reported by Kent and Jacob after eight treatments but the investigators noted most waist reduction was observed after the fourth treatment. None of these studies demonstrated significant weight change following EMMS treatment.

Studies also demonstrate the applicability of EMMS to noninvasive buttock augmentation and lifting. Busso et al. showed esthetically favorable changes in buttocks shape and volume while providing buttocks lifting and reduction in muscle laxity. Patients reported high satisfaction scores, and no treatment-associated discomfort was described. Jacob et al. also showed that EMMS resulted in a lifting effect of the buttocks, improvement in gluteal folds, overall buttocks tightness, and improved patient confidence and satisfaction. Palm used MRI to objectively demonstrate a significant increase in the size of the examined muscles at 1-month ($+10.81 +/- 1.60\%$) and 3-month ($+13.23 +/- 0.91\%$) follow-up. Gluteal adipose tissue and weight were not significantly affected.

Limited data supports the applicability of EMMS to arms and calves. In two patients treated with EMMS, MRI evaluation showed increases in biceps, triceps, and gastrocnemius muscle masses by 17.1%, 10.2%, and 14.6 % respectively with coincident reduction in subcutaneous fat thickness in the arm and calf by 12.8% and 9.9%.

Several studies have explored the microscopic effect of EMMS on muscle and fat with mixed results. Duncan and Dinev used histopathologic assessment to reveal a hypertrophic effect of EMMS application on a cellular level. Histological assessment of biopsied muscle samples obtained from an in-vivo porcine model after four treatments demonstrated an increase in muscle mass density by 20.56% two weeks posttreatment compared to baseline. Similarly, muscle fiber density increased, and the size of individual muscle fibers increased by 12.15%. Weiss and Bernardy used biopsy and blood specimens also from an in-vivo porcine model to show a statistically significant increase in adipocyte apoptosis and biochemical evidence of alteration to fat and muscle metabolism. A follow-up study conducted by Zachary et al. on human subjects did not show histological evidence of fat cell injury or inflammatory response.

EMMS can be combined with other technologies for synergistic effect. Kilmer et al. found one treatment of cyrolipolysis in addition to a four-treatment session using EMMS resulted in superior abdominal circumference reduction and satisfaction scores than EMMS alone and cyrolipolysis alone.

Treatment with EMMS is generally very well tolerated. Side effects to treatment include myalgias, temporary muscle spasm, arthralgias, and erythema at the treatment site. Patients may also experience muscle fatigue which typically resolves within 12–48 hours. Contraindications include metal or electrical devices or implants including but not limited to pacemakers, implanted hearing devices, implanted defibrillators, implanted neurostimulators, drug pumps, and hearing aids. Use of EMMS is not recommended in patients with fever, malignancy, hemorrhagic conditions, epilepsy, recent surgery, pulmonary insufficiency, Graves' disease, or pregnancy. EMMS should not be used over areas of active skin dermatitis or infection, a menstruating uterus, heart or head areas, areas of new bone growth, carotid sinus, neck or mouth sites, or skin with abnormal sensation (Case Study 1).

NEUROMUSCULAR ELECTRICAL STIMULATION

NMES utilizes applied electrical current via surface electrodes on the skin to directly stimulate motor nerves, resulting in contraction of skeletal muscle fibers. In contrast to a voluntary muscular contraction, during which smaller motor units composed primarily of Type I (slow twitch, fatigue-resistant) fibers are recruited first, NMES muscular contraction preferentially recruits Type II

CASE STUDY 1

A 34-year-old female patient presents to discuss options for abdominal firming and toning. She is 6 months postpartum and is otherwise healthy without any implanted metal or devices. She is currently menstruating. The patient states that she is interested in a non-invasive procedure but is worried about pain. She also wonders if she will experience any weight loss from the procedure.

The patient is 5'6" (1.68 m) tall and weighs 141 pounds (64 kg) with a body-mass index (BMI) of 22.8. Localized pockets of excessive adipose tissue in the periumbilical region with some muscle laxity and diastasis recti are appreciated. A pinch test is performed to estimate the thickness of the subcutaneous fat layer and was found to be less than 3 cm.

After evaluation, she is found to be a good candidate for treatment using EMMS. However, EMMS is not recommended over top of an actively menstruating uterus as this can intensify menstrual cramping. She was also counseled that EMMS has not been shown to significantly alter body weight in clinical trials. She elects to proceed with EMMS and returns following completion of her menstrual cycle for treatment.

The patient completes four treatment sessions using EMMS spaced over 2 weeks, each session lasting 30 minutes. She describes the sensation during treatment as "strange" but not painful. Following each treatment, she experiences transient muscle fatigue which resolves within 24 hours of treatment. No other adverse effects are noted. She appreciates improvements in muscle tone and happily notes that her jeans fit better. Objectively, there is reduction of her diastasis recti and corresponding waist circumference.

(fast twitch fibers) first, as the larger diameter of their motor nerves have a relatively low threshold to electrical stimulation. As these fibers begin to fatigue, remote motor units with higher thresholds are recruited.

PEARL 3

NMES produces muscle contractions through high frequency (20–50 Hz) stimulation of motor nerves. In contrast, transcutaneous electrical nerve stimulation (TENS), utilizes low frequencies (2–10 Hz), which target sensory nerve fibers to override pain impulses. TENS does not produce a muscular contraction.

NMES is well established in the literature as a method to increase muscular strength and improve functional performance. The use of NMES is reported as early as 1964 and over the past 6 decades, has been a treatment modality utilized by rehabilitation specialists, orthopedic surgeons, and athletes to improve strength, increase range of motion, and decrease atrophy and pain. Notably, the body of literature regarding NMES originates almost exclusively from these specialties and contains marked heterogeneity in patient populations (baseline body habitus, comorbidities, and levels of physicality), treatment protocols, and frequency capabilities of the devices studied.

A Cochrane review by Jones et al. of 18 studies involving over 900 participants with COPD, chronic heart failure, and cancer demonstrated statistically significant improvements in quadriceps muscle strength compared to control, increase in muscle mass, and statistically significant improvements in exercise performance. The overall GRADE quality of evidence was deemed "low." Other studies evaluating the use of NMES for spinal cord injuries and ICU patients demonstrated equivocal results. In a study of healthy adults, NMES was shown to induce statistically significant increases in muscle size of the rectus abdominus and lateral abdominal wall by magnetic resonance imaging, and in the same study population, improve strength and endurance of abdominal muscles and lumbopelvic stability.

NMES has been rigorously evaluated as a method to expedite recovery following surgery. NMES has an established application for the care of patients post-Anterior Cruciate Ligament (ACL) repair; multiple studies have demonstrated expedited recovery, reduced muscle atrophy, and earlier return to sport. Notable to the field of esthetics, Taradaj et al. found that though NMES led to a statistically significant increase in quadriceps strength compared to exercise-only cohort in soccer players post-ACL reconstruction, only modest increases in quadriceps circumference (+1.4% vs. +0.6% for the exercise-only cohort) were appreciated. This outcome can be explained by Kraemer's observation in 1996 that initial increases in muscular force production is largely mediated by neural factors rather than visible hypertrophy of muscle fibers in healthy adults. Visible hypertrophy of muscle fibers is usually not evident until training is conducted over a longer period of time (greater than 8 weeks). In other words, functional benefits precede appreciable changes in form.

Recently, NMES has emerged as a useful tool for cosmetic shaping and toning. The truSculpt flex® (Cutera,

Brisbane, CA) is the first commercially available, esthetically marketed NMES device. It is FDA-cleared to strengthen, firm, and tone the abdomen, buttocks, and thighs. This device features eight paired (one positive, one negative), color-coded surface electrodes (6 cm × 6 cm). Each of the 16 electrodes are placed on adhesive gel pads applied to bare skin for the simultaneous treatment of up to eight treatment areas (traditionally the rectus abdominus, external abdominal obliques, and rectus femoris; Fig. 11.1 and Video 11.1). Three treatment mode options ("Prep Mode," "Tone Mode," and "Sculpt Mode") create multiple types of muscle contraction that replicate intensified twisting, squatting, and abdominal crunch actions. "Prep Mode" is designed for nonactive patients, whereas "Tone Mode" and "Sculpt Mode" are designed for active patients, with the intent to increase strength and endurance, and build muscle mass, respectively. Tone Mode features a treatment protocol that includes 30 minutes of "initial intensity" followed by 15 minutes of "high intensity interval training" (HIIT). Sculpt Mode starts with 15 minutes of initial intensity, and transitions to 30 minutes of HIIT. Intensity can be manually increased by either the operator or the patient on scale of "0" to "100" throughout each 45-minute treatment session. It is the experience of the authors that a starting intensity of 15–35 is reasonable for most patients, and that this this intensity should be increased at regular intervals over the treatment cycle to continually elicit the maximum muscle contraction without unacceptable discomfort. It is the rare (and very fit) patient who can achieve an intensity of 100 on this device. Most patients will experience mild to moderate tingling or numbness that usually resolves within several hours (but can last up to 24 hours). Other commonly-reported effects are mild to moderate erythema localized to the treatment sites, muscle soreness, and mild random muscle contractions. Rarely reported effects include a mildly increased heart rate, skin hypersensitivity, frequent urination, and increased hunger (all of which resolve in 24 hours).

PEARL 4

Treatment with NMES, though tolerable, should not be "comfortable" to achieve maximal results. The patient should feel like they are doing work. If a patient is happily scrolling on their phone or chatting, it is time to increase intensity by 1–2 points.

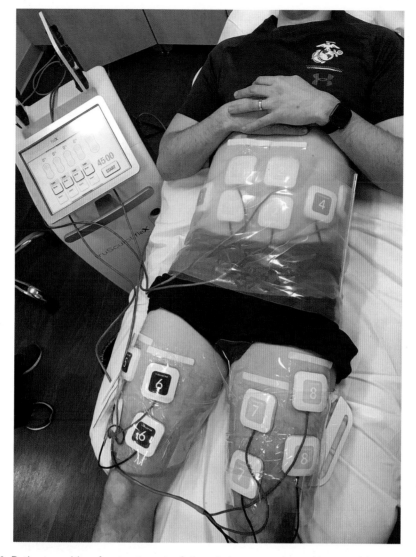

Fig. 11.1 Patient position for treatment of the abdomen and quadriceps with neuromuscular electrical stimulation (NMES).

Preliminary data by Ronan demonstrated an average 30% increase in muscle mass and a modest reduction in overlying adipose thickness on ultrasound imaging following four to six treatment sessions with the truSculpt flex®. Spring et al. conducted a prospective, randomized, controlled pilot trial that evaluated both the functional and esthetic performance of the truSculpt flex®, and found that four treatments led to statistically significant improvements in both abdominal and quadriceps strength and endurance, sustained through 4-weeks posttreatment. Subject satisfaction for both functional and esthetic improvements was reported as "satisfied" or "very satisfied" in 89% and 92% at 4 weeks and 8 weeks posttreatment, respectively. Mean waist circumference decreased, and quadriceps circumference increased nonsignificantly (Figs. 11.2 and 11.3).

Despite modest improvements in muscular esthetics and tone (which is appreciable not in isolation, but in conjunction with the overlying adipose layer), it has been the experience of the authors that our patients

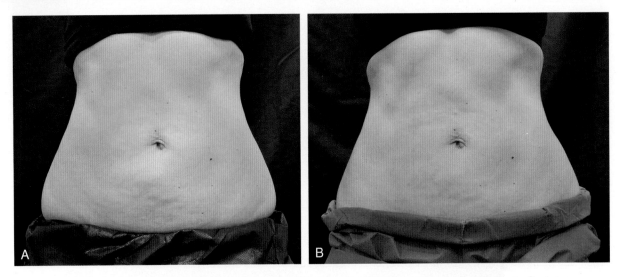

Fig. 11.2 A 43-year-old-woman: (A) before and (B) 4-weeks after four treatments with the truSculpt flex® device. (Photographs courtesy Leah Spring, DO.)

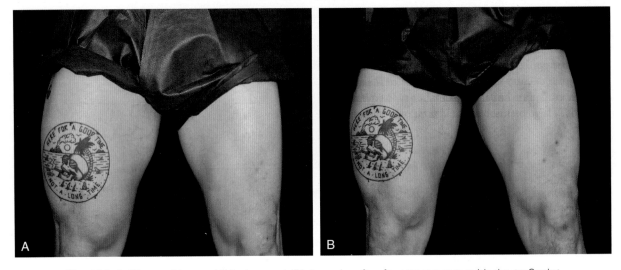

Fig. 11.3 A 27-year-old-man: (A) before and (B) 4-weeks after four treatments with the truSculpt flex® device. (Photographs courtesy Leah Spring, DO.)

more readily remark on increased ease of climbing stairs, reduced fatigue when running, improved ability to perform at the gym, stabilization of their core, and even reduced back pain. Our clinical observation is support by the previously reviewed literature on muscle strength and functional performance following NMES treatment (Case Studies 2 and 3).

PATIENT EVALUATION AND EXPECTATION MANAGEMENT

Visible changes to the muscle can only be appreciated in context with the overlying adipose layer, which can potentially obscure esthetic improvements of muscular hypertrophy. In addition to affecting the esthetic outcome, adipose can affect treatment efficacy. The

CASE STUDY 2

A 32-year-old female who is 5'5" (1.65 m) tall and weighs 168 pounds (76 kg) is interested in a body contouring procedure prior to her wedding next month. She states she wants to look "toned and tight" on her wedding day, does not want to pursue any invasive surgeries, and does not have time for exercise.

This patient's BMI is 28, which is in the overweight range. She does have localized pockets of excess adipose tissue below the umbilicus and lateral thighs, without substantial skin redundancy.

Expectation management and appropriate counseling prior to treatment is paramount. Because of the patient's BMI, a "toned and tight" appearance following EMMS or NMES is an unrealistic goal. These treatments will likely produce modest results she can feel, rather than visually appreciate. This patient may be better served with a CoolSculpting procedure to reduce localized adiposity. If she decides to proceed with your recommendation, she should be aware that the full effect of the treatment will not be visible for 2–3 months.

CASE STUDY 3

A 45-year-old male who is 6'1" (1.85 m) tall and weighs 175 pounds (79 kg) presents to discuss noninvasive muscle building options. He is an avid tennis player, and lifts weights once to twice weekly. He notes occasional back pain, but denies numbness, tingling, or weakness down his extremities. He is interested in a more toned appearance of his abdomen and thighs, and wouldn't mind if treatment helped his backhand.

His BMI is 23, which is in the normal range. There are no localized collections of adipose tissue, and he has an underlying visible muscular tone.

After discussing options, he elects to have his abdomen and quadriceps treated with the truSculpt flex. Sixteen electrodes are placed over the abdomen and quadriceps and intensity is increased over each individual treatment. The patient sees each treatment as a personal challenge, and tries to "beat his score" each time.

The first improvement he notes is a "more stable core." One month after his treatment course, he notes his "jeans fit better" and can visualize a modest, but appreciable improvement in the definition of his abdomen and quadriceps. He is pleasantly surprised that his back pain is markedly improved, and notes decreased fatigue and soreness after a tennis game.

subcutaneous fat separates and insulates the underlying musculature from the magnetic coil of EMMS and the direct current of NMES. Application of EMMS or NMES to patients with an overlying adipose layer greater than 3 cm in thickness may result in a reduction in stimulation intensity experienced by the muscle, and thus reduction in the intensity of muscular contractions.

Maximal esthetic results will thus be achieved by patients who are at or very near their ideal body fat composition. However, it is the belief of the authors that our potential patient base extends beyond this small cohort. Physically inactive patients who desire improved strength, endurance, and stabilization of their core (with reasonable expectations of the very modest, if any, cosmetic benefits that can be achieved) may also benefit from noninvasive muscle toning and contouring.

Pre-treatment assessment should include a history of the patient's current level of physical activity, previous musculoskeletal injuries and surgeries, and their goals of treatment. Body mass index (BMI), a person's weight in kilograms divided by their square of their height in meters, is a helpful guide to screen patients (and set expectations) prior to treatment; however, as BMI has been shown to remain stable during and after treatment with EMMS or NMES, it is not a particularly useful tool to assess response to therapy. It is our experience that photographs and circumference measurements (waist, thigh, and arm, as applicable) more accurately reflect the patient's treatment results.

Patients should be counseled that results are transient, with reports suggesting a duration of effect ranging from 8 to 12 weeks. Additional treatments will likely be required to maintain the desired result. The patient's commitment to a stable diet and regular exercise program should be encouraged.

CONCLUSION

EMMS (EmSculpt® and CoolTone®) and NMES (truSculpt flex®) devices are now in our esthetic armamentarium, allowing us to finally add the enhancement of muscle tone and strength to the noninvasive body contouring pillars of tissue tightening and reduction of fat and cellulite. When EMMS or NMES is used as an adjunct to resistance training, the combination can improve muscle function, strength, and endurance. When these devices are used in combination with a healthy diet and a baseline ideal body mass index (BMI), patients can also achieve optimal cosmetic results in the form of a more firm and toned appearance.

A limitation of both NMES and EMMS is the short term effectiveness (the "use it or lose it" principle). A waning benefit is appreciated 4–12 weeks following treatment discontinuation. Therefore, maintenance treatments will be required for sustained results. The optimal frequency of these treatments have yet to be established in the literature. However, it is the experience of the authors that two to four treatments every 2 months after the initial treatment coupled with a regular strength training program achieves both the patient's and clinician's mutual goals.

Future research will continue to refine treatment protocols, identify patient populations that can benefit from treatment, and further define the esthetic and functional roles of NMES and EMMS—both when used independently or in combination with other noninvasive body contouring treatments.

FURTHER READING

Abulhasan J, Rumble Y, Morgan E, Slatter W, Grey M. Peripheral electrical and magnetic stimulation to augment resistance. *Training. J Funct Morphol Kinesiol.* 2016;1(3):328–342.

Barker AT. An introduction to the basic principles of magnetic nerve stimulation. *J Clin Neurophysiol.* 1991;8(1):26–37.

Bickel CS, Gregory CM, Dean JC. Motor unit recruitment during neuromuscular electrical stimulation: a critical appraisal. *Eur J Appl Physiol.* 2011;111(10):2399–2407.

Busso M, Denkova R. *High-Intensity Focused Electromagnetic (HIFEM) Field Therapy Used for Non-Invasive Buttock Augmentation and Lifting: Feasibility Study.* 2019;5. http://www.imedpub.com/.

Doucet BM, Lam A, Griffin L. Neuromuscular electrical stimulation for skeletal muscle function. *Yale J Biol Med.* 2012;85(2):201–215.

Dowling JJ, Konert E, Ljucovic P, Andrews DM. Are humans able to voluntarily elicit maximum muscle force? *Neurosci Lett.* 1994;179(1-2):25–28.

Duncan D, Dinev I. Noninvasive induction of muscle fiber hypertrophy and hyperplasia: effects of high-intensity focused electromagnetic field evaluated in an in-vivo porcine model: a pilot study. *Aesthet Surg J.* 2020;40(5):568–574.

Gandevia SC. Spinal and supraspinal factors in human muscle fatigue. *Physiol Rev.* 2001;81(4):1725–1789.

Han TR, Shin HI, Kim IS. Magnetic stimulation of the quadriceps femoris muscle: comparison of pain with electrical stimulation. *Am J Phys Med Rehabil.* 2006;85(7):593–599.

Hauger AV, Reiman MP, Bjordal JM, Sheets C, Ledbetter L, Goode AP. Neuromuscular electrical stimulation is effective in strengthening the quadriceps muscle after anterior cruciate ligament surgery. *Knee Surg Sports Traumatol Arthrosc.* 2018;26(2):399–410.

Hwang UJ, Kwon OY, Jung SH, Kim HA, Gwak GT. Effect of neuromuscular electrical stimulation training for abdominal muscles on change of muscle size, strength, endurance and lumbopelvic stability. *J Sports Med Phys Fitness.* 2020;60(2):206–213.

Jacob C, Kinney B, Busso M, et al. High intensity focused electro-magnetic technology (HIFEM) for non-invasive buttock lifting and toning of gluteal muscles: a multicenter efficacy and safety study. *J Drugs Dermatol.* 2018;17(11):1229–1232.

Jacob CI, Paskova K. Safety and efficacy of a novel high-intensity focused electromagnetic technology device for noninvasive abdominal body shaping. *J Cosmet Dermatol.* 2018;17(5):783–787.

Jones DA, Bigland-Ritchie B, Edwards RHT. Excitation frequency and muscle fatigue: mechanical responses during voluntary and stimulated contractions. *Exp Neurol.* 1979;64(2):401–413.

Katz B, Bard R, Goldfarb R, Shiloh A, Kenolova D. Ultrasound assessment of subcutaneous abdominal fat thickness after treatments with a high-intensity focused electromagnetic field device: a multicenter study. *Dermatol Surg.* 2019;45(12):1542–1548.

Kilmer SL, Cox SE, Zelickson BD, et al. Feasibility study of electromagnetic muscle stimulation and cryolipolysis for abdominal contouring. *Dermatol Surg.* 2020;46(1):S14–S21.

Kinney BM, Lozanova P. High intensity focused electromagnetic therapy evaluated by magnetic resonance imaging: safety and efficacy study of a dual tissue effect based non-invasive abdominal body shaping. *Lasers Surg Med.* 2019;51(1):40–46.

Kinney BM, Kent DE. MRI and CT assessment of abdominal tissue composition in patients after high-intensity focused electromagnetic therapy treatments: one-year follow-up. *Aesthet Surg J.* 2020;40(12):NP686–NP693.

Palm M. Magnetic resonance imaging evaluation of changes in gluteal muscles after treatments with the high-intensity focused electromagnetic procedure. *Dermatol Surg.* 2021;47(3):386–391.

Ronan SJ. A novel bio-electric current stimulation device for improvement of muscle tone: the truSculpt flex [White paper]. Cutera. 2019.

Spring, LK, Petrell K, Depina J, Dover JS. Use of neuromuscular electrical stimulation for abdominal and quadriceps muscle strengthening: a randomized controlled trial [abstract]. In: American Society for Dermatologic Surgery Virtual Annual Meeting; October 9–11, 2020.

Taradaj J, Halski T, Kucharzewski M, et al. The effect of neuromuscular electrical stimulation on quadriceps strength and knee function in professional soccer players: return to sport after ACL reconstruction. *Biomed Res Int*. 2013;2013:802534.

Toth MJ, Tourville TW, Voigt TB, et al. Utility of neuromuscular electrical stimulation to preserve quadriceps muscle fiber size and contractility after anterior cruciate ligament injuries and reconstruction: a randomized, sham-controlled, blinded trial. *Am J Sports Med*. 2020; 48(10):2429–2437.

Wakahara T, Shiraogawa A. Effects of neuromuscular electrical stimulation training on muscle size in collegiate track and field athletes. *PLoS One*. 2019;14(11): e0224881.

Weiss RA, Bernardy J. Induction of fat apoptosis by a non-thermal device: mechanism of action of non-invasive high-intensity electromagnetic technology in a porcine model. *Lasers Surg Med*. 2019;51(1):47–53.

Zachary CB, Burns AJ, Pham LD, Jimenez Lozano JN. Clinical study demonstrates that electromagnetic muscle stimulation does not cause injury to fat cells. *Lasers Surg Med*. 2021;53(1):70–78.

12

Radiofrequency Microneedling

Marcus G. Tan, Anne Chapas, Jennifer MacGregor, and Shilpi Khetarpal

SUMMARY AND KEY FEATURES

- Radiofrequency microneedling is a minimally invasive modality that creates perforations in the skin and delivers radiofrequency-generated thermal energy into the underlying tissue
- The perforations created by microneedles improve transcutaneous absorption of topical products and transcutaneous elimination of skin debris
- The mechanical and thermal effects of radiofrequency microneedling cause dermal coagulation, collagen remodeling, and neoelastogenesis via a wound-healing response
- Dermatologic conditions with numerous high-quality evidence supporting its use include skin rejuvenation, acne scars, acne vulgaris, and axillary hyperhidrosis
- Other potential dermatologic indications include striae, rosacea, androgenetic alopecia, cellulite, and melasma.
- Radiofrequency microneedling is a safe option with low risk of postinflammatory hyperpigmention, even in individuals with darker skin phototypes
- Radiofrequency microneedling can be safely combined with several other therapeutic modalities to augment clinical outcomes without significant increase in risk of adverse events

INTRODUCTION

Radiofrequency devices have been used in the medical field for decades to achieve hemostasis, electrocoagulation, and endovenous closure. Within the realm of esthetic medicine, the first radiofrequency device (ThermaCool, Bausch Medical, Bothell, WA) was approved for the treatment of periocular rhytides in 2002, then facial rhytides in 2004, and subsequently extra-facial sites in 2006. Numerous radiofrequency devices for esthetic purposes have since been approved and utilize various methods of delivering radiofrequency energy to the underlying dermis and subcutis (Table 12.1). Radiofrequency energy can be delivered to the underlying dermis and subcutis via noninvasive probe-based electrodes, or minimally invasive needle-based electrodes. This chapter will focus primarily on the needle-based method, also known as radiofrequency microneedling (RFMN).

RADIOFREQUENCY

Radiofrequency energy is within the electromagnetic spectrum with a frequency ranging from 3 kHz to 300 GHz. The typical frequencies used in esthetic medicine is between 0.3 and 10 MHz. Thermal energy is generated from the tissue's intrinsic resistance, known as impedance, to the movement of electrons within the radiofrequency field. The amount of energy delivered is governed by Ohm's law and is relative to the amount of current, exposure time and impedance of target tissue (see Box 7.2).

Various structures of the skin and the underlying tissue exhibit different impedance (see Table 7.2).

TABLE 12.1 FDA-Approved Radiofrequency Microneedling Devices (Nonexhaustive)

Company	Device	Length of Needle (mm)	No. of Needles	Insulation	Fractional or Bulk	Motorized or Manual
Aesthetics Biomedical	Vivace	0.5–3.5	36	Insulated	Fractional	Motorized
Cutera	Secret	0.5–3.5	25 or 64	Noninsulated or insulated	Fractional	Motorized
Endymed	Intensif	0.5–5.0	25	Noninsulated	Fractional	Motorized
Gowoonsesang Cosmetics	AGNES	0.8–2.0	1–3	Insulated	Fractional	Manual
Inmode	Fractora	Up to 3	24, 60, or 126	Noninsulated or insulated	Fractional and bulk	Manual
Inmode	Morpheus8	2–8	25	Insulated	Fractional	Motorized
Jeisys Perigee	Intracel	0.1–2.0	36	Insulated	Fractional	Motorized
Lumenis	Voluderm	0.6–1.0	24 or 36	Noninsulated	Fractional	Manual
Lutronic	Infini	0.25–3.5	49	Insulated	Fractional	Motorized
Lutronic	Genius	0.5–4.5	49	Insulated	Fractional	Motorized
Syneron Candela	Profound	5	10	Insulated	Fractional	Manual
Syneron Candela	eMatrix	0.5	44 or 64	Noninsulated	Fractional and bulk	Manual

Courtesy Steven F. Weiner, MD.

Tissues with higher impedance, such as muscle, cartilage or wet skin, are more susceptible to heating compared to tissues with lower impedance, such as bone, fat and dry skin. The properties of an individual's tissue (thickness of skin, fat and fibrous septa, the number and size of adnexal structures) all contribute to impedance, heat perception and total energy deposited. The tissue impedance is further affected by its current temperature and in general, decreases by 2% for every 1°C increase in temperature.

POLARITY OF RADIOFREQUENCY

Radiofrequency energy can be delivered via monopolar or bipolar configuration. In monopolar configuration, current passes from a single electrode in the handpiece to a grounding pad placed on a patient's distal body part (Fig. 12.1). Monopolar configuration creates a high density of power at the electrode's surface and has the potential to heat deeper tissues such as the reticular dermis and fibroseptal network (Fig. 12.2A). In bipolar configuration, current passes between electrodes within the handpiece (Fig. 12.2B). This configuration allows for

a more controlled distribution of radiofrequency at a higher energy level, but is more limited in the depth of penetration. Other factors affecting the depth of penetration include the frequency of the electrical current, as well as temperature and types of tissues present.

COLLAGEN REMODELING

The optimal temperature to induce partial dermal collagen denaturation, neocollagenesis and neoelastogenesis is approximately 67°C. Dermal temperatures ≥69.5°C or ≤62°C result in suboptimal clinical efficacy due to overdenaturation and underdenaturation of collagen respectively. The amount of collagen denaturation is determined by a combination of temperature and exposure time (Fig. 12.3). Studies have shown that temperatures ≥85°C are needed when shorter exposure times (<1 second) are used, or temperatures 60°C–65°C are needed when longer exposure times (≥1 second) are used. To achieve the optimal treatment outcome, temperature and impedance of the tissues being treated have to be monitored so that the RFMN device delivers the

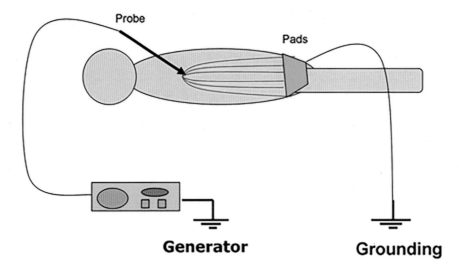

Fig. 12.1 Monopolar radiofrequency circuitry. The patient is part of the electrical circuitry, and tissue conductivity affects the zone of coagulation. (From Hong K, Georgiades C. Radiofrequency ablation: mechanism of action and devices. *J Vasc Interv Radiol.* 2010;21(8 suppl):S179–S186.)

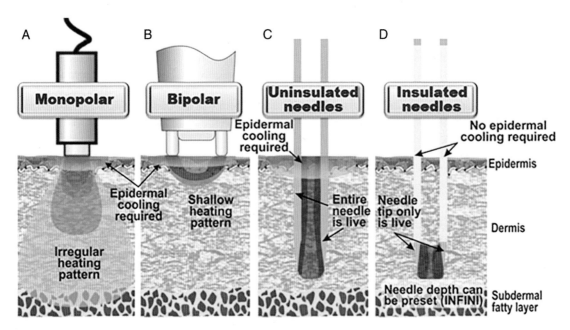

Fig. 12.2 (A) Monopolar radiofrequency. (B) Bipolar radiofrequency. (C) Uninsulated microneedles showing epidermal and dermal coagulation. (D) Insulated microneedles showing dermal coagulation only. (From Weiner SF. A review of radio frequency for skin tightening by Dr. Steven Weiner (Finally! A radiofrequency system that makes sense: the infini from Lutronic; 2013.)

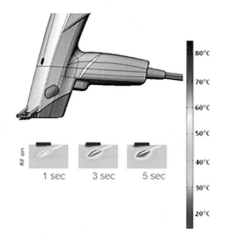

Fig. 12.3 Real-time lesion temperature and impedance feedback and control. A larger area of coagulation is seen with longer exposure times.

precise amount of energy. This monitoring occurs via feedback loops within the handpiece and provides real-time feedback to maintain the temperature during the exposure time.

EPIDERMAL PROTECTION

In contrast to the dermis, the critical heat threshold to avoid epidermal burns is 44°C. Therefore overly aggressive treatment of the deeper tissues without proper protection of the overlying epidermis can lead to epidermal burns and complications such as blistering, scarring, and postinflammatory hyperpigmentation (PIH).

Epidermal cooling, in the form of a cryogen spray or contact cooling plate, can be applied to protect the superficial layers of the skin while heating the deeper tissues (Fig. 12.2A–C). Epidermal cooling also increases tissue impedance and redirects radiofrequency away from the epidermis. Other methods of minimizing epidermal injury may include constant motion of the handpiece or using insulated microneedles. In RFMN using insulated microneedles, the proximal ends of the needles are insulated, and radiofrequency is delivered only at the distal ends that are embedded in the target tissue (Figs. 12.2D and 12.4). The temperature of the epidermis and dermis can be monitored in real-time by sensors within the handpiece or through infrared cameras.

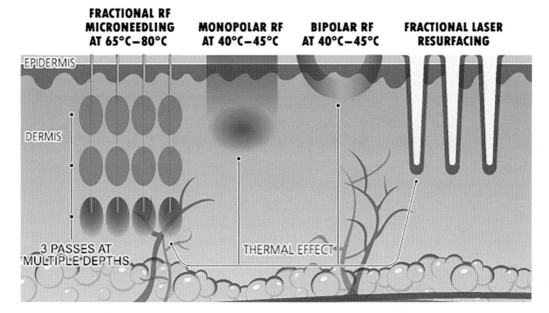

Fig. 12.4 *(Left to right)* Radiofrequency *(RF)* microneedling, monopolar and bipolar noninvasive fractional radiofrequency, and fractional ablative laser. Note: monopolar and bipolar RF are noninvasive fractional radiofrequency devices that deliver dermal coagulation via pin electrodes in contact with the epidermis, rather than microneedles penetrating the skin. (Courtesy Lutronic, Billerica, MA.)

RADIOFREQUENCY VERSUS LASERS

RFMN differs from ablative lasers in several aspects. Lasers function on the theory of selective photothermolysis, whereby chromophores in the skin have different absorption peaks at different wavelengths of light. Ablative lasers selectively target water as the chromophore and creates a temperature gradient that tends to be highest at the epidermis and decreases as it penetrates the deeper layers of the skin. This thermal injury to the epidermis increases the risk of PIH, especially in patients with darker skin phototypes. In contrast, RFMN is dependent on impedance of the target tissue only and is strictly an electrothermal effect. It is not dependent on skin chromophores, thereby rendering RFMN a "color-blind" technology that is not affected by the amount of melanin present in the skin. Radiofrequency energy is directly delivered to the target depth through the microneedle electrodes, thus creating a temperature gradient that is highest in the deeper structures and cooler at the superficial structures. This results in less epidermal heating and reduces the risk of PIH. Compared to lasers, radiofrequency energy can also be delivered to deeper structures of the skin through increasing the depth of penetration or length of microneedle electrodes.

CHARACTERISTICS OF MICRONEEDLES IN RADIOFREQUENCY MICRONEEDLING

The microneedles used in RFMN are wider at the proximal ends connected to the handpiece, and taper to sharp tips at the distal ends to allow for penetration of the skin. They are usually arranged in square arrays of 5 × 5, 6 × 6, or 7 × 7 microneedles, but many other arrangements also exist. The microneedles are delivered to the skin through either mechanical motors, solenoids, or manual operator applications. The length of microneedle and depth of penetration in most modern RFMN devices can be adjusted depending on the indication of treatment (Fig. 12.5). This allows for a more precise targeting of the desired tissue, while avoiding injury to collateral structures. The adjustability is also important given that different anatomic sites have different epidermal and dermal thickness (Figs. 12.6 and 12.7).

An important consideration when deciding on treatment parameters is to note that the desired depth of penetration may not always correspond to the actual depth. In general, the actual depth of penetration tends to be more superficial. Many factors can contribute to this inadvertent targeting of more superficial structures than desired: (1) operator-dependent factors, such as insufficient pressure applied or imprecise holding of the

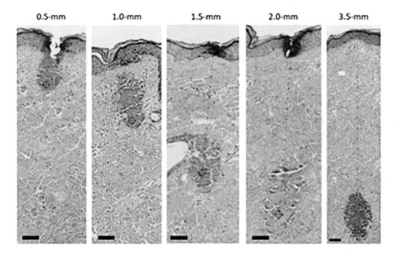

Fig. 12.5 Histologic section of human tissue showing controlled coagulation within the dermis at different depths. (Courtesy Dr. Sung Bin Cho, MD.)

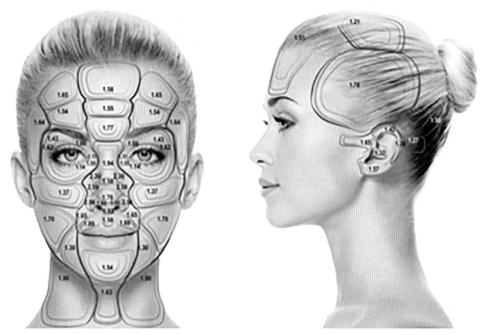

Fig. 12.6 *(Left)* Anterior view of epidermal relative thickness. *(Right)* Lateral view of epidermal relative thickness. (From Chopra K, et al. A comprehensive examination of topographic thickness of skin in the human face. *Aesthet Surg J*. 2015;35(8):1007–1013. Courtesy of Karan Chopra, MD.)

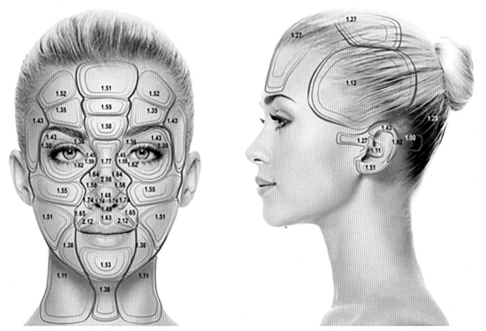

Fig. 12.7 *(Left)* Anterior view of dermal relative thickness. *(Right)* Lateral view of dermal relative thickness. (From Chopra K, et al. A comprehensive examination of topographic thickness of skin in the human face. *Aesthet Surg J*. 2015;35(8):1007–1013. Courtesy Karan Chopra, MD.)

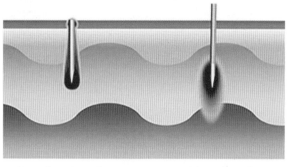

Non-insulated RF   Semi-insulated RF

Fig. 12.8 *(Left)* Noninsulated radiofrequency *(RF)* microneedle delivers radiofrequency throughout the length of the microneedle, resulting in epidermal and dermal coagulation. *(Right)* Semiinsulated RF microneedle delivers radiofrequency only at the distal tip, resulting in only dermal coagulation while protecting the epidermis from thermal injury. (Courtesy of Cutera.)

handpiece resulting non-perpendicular contact with the skin; (2) patient-dependent factors, such as thickened or scarred skin is more difficult to penetrate; (3) device-dependent factors, such as an underpowered motors or solenoids, or dull needles from poor manufacturing quality.

The microneedles can be noninsulated or semiinsulated. In RFMN using noninsulated microneedles, radiofrequency energy is delivered along the entire length of the microneedle electrode (Fig. 12.8 Left). This results in both mechanical and thermal injuries to the epidermis and underlying structures. In RFMN using semiinsulated microneedles, radiofrequency energy is delivered only at the distal end of the microneedle electrode, bypassing the epidermis (Fig. 12.8 Right). Hence, epidermal injury is limited only to the mechanical perforations and this reduces downtime and patient discomfort. When using more aggressive treatment settings however, some degree of heat can still permeate through the insulation.

In addition to radiofrequency-induced thermal injury, the mechanical effects of microneedles creating perforations in the skin also allow for improved transcutaneous absorption and elimination of topical products and skin debris respectively, and further stimulates the wound-healing response and secretion of growth factors that lead to migration and proliferation of fibroblasts for collagen remodeling, neocollagenesis and neoelastogenesis.

INDICATIONS

The most common indications for RFMN are skin rejuvenation, acne scars, acne vulgaris, and axillary hyperhidrosis. Other conditions which may also respond to RFMN include rosacea, male-pattern androgenetic alopecia, and striae. Although RFMN has been successfully used for the treatment of melasma and cellulite, there is still limited evidence to support its use in these conditions.

SKIN REJUVENATION

The complex physiologic aging of skin results in increased skin laxity, rhytides, overall roughness, and uneven dyspigmentation. RFMN delivers radiofrequency energy to underlying dermis to stimulate neocollagenesis and neoelastogenesis to achieve skin tightening and reduced roughness. The mechanical perforations created by microneedles also stimulate the wound healing response, and allow for increased transcutaneous absorption of topical products, as well as transcutaneous elimination of unwanted skin debris and melanin.

Studies evaluating RFMN for facial rhytides, skin laxity and textural roughness reported a 20%–62% improvement after one to three treatment sessions (Fig. 12.9). The earliest and greatest clinical improvements were observed at 1 month and 3 months respectively. At 7 months posttreatment, the skin rejuvenating effects of RFMN remained visible. In contrast to botulinum toxin A, which is often regarded as the gold standard for periorbital rhytides, RFMN had a slower onset, less efficacy and longer downtime. However, the antirhytid and skin tightening effects of RFMN were more durable and continued to improve even 6 months posttreatment, as RFMN stimulated neocollagenesis and neoelastogenesis whereas botulinum toxin A did not.

RFMN has also been compared to fractional ablative Er:YAG laser for facial skin rejuvenation. Er:YAG laser was found to be more effective for periorbital rhytides, while RFMN was more effective for nasolabial, perioral, jawline and neck rhytides. This dichotomy was thought to be due to Er:YAG laser creating a broader but more

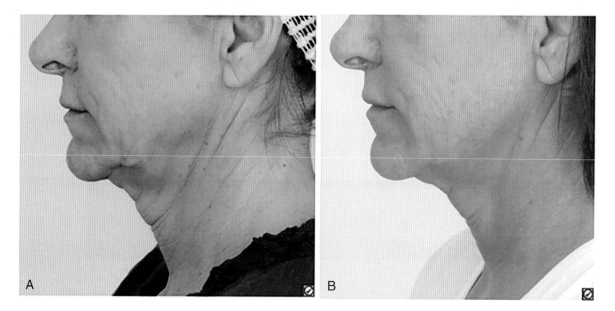

Fig. 12.9 Lower face and neck rejuvenation. (A) Before treatment. (B) 4 months after two radiofrequency microneedling treatments. (Courtesy Shilpi Khetarpal, MD.)

superficial microthermal zones of injury (MTZ) in the upper face with thinner skin, compared to RFMN that creates deeper MTZ for the lower face with thicker skin. RMFN can be safely combined with ablative or nonablative lasers to result in more clinically significant improvements (Fig. 12.10).

One study comparing RFMN to surgical facelift for skin laxity found that RFMN achieved 37% efficacy of a surgical facelift and had no adverse events or scarring. However, two-thirds of patients receiving facelift experienced hypertrophic scarring requiring further scar management.

ACNE SCARS

Check online video (Video 12.1)

Acne scars are among some of the most common complaints presenting to an esthetic practice. Studies evaluating RFMN for acne scars reported 25%–40% improvement in the appearance of acne scars after 3 treatment sessions (Fig. 12.11). RFMN has been found to be similar in efficacy to Er:Glass laser, but patients reported less discomfort, shorter downtime, fewer adverse events and safer in individuals with darker skin phototype. RFMN can be safely combined with

Er:Glass, CO_2, noninvasive fractional radiofrequency or platelet rich plasma to improve outcomes without increased incidence of adverse events (Fig. 12.12).

ACNE VULGARIS

RFMN delivers radiofrequency to destroy the sebaceous glands and reduce its activity, thereby disrupting the pathogenesis of acne vulgaris. Studies evaluating RFMN for acne vulgaris reported 36%–41% mean improvement in acne lesions after two treatment sessions (Fig. 12.13). Microneedling alone, without radiofrequency, actually resulted in worsening of acne vulgaris.

RFMN was found to be superior to 1450-nm diode laser for treating acne vulgaris and had a longer disease remission period. RFMN was either superior, or at least equivalent to, noninvasive fractional radiofrequency. RFMN has a similar efficacy to fractional CO_2 laser but lower risk of PIH.

AXILLARY HYPERHIDROSIS

Axillary hyperhidrosis is due to overactive sweat glands. RFMN can deliver radiofrequency energy to the reticular dermis and subcutaneous fat, where eccrine sweat

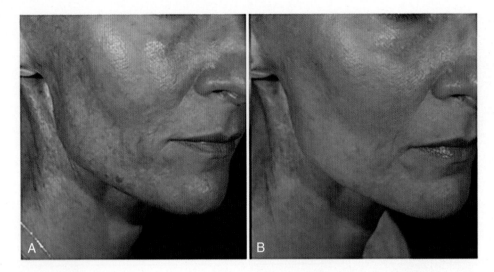

Fig. 12.10 Radiofrequency microneedling (RFMN) can be safely combined with other treatment modalities. This patient had volume loss and radiation dermatitis following parotidectomy and radiation. (A) Before treatment. (B) 1 month following RFMN and 1927-nm Thulium fractional laser performed on the same day. (Courtesy Jennifer MacGregor, MD.)

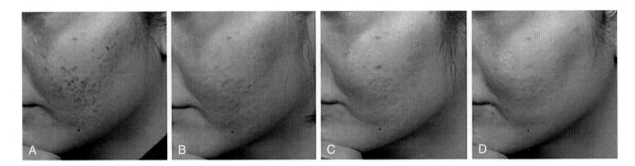

Fig. 12.11 Patient's left profile at (A) baseline, (B) 1 month, (C) 3 months, and (D) 6 months after three treatment sessions of radiofrequency microneedling. (From Vejjabhinanta V, et al. The efficacy in treatment of facial atrophic acne scars in Asians with a fractional radiofrequency microneedle system. *J Eur Acad Dermatol Venereol.* 2014;28(9):1219–1225. Courtesy Voraphol Vejjabhinanta, MD.)

glands reside. Studies evaluating RFMN for axillary hyperhidrosis found a 42%–46% improvement after three treatment sessions (Fig. 12.14).

Two sessions of RFMN were inferior to 50 units of botulinum toxin A for axillary hyperhidrosis at 12 weeks posttreatment. However, the effects of RFMN were more durable and lasted 1-year post-RFMN, compared to 6–7 months duration for botulinum toxin A. RFMN was also compared to surgical subdermal pruning for osmidrosis. Although RFMN was 13.7% less effective, it

also had shorter downtime and fewer treatment-related complications.

In axillary hyperhidrosis, bipolar radiofrequency settings in a multilayered and multipass approach, with lower power but longer conduction time (3 seconds, 4.3 W) has been shown to be more effective while having fewer side effects than settings with high power but shorter conduction time (0.7 seconds, 21.1 W). The former creates broad MTZ that extend into the upper subcutaneous tissue, whereas the latter only creates focal

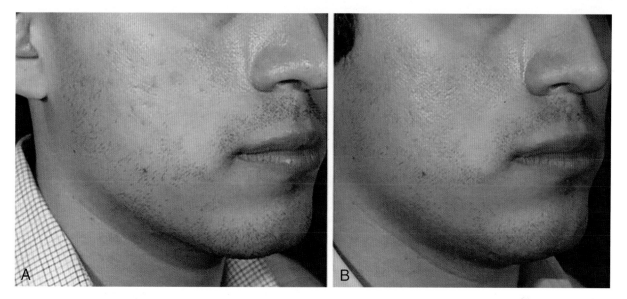

Fig. 12.12 Acne scars. (A) Before treatment. (B) 3 months after the third session of RFMN with platelet rich plasma. (Courtesy Jennifer MacGregor, MD.)

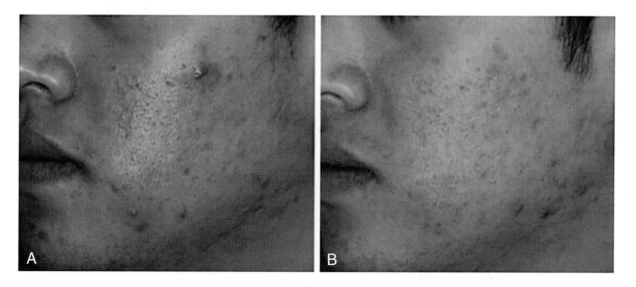

Fig. 12.13 Radiofrequency microneedling for acne vulgaris. (A) Before treatment. (B) 2 months after two sessions of radiofrequency microneedling. (From: Lee SJ, et al. Use of fractionated microneedle radiofrequency for the treatment of inflammatory acne vulgaris in 18 korean patients. *Dermatol Surg.* 2012;38(3):400–405. Courtesy Sang Ju Lee, MD, PhD.)

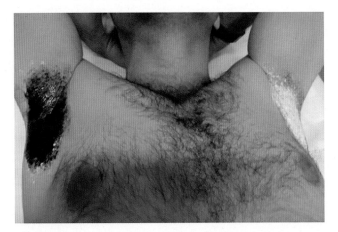

Fig. 12.14 Radiofrequency microneedling for axillary hyperhidrosis. Starch-iodine test shows significant reduction in axillary hyperhidrosis following three treatment sessions in left axilla (treated) compared to right axilla (untreated). (From Fatemi Naeini F, et al. Fractionated microneedle radiofrequency for treatment of primary axillary hyperhidrosis: a sham control study. *Australas J Dermato*. 2015;56:279–284. Courtesy Farahnaz Fatemi Naeini, MD.)

areas of MTZ in the dermal-subcutaneous junction. Insulated needles and epidermal cooling are preferred to protect the upper skin layers.

OTHER INDICATIONS

RFMN has also been employed in several other dermatologic conditions, such as striae, rosacea, and androgenetic alopecia. When used for treating striae, RFMN showed a mean improvement of 30%–45% after three treatment sessions, which is similar in efficacy to fractional CO_2 laser, but lower incidence of PIH and is therefore safer for individuals with darker skin phototypes. RFMN can also be combined with a fractional CO_2 laser to augment its efficacy synergistically, without increasing the risk of adverse events.

Rosacea is an inflammatory disease of the pilosebaceous glands and there is some evidence supporting the use of RFMN for treating rosacea. Patients experienced a mean improvement of 20% after two RFMN treatment sessions and reported moderate reduction in the subjective symptoms of rosacea. The papulopustular variant of rosacea responded better than the erythematotelangiectatic variant of rosacea.

In addition to delivering radiofrequency to the underlying tissue, RFMN also enhances the transcutaneous absorption of topical products through the mechanical channels created by the microneedles. In male-pattern androgenetic alopecia, when 5% minoxidil is applied post-RFMN, the mean hair counts increased by an additional 80% compared to topical 5% minoxidil monotherapy. RFMN also triggers the wound-healing response which has also shown to stimulate hair follicle growth and accelerate hair cycling, leading to better clinical outcomes.

There are some studies evaluating the use of RFMN to treat cellulite and melasma. In cellulite, it is thought that RFMN stimulates the formation of new connective tissue in the subcuticular junction, thereby preventing fat herniation into the dermis and creating the peau d'orange dimpling seen in cellulite. One randomized, evaluated blinded study showed that 86% of participants treated with one session of RFMN achieved a clinically significant improvement in their cellulite appearance.

In melasma, the thermal effects of RFMN are thought to induce remodeling of the dermis, reduce inflammation, and decrease angiogenesis. The mechanical channels created by the microneedles also allow for transcutaneous elimination of melanin and unwanted skin debris. When used in combination with low-fluence Q-switched Nd:YAG laser, RFMN augmented the efficacy for treating melasma and reduced the risk of rebound hyperpigmentation, without any increase in adverse events.

PATIENT SELECTION

To maximum patient satisfaction, clinicians must counsel patients that the results of RFMN are gradual and tend to peak around 3–6 months after treatment. Furthermore, clinicians should emphasize that RFMN is not equivalent to surgical treatment, but rather, should be thought of as an alternative, minimally-invasive, therapeutic modality.

The side effects and potential complications of RFMN are similar to those covered in Chapter 9, Ablative Laser Resurfacing, and include transient erythema, bleeding, itching, purpura, infection, postinflammatory dyschromia, and scarring. Purpura can be quite significant depending on the treatment settings, and pulsed-dye lasers may be used to speed up the recovery process if desired (Figs. 12.15 and 12.16).

One notable complication of RFMN is the appearance of grid-like or tram-track marks following treatment (Fig. 12.17). These marks can be more common with certain RFMN devices at higher settings, and may last up to several weeks depending on the intensity of

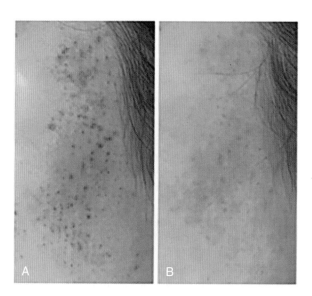

Fig. 12.15 Grid marks and petechiae. (A) Day 1 post-RFMN. (B) 1 day following treatment of petechia with 595-nm pulsed dye laser. (Courtesy Claire Chang, MD.)

treatment. Fortunately, these marks usually resolve spontaneously by 3–4 weeks with a proper posttreatment care regimen. However, if these marks do not resolve by 4 weeks or if accelerated recovery is desired, nonablative fractional lasers such as 1550 Er:Glass laser or 1927-nm thulium laser may be used to treat them. Patients should be counseled about this potential complication prior to treatment, especially if more aggressive settings are used.

In general, it is not recommended to use more aggressive settings than necessary, as this prolongs the downtime and increases the risk of complications without additional clinical benefit. Furthermore, clinicians should take into consideration that patients seeking minimally invasive treatments are typically attracted to them due to the minimal downtime and low risk of complications. Hence, they may not be willing to accept the longer downtime.

ABSOLUTE CONTRAINDICATIONS

Active Infection

RFMN should not be performed in the presence of any active infection, regardless of bacterial, viral, or fungal infections.

Pregnancy and Lactation

Patients who are pregnant or lactating should avoid RFMN treatment as there is limited evidence supporting safety during pregnancy or in lactating women.

Cardiac Pacemaker and Cardiac Defibrillator

Patients with cardiac pacemaker or cardiac defibrillators should avoid RFMN treatment as there is a potential risk of radiofrequency interfering with the proper functioning of the device.

Metal Implants

Patients with metal implants in the immediate vicinity of the area desiring treatment should not be treated with RFMN, due to the potential risk of heating the metal implant and causing thermal burns. For patients with metal implants not within the vicinity of the target area, RFMN using bipolar radiofrequency is strongly advised, as radiofrequency will be limited to the treatment area between the electrodes. Patients with metallic dental implants can receive RFMN.

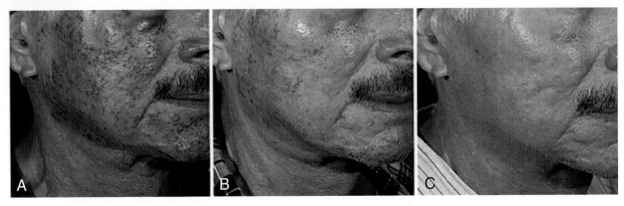

Fig. 12.16 Posttreatment purpura secondary to intentional long exposure duration. Topical vitamin C and topical moisturizer with ceramide was administered twice daily as part of posttreatment care. (A) Day 1 post-RFMN. (B) Day 3 post-RFMN. (C) Day 7 post-RFMN. (Courtesy Jennifer MacGregor, MD.)

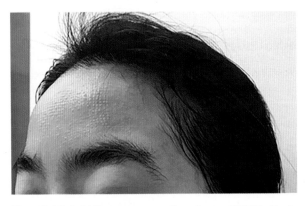

Fig. 12.17 Grid-like pattern on Day 6 post-RFMN. Postcare regimen consisted of white petrolatum, gentle unscented cleanser and physical sunscreen. Lesions resolved by Day 10. (Courtesy Jennifer MacGregor, MD.)

RELATIVE CONTRAINDICATIONS

Unrealistic Patient Expectations

Unrealistic patient expectations are among one of the most common problems experienced by clinicians. RFMN can produce significant clinical improvements, but clinicians should not overstate or oversell the potential benefits of RFMN.

History of Keloid or Significant Scarring

Patients with a history of keloid or abnormal scarring should be counseled about the potential risks of scarring with the procedure.

History of Orolabial Herpes

Patients with a history of orolabial herpes should be counseled about the potential risk of reactivation following RFMN treatment. Patients with significant history of orolabial herpes may benefit from antiviral prophylaxis, especially if treating the perioral region, starting 3 days prior to RFMN and continuing until complete reepithelialization has occurred.

Previous Deep Chemical Peels, Deep Laser Resurfacing, Prior Surgery, or Skin Grafts

Patients with a history of deep chemical peels, deep full-field laser resurfacing or skin grafts may have absent or damaged cutaneous appendages which slows or interferes with the normal skin healing process, hence clinicians should be more cautious in these patients. Clinicians must also be aware of the patient's surgical history, as skin thickness and quality may be affected. For instance, in patients who have undergone face and neck lifts, the thinner skin from the neck would have been transposed over the mandible which previously had thicker skin. Hence, the depth of microneedle penetration would have to be adjusted accordingly.

Isotretinoin Use

Historically, the recommendation has been to avoid ablative procedures in patients with recent or concurrent isotretinoin use due to case reports of keloid or hypertrophic scarring posttreatment. However, more recent studies have shown that RFMN can be used in patients on low-dose isotretinoin safely. Nonetheless, this remains controversial and the final decision should be based on the medical needs of the patient.

Dermatologic Diseases That Exhibit Koebner Phenomenon

Patients with dermatologic diseases that exhibit the Koebner phenomenon, such as psoriasis, vitiligo, or lichen planus, should be cautioned against receiving RFMN until their disease has been well controlled and stable for several months. Otherwise, there is a risk of exacerbating their disease following RFMN treatment.

PRETREATMENT AND POSTTREATMENT REGIMENS

Topical anesthetics applied 30–60 minutes prior to RFMN is encouraged. Nerve blocks or tumescent anesthesia may be administered, especially if treating deeper structures such as in axillary hyperhidrosis or if treatment exposures times ≥ 2 seconds. Anxiolytics, inhaled nitrous mixtures, calming music, "talkaesthesia," or other methods to disrupt the gate control theory of pain can also be utilized to improve patient comfort.

Adherence to photoprotection post-RFMN is also strongly encouraged, especially in individuals with darker skin phototypes to minimize the risk of PIH. Thick emollients, zinc-based barrier creams or serums containing growth factors may also be used post-RFMN to encourage wound healing. Prophylactic topical or oral antibiotics post-RFMN is generally not required. Clinicians must also emphasize that a strict adherence to the recommended posttreatment care regimen is essential. Patients should not deviate from this regimen or use any of their own topical products on treated areas, as these can increase the risk of irritant, allergic, or granulomatous reactions.

CONCLUSION

RFMN can be an effective treatment modality that is safe to use in all skin phototypes. Although the effects of RFMN are slow and gradual, its effects are longer lasting and it can be safely combined with other treatment modalities to augment efficacy without significant increase in risk of adverse events.

FURTHER READING

Abtahi-Naeini B, Naeini FF, Saffaei A, et al. Treatment of primary axillary hyperhidrosis by fractional microneedle radiofrequency: is it still effective after long-term follow-up? *Indian J Dermat.* 2016;61(2):234.

Afify AA, Fawzy HM, Al-Rubaiay NHA, Abdallah M. Fractional microneedling radiofrequency in striae alba: do growth factors add value? *J Cosmet Dermatol.* 2020; 19(10):2583–2590.

Ahn GR, Kim JM, Park SJ, Li K, Kim BJ. Selective sebaceous gland electrothermolysis using a single microneedle radiofrequency device for acne patients: a prospective randomized controlled study. *Lasers Surg Med.* 2020; 52(5):396–401.

Alexiades M, Berube D. Randomized, blinded, 3-arm clinical trial assessing optimal temperature and duration for treatment with minimally invasive fractional radiofrequency. *Dermatol Surg.* 2015;41(5):623–632.

Alexiades M, Munavalli G, Goldberg D, Berube D. Prospective multicenter clinical trial of a temperature-controlled subcutaneous microneedle fractional bipolar radiofrequency system for the treatment of cellulite. *Dermatol Surg.* 2018;44(10):1262–1271.

Alexiades-Armenakas M, Rosenberg D, Renton B, Dover JS, Arndt KA. Blinded, randomized, quantitative grading comparison of minimally invasive, fractional radiofrequency and surgical face-lift to treat skin laxity. *Arch Dermat.* 2010;146(4):396–405.

Alexiades-Armenakas M, Newman J, Willey A, et al. Prospective multicenter clinical trial of a minimally invasive temperature-controlled bipolar fractional radiofrequency system for rhytid and laxity treatment. *Dermatol Surg.* 2013;39(2):263–273.

Al-Muriesh M, Huang C, Ye Z, Yang J. Dermoscopy and VISIA imager evaluations of non-insulated microneedle radiofrequency versus fractional CO_2 laser treatments of striae distensae. *J Eur Acad Dermatol Venereol.* 2020;34(8):1859–1866.

An MK, Hong EH, Suh SB, Park EJ, Kim KH. Combination therapy of microneedle fractional radiofrequency and topical poly-lactic acid for acne scars: a randomized controlled split-face study. *Dermatol Surg.* 2020;46(6):796–802.

Atkins D, Best D, Briss PA, et al. Grading quality of evidence and strength of recommendations. *BMJ (Clinical Research Ed.).* 2004;328(7454):1490.

Chae WS, Seong JY, Jung HN, et al. Comparative study on efficacy and safety of 1550 nm Er:glass fractional laser and fractional radiofrequency microneedle device for facial atrophic acne scar. *J Cosmet Dermatol.* 2015;14(2):100–106.

Cho SB, Park J, Zheng Z, Yoo KH, Kim H. Split-axilla comparison study of 0.5-MHz, invasive, bipolar radiofrequency treatment using insulated microneedle electrodes for primary axillary hyperhidrosis. *Skin Res Technol.* 2019;25(1):30–39.

Faghihi G, Poostiyan N, Asilian A, et al. Efficacy of fractionated microneedle radiofrequency with and without adding subcision for the treatment of atrophic facial acne scars: a randomized split-face clinical study. *J Cosmet Dermatol.* 2017;16(2):223–229.

Fatemi Naeini F, Abtahi-Naeini B, Pourazizi M, Nilforoushzadeh MA, Mirmohammadkhani M. Fractionated microneedle radiofrequency for treatment of primary axillary hyperhidrosis: a sham control study: radiofrequency for treatment of PAH. *Aust J Dermatol.* 2015;56(4):279–284.

Fatemi Naeini F, Behfar S, Abtahi-Naeini B, Keyvan S, Pourazizi M. Promising option for treatment of striae alba: fractionated microneedle radiofrequency in combination with fractional carbon dioxide laser. *Dermatol Res Prac.* 2016;2016:1–7.

Gold M, Taylor M, Rothaus K, Tanaka Y. Non-insulated smooth motion, micro-needles RF fractional treatment for wrinkle reduction and lifting of the lower face: international study. *Lasers Surg Med.* 2016;48(8):727–733.

Hantash BM, Ubeid AA, Chang H, Kafi R, Renton B. Bipolar fractional radiofrequency treatment induces neoelastogenesis and neocollagenesis. *Lasers Surg Med.* 2009;41(1):1–9.

Jeon IK, Chang SE, Park GH, Roh MR. Comparison of microneedle fractional radiofrequency therapy with intradermal botulinum toxin a injection for periorbital rejuvenation. *Dermatol.* 2013;227(4):367–372.

Jung JW, Kim WO, Jung HR, Kim SA, Ryoo YW. A face-split study to evaluate the effects of microneedle radiofrequency with Q-Switched Nd:YAG laser for the treatment of melasma. *Ann Dermatol.* 2019;31(2):133.

Kim JK, Roh MR, Park GH, Kim YJ, Jeon IK, Chang SE. Fractionated microneedle radiofrequency for the treatment of periorbital wrinkles. *J Dermatol.* 2013;40(3):172–176.

Kwon HH, Park HY, Choi SC, Bae Y, Jung JY, Park GH. Novel device-based acne treatments: comparison of a 1450-nm diode laser and microneedling radiofrequency on mild-to-moderate acne vulgaris and seborrhoea in Korean patients through a 20-week prospective, randomized, split-face study. *J Eur Acad Dermatol Venereol.* 2018;32(4):639–644.

Kwon H, Park H, Choi S, et al. Combined fractional treatment of acne scars involving non-ablative 1,550-nm erbium-glass laser and micro-needling radiofrequency: a 16-week prospective, randomized split-face study. *Acta Derm Venereol.* 2017;97(8):947–951.

Kwon HH, Choi SC, Jung JY, Park GH. Combined treatment of melasma involving low-fluence Q-Switched Nd:YAG laser and fractional microneedling radiofrequency. *J Dermatol Treat.* 2019;30(4):352–356.

Kwon SH, Choi JY, Ahn GY, et al. The efficacy and safety of microneedle monopolar radiofrequency for the treatment of periorbital wrinkles. *J. Dermatol Treat.* 2019;32(4):460–464.

Lee SJ, Goo JW, Shin J, et al. Use of fractionated microneedle radiofrequency for the treatment of inflammatory acne vulgaris in 18 korean patients. *Dermatol Surg.* 2012;38(3):400–405.

Lee SJ, Kim JI, Yang YJ, Nam JH, Kim WS. Treatment of periorbital wrinkles with a novel fractional radiofrequency microneedle system in dark-skinned patients. *Dermatol Surg.* 2015;41(4):615–622.

Lin L, Huo R, Bi J, Meng Z, Cao Y. Fractional microneedling radiofrequency treatment for axillary osmidrosis: a minimally invasive procedure. *J Cosmet Dermatol.* 2019;18(1):115–120.

Liu TM, Sun YM, Tang ZY, Li YH. Microneedle fractional radiofrequency treatment of facial photoageing as assessed in a split-face model. *Clin Exp Dermatol.* 2019;44(4):e96–102.

Lu W, Wu P, Zhang Z, Chen J, Chen X, Ewelina B. Curative effects of microneedle fractional radiofrequency system on skin laxity in asian patients: a prospective, double-blind, randomized, controlled face-split study. *J Cosmet Laser Ther.* 2017;19(2):83–88.

Min S, Park SY, Yoon JY, Suh DH. Comparison of fractional microneedling radiofrequency and bipolar radiofrequency on acne and acne scar and investigation of mechanism: comparative randomized controlled clinical trial. *Arch Dermatol Res.* 2015;307(10):897–904.

Park JY, Lee EG, Yoon MS, Lee HJ. The efficacy and safety of combined microneedle fractional radiofrequency and sublative fractional radiofrequency for acne scars in asian skin. *J Cosmet Dermatol.* 2016;15(2):102–107.

Park SY, Kwon HH, Yoon JY, Min S, Suh DH. Clinical and histologic effects of fractional microneedling radiofrequency treatment on rosacea. *Dermatol Surg.* 2016;42(12):1362–1369.

Rummaneethorn P, Chalermchai T. A comparative study between intradermal botulinum toxin a and fractional microneedle radiofrequency (FMR) for the treatment of primary axillary hyperhidrosis. *Lasers Med Sci.* 2020;35(5):1179–1184.

Ryu H-W, Kim S-A, Jung HR, Ryoo Y-W, Lee K-S, Cho J-W. Clinical improvement of striae distensae in korean patients using a combination of fractionated microneedle radiofrequency and fractional carbon dioxide laser. *Dermatol Surg.* 2013;39(10):1452–1458.

Schünemann, H, J Brożek, G Guyatt, and A Oxman. *Handbook for Grading the Quality of Evidence and the Strength of Recommendations Using the GRADE Approach*; n.d.

Seo KY, Kim DH, Lee SE, Yoon MS, Lee HJ. Skin rejuvenation by microneedle fractional radiofrequency and a human stem cell conditioned medium in Asian skin: a randomized controlled investigator blinded split-face study. *J Cosmet Laser Ther*. 2013;15(1):25–33.

Seo KY, Yoon MS, Kim DH, Lee HJ. Skin rejuvenation by microneedle fractional radiofrequency treatment in asian skin; clinical and histological analysis. *Lasers Surg Med*. 2012;44(8):631–636.

Serdar ZA, Tatlıparmak A. Comparison of efficacy and safety of fractional radiofrequency and fractional Er:YAG laser in facial and neck wrinkles: six-year experience with 333 patients. *Dermatol Ther*. 2019;32(5):e13054.

Shin JU, Lee SH, Jung JY, Lee JH. A split-face comparison of a fractional microneedle radiofrequency device and fractional carbon dioxide laser therapy in acne patients. *J Cosmet Laser Ther*. 2012;14(5):212–217.

Sobhi RM, Mohamed IS, Sharkawy DAE, Wahab MAEFAE. Comparative study between the efficacy of fractional micro-needle radiofrequency and fractional CO_2 laser in the treatment of striae distensae. *Lasers Med Sci*. 2019;34(7):1295–1304.

Tan MG, Jo CE, Chapas A, Khetarpal S, Dover JS. Radiofrequency microneedling: a comprehensive and critical review. *Dermatol Surg*. 2021;47(6):755–761.

Tatlıparmak A, Aksoy B, Shishehgarkhaneh LR, Gökdemir G, Koç E. Use of combined fractional carbon dioxide laser and fractional microneedle radiofrequency for the treatment of acne scars: a retrospective analysis of 1-month treatment outcome on scar severity and patient satisfaction. *J Cosm Dermatol*. 2020;19(1):115–121.

Vejjabhinanta V, Wanitphakdeedecha R, Limtanyakul P, Manuskiatti W. The efficacy in treatment of facial atrophic acne scars in asians with a fractional radiofrequency microneedle system. *J Eur Acad Dermatol Venereol*. 2014; 28(9):1219–1225.

Weiner SF. Radiofrequency microneedling: overview of technology, advantages, differences in devices, studies, and indications. *Facial Plast Surg Clin North Am*. 2019;27(3): 291–303.

Yu A-J, Luo Y-J, Xu X-G, et al. A pilot split-scalp study of combined fractional radiofrequency microneedling and 5% topical minoxidil in treating male pattern hair loss. *Clin Exp Dermatol*. 2018;43(7):775–781.

Zeng R, Liu Y, Zhao W, et al. A split-face comparison of a fractional microneedle radiofrequency device and fractional radiofrequency therapy for moderate-to-severe acne vulgaris. *J Cosmet Dermatol*. 2020;19(10):2566–2571.

Zhang M, Fang J, Wu Q, Lin T. A prospective study of the safety and efficacy of a microneedle fractional radiofrequency system for global facial photoaging in chinese patients. *Dermatol Surg*. 2018;44(7):964–970.

13

Laser Treatment of Ethnic Skin

Kachiu Lee, Shraddha Desai, Mara Weinstein Velez, and Deborah Paul

SUMMARY OF KEY FEATURES

- The use of lasers, lights and devices can be safe and effective in ethnic skin.
- Sun protection pre- and posttreatment, together with the use of bleaching agents and topical corticosteroids, may reduce the risks of postinflammatory hyperpigmentation.
- For patients undergoing laser treatment for melasma, sun protection is essential to disease management.
- Lasers and light sources with longer wavelengths target dermal pigmentation and are safer in ethnic skin to minimize damage to epidermal melanocytes.
- Diascopy during treatment of pigmented lesions reduces the risk of collateral vascular damage.
- While the 585/595-nm pulsed-dye laser (PDL) and 532-nm potassium titanyl phosphate (KTP) and lithium triborate (LBO) lasers have been shown to be safe in ethnic skin, the 1064-nm Nd:YAG may be preferred for treating vascular lesions given its longer wavelength because of less pigment absorption.

- Picosecond lasers are effective in targeting dermal pigment (Hori's nevus, Nevus of Ota, tattoo pigment) and can be safe to use in ethnic skin.
- Lower fluences with increased treatment sessions are commonly required when using Q-switched lasers in ethnic skin. Longer treatment intervals are needed to minimize risks of both hyper- and hypopigmentation.
- Microneedling offers a minimally invasive alternative to laser therapy in ethnic skin with lower risks of dyspigmentation. However, multiple treatment sessions may be required.
- Fractional plasma radiofrequency devices are a new and emerging safe alternative to traditional lasers for treating scars, skin laxity and lines.
- Skin tightening devices are "color blind" devices and safe across all skin types with minimum to no direct effect on skin pigmentation.
- An important consideration prior to laser or light treatment is to identify the presence of body dysmorphic disorder.

INTRODUCTION

The 21st century marks a dramatic transformative change in the diversity of the US population. According to the Pew research center, it is estimated that the population will grow to 438 billion, with over 50% representing traditionally ethnic minorities (Asian, Black, and Hispanics) as a result of immigration and intermarriage. In dermatology, this is of particular importance in the care of ethnic skin patients. This diverse group more

broadly encompasses African, African-American, Afro-Caribbean, Asian, Indian, Middle Eastern, Latin-X, and biracial/multiracial individuals. Their skin color falls into the Fitzpatrick skin type scale IV–VI, distinguished by their lower response to UV sun exposure.

Special consideration is needed in the treatment of cutaneous disease in patients with ethnic skin. Unique differences exist compared to skin types I–III patients. Ethnic skin contains numerous larger melanosomes with more melanin and stability that is dispersed broadly to individual keratinocytes compared to skin types I–III, where the melanosomes are smaller, less stable and are clustered close together. This difference in melanosome biology results in increased photoprotection in ethnic skin. It also creates a therapeutic challenge in managing skin disease in ethnic skin, where dyspigmentation is a significant concern and not uncommon complication of lasers.

Careful selection of lasers and settings is essential to preventing unwanted dyspigmentation as melanin is a bystander chromophore that challenges treatment in ethnic skin. The aim of this chapter is to explore the challenges of using laser and light-based therapies in ethnic skin and to provide guidance to the practicing dermatologist on how to optimize its safe use in ethnic skin. Clinical pearls, prevention, and management of complications will also be highlighted in this chapter.

EVALUATING THE ETHNIC SKIN PATIENT

It is critical that all patients undergo a complete history and exam prior to treatment. The history should include past experiences with procedures, any treatment complications, current practices for UV protection and most importantly, evaluate patient expectations for treatment. On exam, it is important to assess the skin in both the desired treatment area and to look for any signs of hyperpigmentation or keloid formation after surgical or traumatic injury in other areas which can be helpful in guiding expectations. The initial appointment should focus on correct diagnosis and evaluating whether the condition of concern can be treated appropriately with laser. Complementary tools can be helpful in confirming the diagnosis. Woods lamp or UV photography can be a useful tool to differentiate between epidermal and dermal pigment in patients with melasma. Diascopy and a dermatoscope may have a role in evaluating ambiguous lesions. For solitary lesions with concerning features on dermoscopy, a biopsy should be considered before proceeding with treatment.

Once the diagnosis is confirmed, a discussion on laser/light options and alternative treatment (neuromodulators, injectables) if appropriate should be completed. The decision to proceed with laser/light treatment is one that should be arrived at after considering patient expectations and the clinical diagnosis. Patient expectations include their primary concern, timeline for treatment

results, costs, expected downtime and complications. A common patient misconception is that acne scars can only be treated when there are no active acne lesions. However, certain lasers such as the 650-millisecond 1064 nm Nd:YAG laser, are indicated for the treatment of active acne lesions.

Another challenge is management of melasma. The patient seeking treatment for melasma should be counseled that topical lightening agents and sun protection are primary therapies for melasma whereas laser is a secondary sometimes even tertiary treatment option after chemical peeling. The topical regimen remains a critical part of the treatment and maintenance of results. After these expectations are reviewed and there is an understanding of treatment goals, a detailed review of treatment and related complications should be completed during the informed written consent process. Patients should also be given an opportunity to have all questions answered and additional time to reflect if desired.

The history and initial evaluation also provide an opportunity to evaluate for any absolute or relative contraindications. An important consideration and possible contraindication is a patient with an excessive and pervasive preoccupation with imagined deformities or exaggeration of actual disease, meeting the criteria for body dysmorphic disorder (BDD). The nature of the contraindication should be evaluated on a case-by-case basis. In a review of 401 Caucasian, Asian, and black women by Marques et al., no statistically significant difference was found in preoccupations among Caucasians and black patients. However, when compared to Caucasians, Asian patients reported less concern with body shape and increased concern with skin color and hair type. Physician awareness of these unique differences is important in managing the ethnic skin cosmetic patient. Referral to a psychiatrist for treatment is often needed.

Relative contraindications to laser therapy include a recent history of keloids or hypertrophic scarring, active pregnancy, active inflammatory disease or infection at the treatment site, and immunocompromised state. Recent systemic retinoid use within the past 6 months should be considered for patients undergoing fully ablative laser resurfacing.

During the initial visit, a key part of the discussion should include patient expectations. During the examination, patients should be given an opportunity to highlight their concerns as those may differ from that of the physician. Realistic treatment goals should be set to address these patient concerns. This should include an estimate on the number of treatments needed to meet expectations. Additionally, counseling on post-procedure care should be completed. This should focus on sun protection during and up to 6 weeks after treatment given the higher risk of dyspigmentation in ethnic skin patients. Written guidelines on post-procedure care should be given, reinforcing the need for regular sunscreen use and topical steroids or bleaching agents if indicated. For patients undergoing laser treatment for melasma, sun protection is essential to disease remission.

After a formal evaluation and setting treatment goals, informed written consent should be obtained. This includes a review of procedure risks and benefits with an opportunity for the patient to have all questions answered. Treatment alternatives and complications can be reviewed at this time. Taking the consent form home before treatment allows for additional review time and can be reassuring for some patients.

POSTINFLAMMATORY HYPERPIGMENTATION

Postinflammatory hyperpigmentation (PIH) frequently ranks among the top 10 concerns in ethnic skin patients. It commonly occurs after inflammatory cutaneous eruptions including acne, folliculitis or various rashes. However, it can also be iatrogenic from minimally invasive interventions such as laser and other energy-based therapies. Patients typically present with ill-defined hyperpigmented macules or patches in the same distribution as the inciting inflammatory cutaneous eruption or in the same shape or pattern as the culprit device. Topical treatment remains the gold standard for treating PIH in ethnic skin patients. Initial treatment discussions should focus on ultraviolet (UV) sun protective measures with frequent application of a broad-spectrum sunscreen with SPF 30 or higher and strict sun avoidance during the treatment period and immediate post-treatment period. Physical blocking agents containing zinc oxide, titanium dioxide, and iron oxides are preferred as they also block visible light.

After a discussion on sun protective measures, topical lightening medications should be considered. Topical lightening agents commonly include retinoids,

hydroquinone, topical corticosteroids, azelaic acid, tranexamic acid, and may also include brightening ingredients like kojic acid (authors' choice of an over counter topical), niacinamide, ascorbic acid, or ferulic acid. Hydroquinone is the most commonly used lightening agent with the best evidence in ethnic skin. It can be used as monotherapy in formulations of 4% or higher as a prescription or 2% over the counter and it is well tolerated. Rare side effects include exogenous ochronosis, usually at higher concentrations, and with prolonged use. Today, hydroquinone is traditionally used in combination therapy in the triple cream (Kligman's formula: 4% hydroquinone, mild-mid potency topical steroid and tretinoin).

Chemical peels and systemic medications (oral tranexamic acid) can also be used as a tertiary treatment after a patient has failed first- and second-line treatments with sun protection and topical lightening agents, respectively. In ethnic skin, superficial peels are preferred because of its low risk since injury is limited to epidermis. There are a wide variety of treatment options for procedure related hyperpigmentation in ethnic skin. It is paramount for clinicians to be familiar with the treatment options available for treating hyperpigmentation in ethnic skin given the not infrequent complication of PIH in ethnic skin patients treated with lasers and light therapy. This chapter will highlight ways to minimize risks of hyperpigmentation in ethnic skin patients through proper laser selection and settings.

Authors' choice of treatment for procedure-related PIH:

- Superficial chemical peels: salicylic acid or mandelic acid every 3–4 weeks until resolution or until maximal effects have reached a clinical plateau
- Pretreating with 4% hydroquinone at least 2 weeks prior to treatment
- Posttreatment: a mid-potency topical corticosteroid for at least 3 days after treatment or a high-potency topical steroid for 2 days after treatment

INTRODUCTION TO LASERS AND LIGHTS IN ETHNIC SKIN

Lasers and energy-based therapy can offer an effective and fairly noninvasive method for treating signs of photoaging, dyspigmentation, scarring, and overall facial rejuvenation. In ethnic skin patients, unique challenges exist due to the not infrequent risk of post-procedure dyspigmentation because of the melanin-rich epidermis compared to nonethnic skin (skin types I–II). Procedure-related dyspigmentation can be a result of accidental melanin injury as a competing bystander chromophore or patient specific risk for PIH as part of the normal healing process. With proper training, more spaced-out treatment sessions and conservative laser settings, similar cosmetic outcomes are achievable for ethnic skin patients with the full spectrum of lasers being a safe and effective treatment option.

Laser selection should focus on identifying the proper target chromophore: water, hemoglobin or melanin, to achieve clinical goals. Other considerations for laser selection include the ability to modify settings for minimally invasive treatment. This can be achieved by using lower fluences. Another example of this includes the selection of ablative versus nonablative lasers. Ablative lasers offer quicker and more remarkable results but come with an increased risk of dyspigmentation due to the uniform sheet like destruction of the epidermis when compared to nonablative lasers that create microthermal zones, keeping most of the epidermis intact. Adjunctive tools can also be beneficial in minimizing dyspigmentation. The use of simple diascopy (glass slide compression of a blood vessel) moves blood away from the vessel lumen during vascular laser treatment (585/595-nm PDL) to decrease purpura and hyperpigmentation in ethnic skin patients without compromising treatment efficacy. With proper settings, adjunctive tools and appropriate laser selection, a wide spectrum of lasers can be available to ethnic skin patients including intense pulsed light (IPL). For IPL, lower energies with multiple passes and combining treatment with a cooling device can make it a safe option in these patients.

Ablative Fractionated Lasers

Lasers: 2940-nm Er:YAG, 10600-nm CO_2.

Indications: Atrophic acne scarring, traumatic or surgical scars, and skin rejuvenation.

Ablative fractionated lasers (AFLs) are the classic resurfacing laser. Ablative fractionated lasers differ from fully ablative lasers in that fractionated lasers stimulate collagen by causing small punctate holes with a specific depth in the dermis instead of a uniform sheet like removal of skin. They target water as a chromophore, vaporizing the skin to induce collagen regeneration. Significant improvement can be achieved in

one or two treatments compared to their nonablative counterpart. Caution is needed given the risks of dyspigmentation from the high coagulation temperatures. The risk of hyperpigmentation in ethic skin is at least 30%. Additional risks include infection, prolonged down times, and scarring. While most safe in skin types I–III, it has been proven to be a safe and effective treatment option in ethnic skin. Manuskiatti et al. showed significant improvement in atrophic scars in 24 Asian patients treated with the combined 2940-nm Er:YAG and 10600-nm CO_2 laser after just two treatment sessions. Success has also been seen in skin type IV–V (Gold 2012).

PEARL 1

- Choose lower densities for darker skin types, especially when treating with higher energies to achieve a greater depth for scars or deep rhytids.
- Reducing the number of passes can help to prevent hyperpigmentation, instead, plan for more treatment sessions to achieve the desired results safely.
- Pretreating with 4% hydroquinone at least 2 weeks prior to treatment and posttreating with a mid-potency topical corticosteroid for at least 3 days after treatment has been effective in reducing dyspigmentation in the authors' personal experiences.
- High potency topical corticosteroids applied twice a day for 2 days posttreatment decreases the risk of hyperpigmentation.

Nonablative Fractionated Lasers

Lasers: 1927/1550-nm, 1927-nm thulium, 1927-nm diode, 1064-nm Nd:YAG, 1550-nm erbium, 1440-nm diode, 755-nm and 1064-nm fractional picosecond lasers.

Indications: Melasma, skin rejuvenation, scars, hyperpigmentation.

Nonablative fractionated lasers (NAFLs) provide a safer alternative to ablative lasers in darker skin types since the stratum corneum remains mostly intact with the use of grid-like microthermal zones and only fractional dermal damage is produced. A series of NAFL procedures produces similar cosmetic outcomes to a single ablative fractionated laser procedure with less recovery time. Kono et al. compared the efficacy and safety of the 1550-nm nonablative fractional laser in 30 Asian patients treated for skin rejuvenation. Patients were split into three groups with a split face technique where each group received different levels of fluences and densities. Findings suggested that higher densities are associated with increased risk of hyperpigmentation and decreased patient satisfaction compared to higher fluences. Safe and effective use of fractionated resurfacing lasers should incorporate lower densities to minimize risks of hyperpigmentation.

The most common use of NAFL in ethnic skin patients is in the treatment of acne scarring and for skin rejuvenation. Marmon et al. reported 10 Asian patients treated with the 1440-nm diode had clinical improvement in fine rhytids, pore size, and roughness after four treatments spaced every 2 weeks. Lee et al. had similar results in 27 patients, treated with the 1550-nm erbium laser for photoaging related hyperpigmentation.

NAFL can also be a safe alternative to topical bleaching agents and chemical peels for patients with recalcitrant melasma. Success has been seen using the 1927-nm thulium and 1550-nm erbium in ethnic skin patients. Laser treatment is often used in combination with a strict sun protection regimen and topical corticosteroids to minimize hyperpigmentation risks. It is important that the sun protection be maintained well after treatment given the risk of rebound hyperpigmentation.

Modest laser settings, appropriate cooling, longer treatment intervals and sun protection are all critical to safely using NAFL and AFL lasers.

PEARL 2

- If higher fluences are being used when treating scarring, use lower densities to decrease the risk of hyperpigmentation (Video 13.1).
- Overlap minimally when completing each pass. For example, in an eight pass per area protocol, complete four passes initially per area and then go back and complete the next four passes. It is also wise to start with four to six passes per area for initial treatments and increase based on the patient's response.

Vascular Lasers

Lasers: 585/595-nm pulsed dye laser (PDL), combined 532-nm KTP/1064-nm Nd:YAG, 1064-nm Nd:YAG, 532-nm KTP or LBO.

Indications: Port-wine stain (PWS), facial erythema, telangiectasia, and scars.

Vascular lasers target hemoglobin to induce vessel injury with absorption peaks of oxyhemoglobin being primarily at 577 nm and 700–1100 nm to a lesser extent. The 585-nm PDL is the classic vascular laser used because of the close relationship with hemoglobin absorption peaks. Use of the 585/595-nm PDL and 532 KTP or LBO lasers in darker skin patients can be challenging due to the overlap with melanin absorption, increasing risks for procedure related dyspigmentation. The 1064-nm Nd:YAG laser is considered to be a safer alternative in the treatment of vascular lesions in ethnic skin patients because of its longer wavelength.

Asahina et al. evaluated the use of 595-nm PDL (7 mm spot size, 10 milliseconds pulse duration, 12 J/cm^2) in the treatment of PWS in skin type IV patients and found 67% of patients achieved good or excellent results after four treatments at 8-week intervals. Hyper- and hypopigmentation was seen in up to 17% and 14% of patients, respectively. Bae and Geronemus reported similar results without hyperpigmentation in the treatment of port wine stains in African-American children, skin types V and VI treated with the 585-nm PDL.

Vascular lasers are often underutilized in clinical practice for ethnic skin patients due to a combination of underdiagnosis of vascular neoplasms and physician reluctance given risks of hyperpigmentation. However, modest settings and use of longer wavelengths with the 1064-nm Nd:YAG should be considered in ethnic skin patients. In the authors' experience, the 585-nm PDL laser can also be used with great success with conservative settings and multiple sessions in port wine stains of adult patients (Fig. 13.1).

PEARL 3

- Vascular lesions can be safely treated in ethnic skin with the 585/595-nm PDL, 532-nm KTP or LBO, and 1064-nm Nd:YAG.
- Due to the lower risk of melanin absorption with the 1064-nm Nd:YAG, this may be the safest wavelength to use in ethnic skin patients.
- Adjusting fluence settings based on location can maximize clinical outcomes (Video 13.2)

Hybrid Laser

Lasers: 1470/2940-nm combined laser.

Indications: Skin resurfacing, skin rejuvenation, scarring.

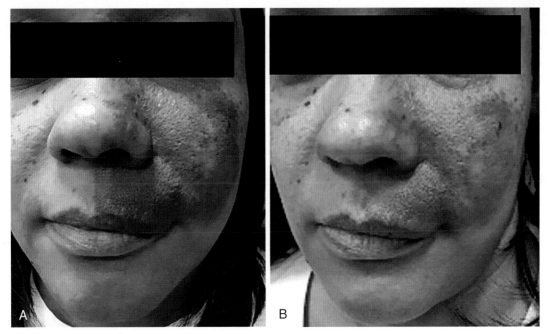

Fig. 13.1 Treatment of a port wine stain in a skin type IV patient after 10 sessions of a 595-nm pulsed-dye laser.

The 1470/2940-nm hybrid laser is the first hybrid laser that delivers nonablative (1470 nm) and ablative (2940 nm) wavelengths sequentially to a treatment area. The 1470 nm wavelength creates focused dermal coagulation to stimulate collagen, while the 2940 nm wavelength provides ablation reaching cutaneous depths of 700 micrometers and 100 micrometers respectively. Waibel et al. studied the efficacy and safety of the 1470/2940-nm hybrid laser in 34 female patients with skin types I–IV, including Asian and Hispanic patients. In this study, 83% of participants had improved pores and 63% had improved skin texture after two laser treatments, 1 month apart. In ethnic skin, lower densities and energies are needed to safely treat patients.

PEARL 4

- Similar to ablative fractional lasers, pretreatment with 4% hydroquinone for at least 2 weeks prior and use of a mid-potency topical corticosteroid for at least 3 days following treatment can decrease dyspigmentation in the authors' experience
- Low densities and completing the passes slowly but continually moving allows for even distribution of heat (Video 13.3)

Laser Hair Removal

Lasers: 694-nm ruby, 755-nm alexandrite, 810-nm diode, and 1064-nm Nd:YAG lasers, and IPL.

Hair removal lasers target follicular melanin, most sensitive during the anagen phase of hair growth to induce apoptosis. This is a safe and effective alternative to electrolysis and traditional methods for hair removal (shaving, waxing, other chemical destruction) and is favored in patients with recurrent folliculitis or hyperpigmentation as a complication of other methods of hair removal. The devices target dermal follicular melanin. Careful consideration is needed given the competing epidermal melanin that the laser must past to reach the follicle. In ethnic skin, conservative settings with adequate cooling, longer wavelengths and longer pulse duration is necessary to decrease the risks of hyperpigmentation and scarring.

Longer wavelengths allow for more targeted treatment. To date, two laser devices are approved by the Food and Drug Administration (FDA) for laser hair removal in ethnic skin, the 810-nm diode, and the 1064-nm Nd:YAG. Both lasers have long wavelengths which penetrate into the dermis, long pulse durations (100 milliseconds or longer for the 810-nm diode and over 30 milliseconds for the 1064-nm Nd:YAG) and concurrent epidermal cooling. In ethnic skin, the 1064-nm Nd:YAG is considered the gold standard for hair removal in skin type IV–VI. Because of its long wavelength, the energy is less well absorbed by melanin (Video 13.4) and the fluence is adjusted to reach the target endpoint of peri-follicular erythema (Video 13.5). A disadvantage of the 1064-nm Nd:YAG is that the longer wavelength and slightly melanin absorption decreases its efficacy when compared to the 810-nm diode laser. Galadari reported a 40% and 35% decrease in hair density with a series of 810-nm diode and 1064 Nd:YAG laser treatments, respectively. Nevertheless, the slightly decreased efficacy must be weighed against the safety. For small treatment areas, one session can provide significant improvement (Fig. 13.2).

Further comparisons of the 755-nm alexandrite, 810-nm diode, and 1064-nm Nd:YAG lasers, and IPL in darker skin types have demonstrated minimal differences in efficacy and safety. Dorgham reviewed these differences in a systematic review of 237 patients with skin types III–VI. In this large review statistically significant similar safety and efficacy profiles were seen across laser groups when compared with IPL and within lasers. A notable exception was an increase in transient acute post-procedure pain which was seen in the laser arms when compared with IPL, with the 1064-nm Nd:YAG being implicated most frequently. However, the overall incidence of dyspigmentation was lower in the 1064-nm Nd:YAG treated group.

> **PEARL 5**
> - The 755-nm alexandrite laser can be an effective and safe alternative to the 1064-nm Nd:YAG in darker skin types when used with the largest spot size at very low fluences.
> - A test treatment area prior to full treatment is recommended.
> - Caution should be used with IPL in darker skin types for hair removal given the nonspecific wavelength and high risk of dyspigmentation.

650-Microsecond 1064-nm Laser

Indications: Active acne, hyperpigmentation, melasma, hair removal, pseudofolliculitis barbae.

The 650-microsecond 1064-nm Nd:YAG laser is considered to be one of the safest lasers in ethnic skin given the long wavelengths, bypassing melanin chromophores. It has revolutionized the use of the Nd:YAG laser in ethnic skin given its relatively short pulse duration of 0.65 ms and long wavelength. In hair removal, the pulse duration is less than the thermal relaxation time of 0.8 ms for skin around the hair follicle. This allows for painless treatment sessions that do not require cooling. It is also unique in that it is contactless since a collimated beam is used, unchanged by fluence or spot size.

Common uses include the treatment of active acne, acne scars and hyperpigmentation. In acne scars, it has been used with great success in the treatment of patients with moderate–severe acne and atrophic scars in combination with low-dose isotretinoin. In melasma, it has successfully

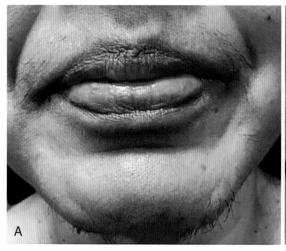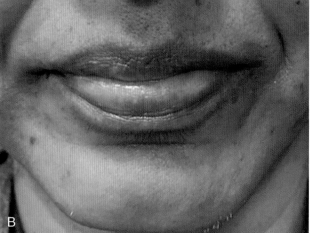

Fig. 13.2 Treatment of hirsutism in a skin type IV patient after one session of an 1064-nm Nd:YAG laser.

targeted dermal pigment in ethnic skin patients when used in combination with cysteamine cream. In one preliminary study by Wong et al. three patients underwent four laser treatments, 1 month apart without complications of dyspigmentation or procedure related pain for melasma with significant improvement.

PEARL 6

- The use of the 650 microsecond 1064-nm laser can be used to effectively treat melasma in ethnic skin by targeting dermal pigmentation in combination with traditional lightening agents to target epidermal pigment

---

Picosecond Lasers

Lasers: Wavelengths include 532 nm, 670 nm, 730 nm, 785 nm, 1064 nm.

Indications: Melasma, PIH, tattoo removal, benign pigmented lesions, skin rejuvenation, acne scarring, reducing pore size

Picosecond lasers deliver very short pulse durations (300–750 picoseconds) which can be used to target endogenous (lentigines and nevus of Ota) and exogenous pigment (tattoos) and pigmentary disorders such as melasma. Anecdotally, low energy, high frequency treatments have been used to treat erythema dyschromicum perstans (Fig. 13.3). These ultrashort pulses produce more mechanical than thermal injury, resulting in minimal collateral damage. When fractionated these lasers are particularly effective in improving photoaging associated pigmentation and treating mild acne scarring and fine wrinkling.

Studies have shown success in the treatment of Hori's nevus in ethnic skin. Ding et al. completed a retrospective review of 225 Chinese patients (skin types III–IV). 66% of patients treated saw clinical improvement in the appearance of their Hori's nevus. Average laser settings included a pulse duration of 750 picoseconds, spot sizes of 2.0–4.5 mm, 5 Hz frequency, and a fluence of 1.26–6.37 J/cm^2. Patients received one to four treatments, with a higher number of treatments correlating with increased efficacy, although 38% of patients had notable improvement after just one treatment. This highlights the rapid onset and efficacy of picosecond lasers. Less treatment sessions are often needed for clinical improvement when compared to Q-switched counterparts.

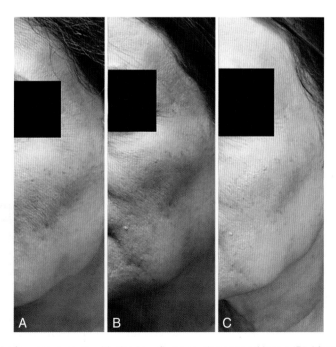

Fig. 13.3 (A) before treatment with the low fluence picosecond laser, (B) After first treatment, of the low fluence picosecond laser (C) After 2 treatments with the low fluence picosecond laser.

The addition of a diffractive lens array transforms the picosecond laser to a nonablative fractionated laser. With this modification, Haimovic et al. demonstrated improvement in acne scarring and striae in darker skin types (VI). Patients were treated with spot size of 6 mm, fluence of 0.71 J/cm^2, and pulse width of 750–850 picoseconds. Treatment was well tolerated with mild post-procedure erythema that self-resolved.

Picosecond lasers are also emerging in the removal of tattoo pigmentation. Kono and Chan compared the 532- and 1064-nm picosecond lasers to nanosecond Q-switched lasers. The 1064-nm picosecond laser was proven effective for black tattoos, the 532-nm picosecond laser for red and green tattoos. Treatments were complicated by a 5.4% incidence of paradoxical darkening.

PEARL 7

- The diffractive lens array or micro lens array handpiece fractionates picosecond laser light through a holographic lens to induce nonthermal optical breakdown and can be highly safe and effective using the 1064-nm wavelength to treat acne scarring and textural irregularities in darker skin. It is a great alternative treatment with little to no downtime, compared to NAFL or AFL.
- Although more treatments are required, the risk of hyperpigmentation is minimal.
- These procedures do not usually require topical anesthesia.
- Low fluence and low energies are recommended in ethnic skin (Video 13.6)

Q-Switched Lasers

Lasers: QS 1064-nm Nd:YAG, 755-nm QS alexandrite, and 694-nm QS Ruby.

Indications: Tattoo removal, freckles and lentigines, nevus of Ota/Ito, Hori's nevus, Becker nevus.

Q-switched lasers deliver high powered, short pulses (nanoseconds). In ethnic skin, lower fluences are recommended. As a result, more treatment sessions are needed to have comparable results to nonethnic skin. Low fluence 1064-nm Nd:YAG, often termed laser toning is well tolerated and effective in skin types III and IV. Kaminaka et al. studied the efficacy of the 1064-nm Nd:YAG in 22 Japanese patients treated with 10 sessions for melasma and solar lentigines. All patients improved. Although

lower fluences allow for the use of Q-switched lasers in ethnic skin, hypopigmentation is a significant concern. Shah and Aurangabadkar reviewed the technique of laser toning in 10 studies with the 1064-nm Q-switched Nd:YAG for melasma. Ten to twelve weekly sessions were performed with fluences between 0.8 and 2 J/cm^2. While melasma was improved, treatment side effects included mottled hypopigmentation, seen 2 months post the final treatment. Other complications included rebound melasma, punctate leukoderma, acneiform eruptions, and petechiae. This risk can be reduced or eliminated by reducing the frequency and number of treatments and the fluence.

Q-switched lasers are also effective for removing tattoos in ethnic skin patients. In a study of 20 female Arabic patients (skin types III–IV) treated with the Q-switched 755-nm alexandrite laser with an average fluence of 6 J/cm^2 (range $4.0\text{–}7.5 \text{ J/cm}^2$) for three to six sessions at 6- to 12-week intervals, Bukhari et al. found that blue-black tattoo pigment was successfully removed without major complications. Longer wavelengths are less well absorbed by melanin and decrease the pigmentary risks.

PEARL 8

- Laser toning should be used with caution in ethnic skin given the sometimes-permanent risk of mottled hypopigmentation.
- Increasing treatment intervals and less total treatments can minimize this risk.

INTENSE PULSED LIGHT

Indications: Skin rejuvenation, lentigines, facial redness and telangiectasia, and hair removal.

IPL is a nonablative, broadband, nonlaser light (515–1200 nm) source that transmits high intensity pulses of mostly visible light. IPL is different from lasers in that it is not monochromatic and delivers a broad range of wavelengths. By using a variety of filters to limit the spectrum of emitted light a long list of entities can be effectively treated including vascular and pigmented targets and unwanted hair.

Shin et al. completed a study of 26 Korean patients with facial dyschromias. Three IPL sessions were performed

4 weeks apart. Eighty-four percent of patients reported improvement in the appearance of pigmented lesions and 58% noted improvement in rhytids. We recommend using longer pulsed durations when treating ethnic skin and limiting the use of IPL to skin types IV and lower.

PEARL 9

- It is paramount that the device remains in full contact with the skin while firing to prevent burns. If the handpiece is not flush with the skin, the heat is delivered unevenly which can lead to complications, especially in darker skin.
- It is safer to perform multiple passes to reach your desired endpoint at very low energies, than to use a higher energy with higher risk.
- Combining the treatment with a cooling device in addition to contact cooling can help with patient comfort and also protect the skin to reduce pigmentary risk.
- Ice immediately after treatment. We usually apply a thin layer of a mid-potency topical corticosteroid immediately after treatment.

MICRONEEDLING

Indications: Melasma, acne, scars, skin rejuvenation, hyperpigmentation.

Microneedling is a safe and minimally invasive procedure for skin resurfacing. It creates numerous superficial micro-punctures in the epidermis and into the superficial dermis. Blood vessel disruption is thought to initiate activation of various platelet-derived growth factors that promote skin remodeling and regeneration. Microneedling devices can either be automated or used manually in a rolling fashion to make numerous punctures in the skin that can allow transdermal delivery of topical medications to better penetrate the stratum corneum, further enhancing rejuvenation. Modified microneedling devices are also emerging with increased use among dermatologists. They include radiofrequency (RF) microneedling (see Chapter 12) and microplasma RF (see below), using high frequency energy to stimulate neocollagenasis.

In ethnic skin, microneedling is generally considered safer than traditional resurfacing light therapies, dermabrasion and chemical peels because the epidermis remains largely intact, resulting in faster recovery.

Furthermore, no chromophores are targeted, and the risk of dyspigmentation is minimal. Given the superficial epidermal penetration, multiple treatment sessions are often needed for significant clinical results (Fig. 13.4).

Microneedling has been used with success in the treatment of acne scars, acne, melasma, and skin rejuvenation in all skin types. Fabbrocini et al. reported a 31% decrease in uneven skin texture after three treatments 4 weeks apart in 50 skin types III–VI patients. In acne vulgaris, Kim et al. reported a decrease in both the amount of sebum production and number of active acne lesions have been reported in skin type III–V patients treated with three sessions, 4 weeks apart. In melasma, microneedling has been used more frequently to enhance the delivery of a topical lightening agent, resulting in decreases in the Melasma Area Severity Index score. Tranexamic acid and other compounded lightening agents have been used with success in conjunction with microneedling.

PEARL 10

- Microneedling is safe in darker skin types because there is no emission of heat, therefore reducing posttreatment erythema and inflammation.

MICROPLASMA RADIOFREQUENCY

Indications: Skin rejuvenation, acne scars.

Microplasma RF is an FDA-cleared micro-ablative high-frequency (>40 MHz) unipolar device, combining RF with plasma. It functions as a fractional resurfacing device using metal pins that transmit RF energy to the skin in a grid like pattern. It provides a quick (<20 minutes) alternative to traditional lasers with comparable results with a smaller number of treatments and minimal recovery time.

In a comparative split face study evaluating the efficacy of the microplasma RF device with the 10,600 CO_2 laser in 33 Asian patients (skin types III–IV) with atrophic acne scars by Zhang and Fei et al., comparable results were seen with fewer side effects in the RF group. In this study, participants received 3 treatments, with an average of 8 weeks apart (range 6–12 weeks). Laser settings for the CO_2 group included an energy output of 20–25 mJ and density of 2–4 (10%–20% coverage/cm² per pass) with one unoverlapping pass. Participants in the fractional microplasma RF group

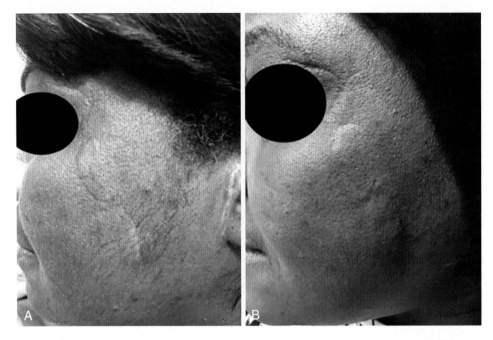

Fig. 13.4 Skin type V patient with scar microneedling before (A) and after (B) four treatments.

completed four passes of the roller tip (50–60 W). Similar clinical improvement was noted 6 months posttreatment (no statistically significant difference) with less procedural erythema in the RF group and no evidence of PIH in the RF group (one-third of the CO_2 group experienced PIH).

Fractional microplasma RF devices can provide a safer and equally effective alternative to traditional ablative lasers in ethnic skin where risks of PIH are high and where conservative laser settings are necessary given this risk of PIH, resulting in less clinical improvement compared to nonethnic skin where more aggressive settings can be tolerated. Fractional plasma can also be customized to provide a chemical peel-like effect or approaching a fractional CO_2-like effect with minimal downtime (Videos 13.7 and 13.8, Fig. 13.5).

PEARL 11

- Remove topical anesthetic in sections and use forced cold air for patient comfort.
- Do not apply pressure to the skin when using the glide tip. Gently roll over the treatment zone.
- Maintain contact with the skin for the entire pulse when using the focus tip.
- Avoid treatment if the patient has metal implants in the underlying treatment zone.

SKIN TIGHTENING DEVICES

Infrared lasers, high-intensity focused ultrasound (HIFU), and radiofrequency devices.

Skin tightening devices are nonsurgical, non to minimally invasive therapies for improving skin laxity. Commonly used devices include infrared lasers, high-intensity focused ultrasound (HIFU), and monopolar and bipolar RF. They are safe and well tolerated in all skin types because IR, ultrasound, and RF are not absorbed by skin pigment. They work by heating dermal collagen to stimulate neocollagenesis, leading to the regeneration of collagen to improve skin laxity. Treatments are very well tolerated and side effects rare. Swelling and erythema are uncommon and thermal burns, subcutaneous nodules and scarring are rare.

Infrared lasers have been used with success in skin types IV–V. Chua et al. completed a study of 21 patients with skin types IV–V for three sessions with 87% improvement in skin laxity. The rare complication of transient dyspigmentation related to treatment was noted in just 7 of the 63 sessions. Similar results have been reported with HIFU in patients with one to two treatment sessions adequate for noticeable clinical improvement.

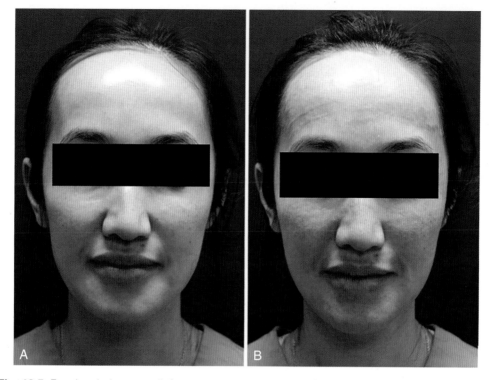

Fig. 13.5 Fractional plasma radiofrequency pretreatment (A) and immediately posttreatment (B) in a skin type IV patient.

CONCLUSION

The changing ethnic demographics globally, creates an increased demand for esthetic treatments in the ethnic patient. Lasers and energy-based therapies have long been used with great efficacy and safety in skin types I–III. Challenges however arise when lasers are applied to ethnic skin patients; skin types IV–VI given the not uncommon risk of PIH and less commonly hypopigmentation. Physician understanding of this unique challenge, patient factors in prevention (sun protection) and appropriate and conservative treatment parameter settings allow these devices to be used safely and effectively in ethnic skin patients.

FURTHER READING

Alexis AF, Obioha JO. Ethnicity and aging skin. *J Drugs Dermatol.* 2017;16(6):s77–s80.

Alster TS, Bryan H, Williams CM. Long-pulsed Nd:YAG laser-assisted hair removal in pigmented skin: a clinical and histological evaluation. *Arch Dermatol.* 2001;137(7):885–889.

Asahina A, Watanabe T, Kishi A, et al. Evaluation of the treatment of port-wine stains with the 595-nm long pulsed dye laser: a large prospective study in adult Japanese patients. *J Am Acad Dermatol.* 2006;54(3):487–493.

Bae YS, Ng E, Geronemus RG. Successful treatment of two pediatric port wine stains in darker skin types using 595 nm laser. *Lasers Surg Med.* 2016;48(4):339–342.

Battle E, Suthamjariya K, Alora M. Very long pulses (20-200 ms) diode laser for hair removal on all skin types. *Lasers Surg Med.* 2000(12 suppl):21–24.

Battle EF, Jr. The 810 nm diode laser: a safe, effective modality to meet a growing population need. *J Drugs Dermatol.* 2011;10(12 suppl):s8–s9.

Battle F, Battle S. Clinical evaluation of safety and efficacy of fractional radiofrequency facial treatment of skin type VI patients. *J Drugs Dermatol.* 2018;17(11):1169–1172. 1.

Budamakuntla L, Loganathan E, Suresh DH, et al. A randomised, open-label, comparative study of tranexamic acid microinjections and tranexamic acid with microneedling in patients with melasma. *J Cutan Aesthet Surg.* 2013;6(3):139–143.

Bukhari IA. Removal of amateur blue-black tattoos in Arabic women of skin type (III-IV) with Q-switched alexandrite laser. *J Cosmet Dermatol.* 2005;4:107–110.

Chan CS, Dover JS. Nd:YAG laser hair removal in Fitzpatrick skin types IV to VI. *J Drugs Dermatol.* 2013;12(3):366–367.

Chandrashekar BS, Sriram R, Mysore R, Bhaskar S, Shetty A. Evaluation of microneedling fractional radiofrequency device for treatment of acne scars. *J Cutan Aesthet Surg.* 2014;7(2):93–97.

Chua SH, Ang P, Khoo LS, Goh CL. Nonablative infrared skin tightening in Type IV to V Asian skin: a prospective clinical study. *Dermatol Surg.* 2007;33(2):146–151.

Cohen BE, Elbuluk N. Microneedling in skin of color: A review of uses and efficacy. *J Am Acad Dermatol.* 2016;74(2):348–355.

Cook-Bolden F. A novel 0.65 millisecond pulsed 1064 nm laser to treat skin of color without skin cooling or anesthetics. *J Drugs Dermatol.* 2011;10(12 suppl): s10–s11.

Ding H, Yang Y, Guo L, Lin T. Use of a picosecond alexandrite laser for treating acquired bilateral nevus of ota-like macules in chinese patients. *Lasers Surg Med.* 2020;52(10):935–939.

Dorgham NA, Dorgham DA. Lasers for reduction of unwanted hair in skin of colour: a systematic review and meta-analysis. *J Eur Acad Dermatol Venereol.* 2020;34(5):948–955.

Fabbrocini G, De Vita V, Monfrecola A, et al. Percutaneous collagen induction: an effective and safe treatment for post-acne scarring in different skin phototypes. *J Dermatolog Treat.* 2014;25(2):147–152.

Galadari I. Comparative evaluation of different hair removal lasers in skin types IV, V, and VI. *Int J Dermatol.* 2003;42(1):68–70.

Goel A, Krupashankar DS, Aurangabadkar S, Nischal KC, Omprakash HM, Mysore V. Fractional lasers in dermatology--current status and recommendations. *Indian J Dermatol Venereol Leprol.* 2011;77(3):369–379.

Gold MH, Manturova NE, Kruglova LS, Ikonnikova EV. Treatment of moderate to severe acne and scars with a 650-microsecond 1064-nm laser and isotretinoin. *J Drugs Dermatol.* 2020;19(6):646–651. 1.

Gold MH. Clinical evaluation of the safety and efficacy of a novel superficial and deep carbon dioxide fractional system in the treatment of patients with skin of color. *J Drugs Dermatol.* 2012;11(11):1331–1335.

Goldberg DJ. Current trends in intense pulsed light. *J Clin Aesthet Dermatol.* 2012;5(6):45–53.

Haimovic A, Brauer JA, Cindy Bae YS, Geronemus RG. Safety of a picosecond laser with diffractive lens array (DLA) in the treatment of Fitzpatrick skin types IV to VI: a retrospective review. *J Am Acad Dermatol.* 2016;74(5):931–936.

Halachmi S, Orenstein A, Meneghel T, Lapidoth M. A novel fractional micro-plasma radio-frequency technology for the treatment of facial scars and rhytids: a pilot study. *J Cosmet Laser Ther.* 2010;12(5):208–212.

Hu S, Yang CS, Chang SL, Huang YL, Lin YF, Lee MC. Efficacy and safety of the picosecond 755-nm alexandrite laser for treatment of dermal pigmentation in Asians—a retrospective study. *Lasers Med Sci.* 2020;35(6): 1377–1383.

Ismail SA. Long-pulsed Nd:YAG laser vs. intense pulsed light for hair removal in dark skin: a randomized controlled trial. *Br J Dermatol.* 2012;166(2):317–321.

Johnson B, Marrone S, Om A. Novel combination of a 650-microsecond neodymium-doped yttrium aluminium garnet 1,064-nm laser and cysteamine cream for the treatment of melasma: a case study. *J Clin Aesthet Dermatol.* 2020;13(3):28–30.

Kaminaka C, Furukawa F, Yamamoto Y. The clinical and histological effect of a low-fluence Q-switched 1,064-nm neodymium: yttrium-aluminum-garnet laser for the treatment of melasma and solar lentigenes in asians: prospective, randomized, and split-face comparative study. *Dermatol Surg.* 2017;43(9):1120–1133.

Kasai K. Picosecond laser treatment for tattoos and benign cutaneous pigmented lesions (secondary publication). *Laser Ther.* 2017;26(4):274–281. 31.

Kim M, Shin JY, Lee J, Kim JY, Oh SH. Efficacy of fractional microneedle radiofrequency device in the treatment of primary axillary hyperhidrosis: a pilot study. *Dermatology.* 2013;227(3):243–249.

Kim ST, Lee KH, Sim HJ, Suh KS, Jang MS. Treatment of acne vulgaris with fractional radiofrequency microneedling. *J Dermatol.* 2014;41(7):586–591.

Kolinko VG, Littler CM, Cole A. Influence of the anagen:telogen ratio on Q-switched Nd:YAG laser hair removal efficacy. *Lasers Surg Med.* 2000;26(1):33–40.

Kono T, Chan HH, Groff WF, et al. Prospective direct comparison study of fractional resurfacing using different fluences and densities for skin rejuvenation in Asians. *Lasers Surg Med.* 2007;39(4):311–314.

Kono T, Chan HHL, Groff WF, Imagawa K, Hanai U, Akamatsu T. Prospective comparison study of 532/1064 nm picosecond laser vs 532/1064 nm nanosecond laser in the treatment of professional tattoos in asians. *Laser Ther.* 2017;29(1):47–52. 20.

Lee HS, Lee JH, Ahn GY, et al. Fractional photothermolysis for the treatment of acne scars: a report of 27 Korean patients. *J Dermatolog Treat.* 2008;19(1):45–49.

Mahmoud BH, Srivastava D, Janiga JJ, Yang JJ, Lim HW, Ozog DM. Safety and efficacy of erbium-doped yttrium aluminum garnet fractionated laser for treatment of acne scars in type IV to VI skin. *Dermatol Surg.* 2010;36(5):602–609.

Manuskiatti W, Iamphonrat T, Wanitphakdeedecha R, Eimpunth S. Comparison of fractional erbium-doped yttrium aluminum garnet and carbon dioxide lasers in resurfacing of atrophic acne scars in Asians. *Dermatol Surg.* 2013;39 (1 Pt 1):111–120.

Marmon S, Shek SY, Yeung CK, Chan NP, Chan JC, Chan HH. Evaluating the safety and efficacy of the 1,440-nm laser in the treatment of photodamage in Asian skin. *Lasers Surg Med.* 2014;46(5):375–379.

Marques L, LeBlanc N, Weingarden H, et al. Body dysmorphic symptoms: phenomenology and ethnicity. *Body Image.* 2011;8(2):163–167.

Mirza FN, Mirza HN, Khatri KA. Concomitant use of isotretinoin and lasers with implications for future guidelines: an updated systematic review. *Dermatol Ther.* 2020;33(6):e14022.

Mojeski JA, Almashali M, Jowdy P, et al. Ultraviolet imaging in dermatology. *Photodiagnosis Photodyn Ther.* 2020;30:101743.

Mulholland RS. Radio frequency energy for non-invasive and minimally invasive skin tightening. *Clin Plast Surg.* 2011;38(3, vi):437–448.

Passel J. Cohn D. U.S. Population projections: 2005-2050. Pew Research Center, Washington, DC; 2008. https://www.pewresearch.org/hispanic/2008/02/11/us-population-projections-2005-2050/.

Preissig J, Hamilton K, Markus R. Current laser resurfacing technologies: a review that delves beneath the surface. *Semin Plast Surg.* 2012;26(3):109–116.

Puiu T, Mohammad TF, Ozog DM, Rambhatla PV. A comparative analysis of electric and radiofrequency microneedling devices on the market. *J Drugs Dermatol.* 2018;17(9):1010–1013. 1.

Rokhsar CK, Fitzpatrick RE. The treatment of melasma with fractional photothermolysis: a pilot study. *Dermatol Surg.* 2005;31(12):1645–1650.

Shah SD, Aurangabadkar SJ. Laser toning in melasma. *J Cutan Aesthet Surg.* 2019;12(2):76–84.

Shin JW, Lee DH, Choi SY, et al. Objective and non-invasive evaluation of photorejuvenation effect with intense pulsed light treatment in Asian skin. *J Eur Acad Dermatol Venereol.* 2011;25(5):516–522.

Sommer S, Sheehan-Dare RA. Pulsed dye laser treatment of port-wine stains in pigmented skin. *J Am Acad Dermatol.* 2000;42(4):667–671.

Trivedi MK, Yang FC, Cho BK. A review of laser and light therapy in melasma. *Int J Womens Dermatol.* 2017;3(1):11–20. 21.

Waibel S, Pozner J, Robb C, Tanzi E. Hybrid fractional laser: a multi-center trial on the safety and efficacy for photorejuvenation. *J Drugs Dermatol.* 2018;17(11):1164–1168.

Wall TL. Current concepts: laser treatment of adult vascular lesions. *Semin Plast Surg.* 2007;21(3):147–158.

Wanitphakdeedecha R, Sy-Alvarado F, Patthamalai P, Techapichetvanich T, Eimpunth S, Manuskiatti W. The efficacy in treatment of facial melasma with thulium 1927-nm fractional laser-assisted topical tranexamic acid delivery: a split-face, double-blind, randomized controlled pilot study. *Lasers Med Sci.* 2020;35(9):2015–2021.

Wind BS, Kroon MW, Meesters AA, et al. Non-ablative 1,550 nm fractional laser therapy versus triple topical therapy for the treatment of melasma: a randomized controlled split-face study. *Lasers Surg Med.* 2010;42(7):607–612.

Wong CSM, Chan MWM, Shek SYN, Yeung CK, Chan HHL. Fractional 1064 nm picosecond laser in treatment of melasma and skin rejuvenation in asians, a prospective study. *Lasers Surg Med.* 2021;53(8):1032–1042.

Zhang Z, Fei Y, Chen X, Lu W, Chen J. Comparison of a fractional microplasma radio frequency technology and carbon dioxide fractional laser for the treatment of atrophic acne scars: a randomized split-face clinical study. *Dermatol Surg.* 2013;39(4):559–566.

14

Treatment of Acne With Light and Energy-Based Devices

Mitchel P. Goldman, Emily Wood, Rawaa Almukhtar, and Steven Krueger

SUMMARY OF KEY FEATURES

- Around 85% of 12- to 24-year olds are affected by acne, while many patients continue to struggle with acne even into adulthood.
- Acne is extremely frustrating for patients and causes depression and anxiety, poor self image, as well as, lasting physical scarring.
- Many patients struggle to achieve long lasting results with standard acne therapy which makes lasers and lights an important modality to consider when treating a patient refractory to treatment.
- Lasers and light-based devices have the ability to not only treat acne in a more expedited manner but also to simultaneously improve acne scars.

INTRODUCTION

Affecting up to 50 million Americans annually, acne is the most common skin condition in the United States. Eight five percent of those aged 12–24 are affected by acne and it in can continue well into adulthood. Lasers and light devices offer many benefits over traditional acne therapy including fewer adverse effects compared to topical and systemic therapies, decreased risk for antibiotic resistance, faster onset of action, minimizing scaring as well as decreased need for continuous therapy (Table 14.1).

Laser and light sources for treatment of acne fall into two broad categories, those that destroy *Cutibacterium acnes* which include: blue light, red light, green light laser, yellow light laser, and intense-pulsed light (IPL) and the second category which include devices that directly destroy sebaceous glands (infrared lasers). We discuss the rationale for using various laser- and light-based devices and their role in treating acne as well as which devices prove to be the most helpful clinically. Further, we detail the use of sequential lasers and lights to activate aminolevulinic acid (ALA) in photodynamic therapy.

PHOTODYNAMIC THERAPY

Historically, the use of light in treatment of acne dates back to the 1940s. Different types of ultraviolet lights have been used to destroy follicular bacteria and expedite resolution of acne lesions. No longer are carcinogenic UVB and UVA light sources used for the treatment of acne, rather, a safer range of light delivery systems are now used. Every living cell synthesizes protoporphyrins, including protoporphyrin IX (PpIX) from endogenous ALA. When ALA is administered exogenously, premalignant and malignant cells, as well as, blood vessels and sebaceous glands, produce increasing amounts of photoactive porphyrins, including PpIX.

Photodynamic therapy requires light, a photosensitizer, and oxygen. ALA is the first compound synthesized in the porphyrin-heme pathway and is converted endogenously into the photosensitizer PpIX. Application of topical ALA bypasses the rate limiting enzyme in heme formation, ALA synthase, creating accumulation of PpIX in target tissue due to increased activity of porphobilinogen deaminase

TABLE 14.1 Laser and Light Therapies Used to Treat Acne Vulgaris

Laser	Wavelength
Blue light	415 nm
Red light	630 nm
Pulsed-dye laser (PDL)	585–595 nm
Intense-pulsed light (IPL)	500–1200 nm
Potassium titanyl phosphate (KTP)	532 nm
Nd:YAG	1064 nm
Nd:YAG	1320 nm
Erbium glass	1540 nm
Erbium glass	1550 nm
Other	1726 nm

and decreased activity of ferrochelatase (Fig. 14.1). Upon exposure to its visible light action spectra (400–410 nm and 635 nm), PpIX is oxidized and produces reactive oxygen species which destroy the target cell (Fig. 14.2). *C. acnes* produces endogenous porphyrins, including PpIX and coprophorphyrin III, which makes it an excellent target for treatment with photodynamic therapy (PDT).

5-Aminolevulinic acid (5-ALA) is the most commonly used photosensitizer with methyl aminolevulinate (MAL), the most common derivative of 5-ALA. 5-ALA has a low-molecular weight allowing it to easily penetrate the stratum corneum. Topical ALA is available in the United States as a 20% solution and is marketed under the trade name Levulan Kerastick (DUSA Pharmaceuticals, Inc., Wilmington, MA). It is FDA approved since 1999 for the treatment of nonhyperkeratotic actinic keratosis (AKs) on the face, scalp, or upper extremities in conjunction with a blue light source. ALA in a 10% gel formulation is designed to be used with red light and is marketed under the name Ameluz (Ameluz; Biofrontera, Inc., Wakefield, MA). The gel formulation offers the advantage of enhancing skin penetration via nanoemulsion technology, longer shelf life (up to 12 weeks in the refrigerator) and the ability to illuminate the treatment area after 3 hours of application. The 20% solution must be discarded 2 hours after mixing ALA with the vehicle.

The addition of a methyl ester group makes MAL more lipophilic and enhances penetration but must be demethylated back to ALA by intracellular enzymes. MAL is no longer available in the United States; however, it is widely used in Europe. It was available in the United States as a 16.8% cream and marketed under the trade name Metvixia (Galderma Laboratories, L.P., Ft. Worth, TX).

Pretreatment

Patients with history of photosensitizing disorders, porphyrias, or documented allergy to ALA should not be treated with PDT. Since wavelengths in the visible light spectrum are used for activation, concurrent use of photosensitizing medications should not be a concern. Degreasing the skin prior to application of ALA allows for even distribution. Traditionally, acetone was used; however, due to its low flash point and pain associated with eroded skin alternative methods are used. Peikert and colleagues showed equal degreasing capability between acetone and hibiclens for prepping skin before chemical peeling of the scalp. Isopropyl alcohol, soap, alpha-hydroxy/salicylic acid cleansers, or cleansing towelettes can also be used.

After degreasing the skin, numerous techniques can be used to disrupt the stratum corneum to increase penetration of ALA. Heavy-handed abrasion with a 4×4 gauze is one of the simplest and cost-effective methods of increasing ALA uptake into the skin. Lee et al. demonstrated a 40- to 50-fold increased uptake of ALA using a microabrasion device (Pepita-C, Mattioli Engineering, Florence, Italy). This device sprays aluminum oxide crystals via a nozzle with a variably programmed pressure (15–25 cm Hg), producing an abrasive effect on the stratum corneum. Similarly Zhou and Banga demonstrated increased penetration of nicotinamide, a hydrophilic molecule, using microdermabrasion with 15 in Hg aluminum oxide crystals on hairless rats (Microclear Vortx System, Lasermax services, Inc., Atlanta, GA). Increased penetration was not seen with lipophilic molecules. Pretreating the skin with microneedling prior to application of ALA has also been shown to increase penetration of ALA without increasing pain and erythema. In the authors practice, we find a non-particulate stainless steel vibratory paddle to be an efficient method of removing the stratum corneum in preparation for applying topical ALA (Vibraderm, Esthetica Inc, Allentown, PA).

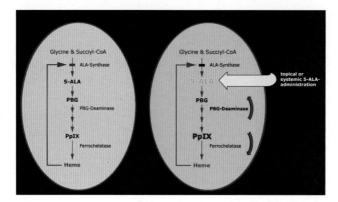

Fig. 14.1 Application of aminolevulinic acid *(ALA)* bypasses the rate-determining action of heme on ALA-synthase. Increased PBG-deaminase and decreased ferrochelatase activities in rapid proliferating cells result in high accumulation of protoporphyrin IX in these tissues. *PpIX*, protoporphyrin IX.

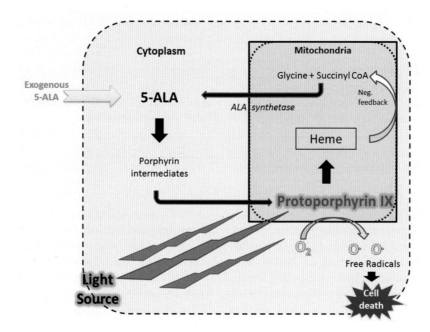

Fig. 14.2 Mechanism of photodynamic therapy (PDT). Exogenous aminolevulinic acid *(ALA)* enters the porphyrin-heme pathway and is converted endogenously into the protoporphyrin IX (PpIX). Once PpIX is activated by the proper wavelength of light production of singlet oxygen free radicals occurs, which destroy the target cell. (From Ozog DM, Rkein AM, Fabi SG, et al. Photodynamic therapy: a clinical consensus guide. *Dermatol Surg.* 2016;42(7):804-827.)

Treatment

Different lasers and lights can be used to activate porphyrins in PDT. Blue and red lights, as well as, IPL (500–1200 nm) and pulsed-dye laser (PDL) (585–595 nm) target the absorption peaks of PpIX. The major absorption peak of PpIX is 415 nm, otherwise known as the soret band, which lies within the blue range of the visible light spectrum (Fig. 14.3).

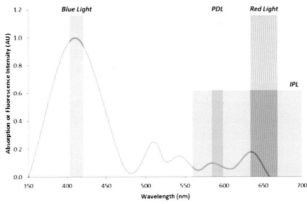

Fig. 14.3 The absorption peaks of protoporphyrin IX, the major absorption peak is seen at 415 nm, otherwise known as the soret band. There are also smaller absorption peaks at 505, 540, 580 nm and 630 nm. (From Friedmann DP, Goldman MP, Fabi SG, Guiha I. The effect of multiple sequential light sources to activate aminolevulinic acid in the treatment of actinic keratoses: a retrospective study. *J Clin Aesthet Dermatol.* 2014;7(9):20–25.) 25276272

A second peak at 630 nm exists within the red range. There are also smaller absorption peaks at 505, 540, and 580 nm. IPL has the benefit of targeting blood vessel, pigment, and even collagen. PDL primarily targets oxyhemoglobin which makes it effective for targeting individual erythematous inflammatory lesions.

In 2000, Hongcharu et al. published the first clinical trial using ALA for the treatment of acne vulgaris. Twenty-two subjects received four different types of treatment (20% ALA plus red light, ALA alone, red light alone, and untreated control). Subjects were divided randomly into two groups, groups received either a single treatment or four treatments of Levulan Kerastick applied under occlusion for 3 hours followed by broadband (550–700 nm) light to a total fluence of 150 J/cm². Only the group treated with ALA plus red light demonstrated statistically significant improvement in acne and those treated with 4 weekly treatments experienced greater improvement than those receiving a single treatment. Biopsies demonstrated reduction in the size of sebaceous glands in both the single and multitreatment groups. In the multitreatment group, continued improvement occurred with complete destruction of sebaceous gland noted at 20 weeks posttreatment. Bacterial fluorescence was also diminished.

Many studies have been conducted since the first clinical trial conducted by Hongcharu et al. Gold et al. performed a study in 2003 in patients with moderate to severe acne in which ALA was applied to patients and allowed to incubate for 30–60 minutes with high intensity blue light applied once a week for 3 months. Results showed 60% improvement in those treated with ALA and blue light (compared with 43% improvement with blue light alone). Goldman and Boyce used ALA and blue light in the treatment of mild to moderate acne. Greater improvement was seen in those treatment with ALA and blue light compared with blue light alone.

Gold et al. published another study in 2004, in which ALA was incubated for 1 hour followed by activation with IPL (430–1100 nm, pulse duration 35 milliseconds, fluence 3–9 J/cm²) once weekly for four consecutive weeks. Treatments were well tolerated and on average patients achieved 72% reduction in acne lesions 12 weeks after the final treatment. Rojanamatin and Choawawanich treated 14 patients with 20% ALA solution applied under occlusion for 30 minutes followed by IPL on one half of the face versus the other half of the face was treated with IPL alone. The ALA-pretreated side demonstrated 87.7% reduction in lesion counts 12 weeks after treatment versus 67% on the side treated with IPL alone (Quantum SR, ESC Medical Systems Ltd., now Lumenis, Yokneam, Israel) settings included a cutoff filter of 560–590 nm with total fluence between 25 and 30 J/cm², in double-pulse mode (first pulse between 2.4 and 3.6 milliseconds; second pulse between 4 and 6 milliseconds) with delayed time of 20–40 milliseconds.

Alexiades-Armenakas demonstrated 100% clearance of acne lesions in the PDT activated by long-pulsed

PDL (LP PDL) with an average of 2.9 treatments, complete clearance was maintained up to 13 months. ALA was applied for 45 minutes followed by one pass with LP PDL (595 nm, 7.0–7.5 J/cm², 10 milliseconds pulse duration, 10 mm spot size, and dynamic cooling spray of 30 milliseconds followed by 30 milliseconds delay). Clearance per treatment was 77% in those treated with ALA and LP PDL compared with only 32% in the two controls treated with LP PDL alone and 20% in the two controls treated with conventional acne therapy (oral antibiotics, oral contraceptives, and topicals).

Regarding optimal ALA incubation times, Sakomoto and colleagues examined the accumulation of ALA under occlusion on porcine ears at different time intervals. Biopsies demonstrated eccrine gland fluorescence after 30 minutes; hair follicle fluorescence at 30 minutes; sebaceous gland showed fluorescence starting at 45–75 minutes. Fluorescence in all sites reached maximum intensity at 3 hours. Oh et al conducted a randomized split face study comparing 30 minute versus 3 hour ALA incubation time followed by IPL on one half of the face compared to IPL alone. Subjects were either treated with a 30-minute ALA incubation or 3-hour ALA incubation time on one-half of the face followed by IPL versus IPL alone. Three consecutive treatments were completed at monthly intervals. The only statistical significance in reduction of acne lesions was noted between the 3-hour incubation group versus IPL alone. Thirty-minute incubation time was not sufficient to reduce acne lesions. There was decreased sebum production in all three groups. Prolonged incubation did not results in increased side effects.

Due to the presence of multiple porphyrin absorption peaks, the use of multiple laser and light devices to activate ALA can increase the efficacy of PDT for treatment of acne. High peak power of pulsed lasers allows for increased efficacy and decreased pain due to short exposure time. Friedmann et al. published a retrospective review demonstrating the safety and efficacy of multiple sequential light sources to activate ALA in patients with moderate to severe acne of the face and/or trunk. Although not statistically significant, greater improvement in acne was seen in patients treated with blue light + PDL + IPL, compared to blue light only or blue light + IPL or blue light + PDL. Importantly, increased number of lasers and light devices did not increase adverse events. Palm and Goldman found red and blue light to be equally efficacious in treatment of patients with MAL-PDT for photorejuvenation. In the authors practice, after prepping and degreasing the skin ALA is applied and allowed to incubate for 1 hour, followed by individual spot treatment with PDL and treatment of non-hair bearing areas of the face with IPL. Finally, the patient is treated simultaneously with red and blue light. Both are used as red light penetrates deeper within the tissue while blue light decreases keratinocyte inflammation (Fig. 14.4). Treatments are performed every 4–8 weeks until clear (see Table 14.2, Video 14.1). Notably, PDL and IPL also have an added benefit of improving acne scars.

Posttreatment

It is critical for patients to remain indoors from dawn to dusk 36 hours after treatment. Zinc oxide or titanium dioxide sunscreen is applied immediately posttreatment. It should be noted, most UV blocking sunscreens including those with zinc oxide or titanium dioxide will not block visible light unless applied in a thick opaque layer. If patients feel tingling or stinging after treatment, they are most likely being exposed to visible light, usually fluorescent light or sunlight penetrating a window. The most common side effects of PDT are erythema, crusting, itching, and mild edema which typically last about 5–7 days (Figs. 14.5 and 14.6).

VISIBLE LIGHT PHOTOTHERAPY

Blue Light Alone

C. acnes, an anaerobic bacterium, produces a large amount of coproporphyrin III and protoporphyrin IX within its cell. Both porphyrins are photosensitized when they absorb blue light. Visible blue light therapy exerts an anti-microbial effect on *C. acnes* by photoactivation of endogenous porphyrins produced by the organism. Furthermore, blue light reduces keratinocyte inflammation. Several studies using visible blue light by itself have shown it to be successful in the treatment of acne. A study by Kawada et al. investigated the efficacy of high-intensity, narrow-band, blue light source phototherapy in patients with mild to moderate acne. Patients were treated in this open label study twice a week for up to 5 weeks. Acne lesions were reduced by 64%. Two patients experienced dryness. No patient discontinued treatment due to adverse effects. Furthermore, in vitro investigation revealed that

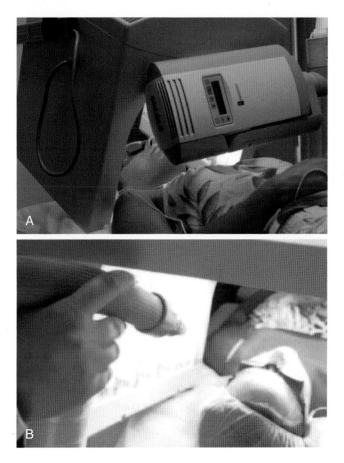

Fig. 14.4 Simultaneous treatment with red and blue light (A). Cool air is directed at the patient to maintain comfort (B). (Courtesy Dr. Goldman.)

irradiation with blue light reduced the number of *C. acnes*. Another study investigated the twice weekly use of a high intensity blue light in 35 patients with acne for 4 weeks. Treatment resulted in 68% reduction of inflammatory and noninflammatory papule count. There were no adverse events were reported in this study. A study by Gold et al. evaluated 25 patients with mild to moderate acne who were randomized to 1% clindamycin versus blue light (Fig. 14.7). Blue light therapy reduced inflammatory acne vulgaris lesions by an average of 34%, as compared to 14% for topical 1% clindamycin solution. A study of daily self-applied blue light therapy for 8 weeks showed 20%–30% reduction in both inflammatory and noninflammatory lesions.

Red Light Alone

Red light is less effective in photoactivating porphyrins, however is able to penetrate deeper within the skin targeting the sebaceous glands directly. Red light also has antiinflammatory effects. Na et al. performed a split-face study to investigate the efficacy of red light in the treatment of mild to moderate acne. 28 patients were treated for 15 minutes twice a day for 8 weeks. Treatment resulted in a significant reduction of inflammatory and noninflammatory lesions and a reduction of visual analog scale from 3.9 to 1.9.

Red and Blue Light

Blue and red light differ in their mechanism of action and level of penetration. Several studies have demonstrated

TABLE 14.2   Photodynamic Therapy Treatment Protocol

Pretreatment	• Exfoliate with microdermabrasion using a non-particulate superficial abrasion with stainless steel for 5 minutes (Vibraderm, Esthetica Inc.) • Degrease with alcohol
Treatment	• Apply ALA • Activate ALA with the following light sources:

A Pulsed-dye laser	B Intense-pulsed light
• Cynergy or VBeam • Wavelength: 595 nm • Spot-size: 5–7 mm • Pulse duration: 10–40 ms • Fluence: 5–12 J/cm² • Cooling: Cryogen (30–40 ms/20 ms; VBeam) vs. forced cold air (Cynergy) 2 passes, primarily as spot-treatment	• Lumenis 1 or M22, Lumenis Inc., San Jose, CA • Cutoff filter: 560 nm (for Fitzpatrick skin types I-III) • Pulse duration: 3–5 ms, double pulsed with 10–30 ms delay • Fluence: 15–22 J/cm² • Cooling: Chilled sapphire crystal (15 × 35 mm), cold coupling gel + forced cold air post-treatment

C Blue light	D Red light
• BLU-U, DUSA Pharmaceuticals Inc., Wimington, MA • Peak wavelength: 417 nm • Duration: 16 min, 40 s • Fluence dose: 10 J/cm²	• Aktilite CL128, Photocure Inc., Princeton, NJ • Peak wavelength: 630 nm • Duration: 8 min • Fluence dose: 37 J/cms

C and D often performed simultaneously, with adjuvant forced air cooling

Posttreatment	• Immediate application of a physical sunscreen • Strict sun protection of treated areas for 24–36 h • Follow-up at 1 week, per our standard protocol

a synergistic effect of both modalities in treatment of acne. Papageorgiou and colleagues reported that the simultaneous use of red and blue light, which was used daily for 12 weeks, was significantly more effective than blue light alone or 5% benzoyl peroxide. A study investigating at home mask using 455 nm blue and 630 nm red light applied for 15 minutes daily for 12 weeks versus mask with salicylic acid (1%) and retinol versus benzoyl peroxide (2.5%) showed superiority of the mask alone in the reduction of inflammatory lesions (24%).

Intense-Pulsed Light

IPL was investigated in the treatment of acne vulgaris in several studies either as a treatment option by itself, or as an activator of PDT. There are several proposed mechanisms of action by which IPL can impact acne. One is thermolysis of blood vessels supplying sebaceous glands. This is associated with reduction of sebum production and gland size. This is supported by findings of Barakat

et al who performed histopathological examination and measurement of surface area of sebaceous glands at baseline and 2 weeks after six treatment sessions with IPL. The study showed a significant reduction in surface area of sebaceous gland following IPL treatment. IPL has also an antiinflammatory effect by downregulating tumor necrosis factor alpha (TNF-α) and upregulating transforming growth factor beta (TGF-β) 1/smad3 signaling pathway.

Chang and colleagues conducted a split-face, open-label, prospective trial in 30 Korean women with mild to moderate acne and found that IPL treatment equipped with a 530- to 750-nm acne filter resulted in improvement of acne red macules, irregular pigmentation, and skin tone but did not affect inflammatory acne lesion counts. Those results were replicated by and Yeung and colleagues in 30 Chinese patients treated with IPL.

The vast majority of studies of IPL in acne patients resulted in reduction of both inflammatory and

LEVULAN

1 WEEK PROGRESSION

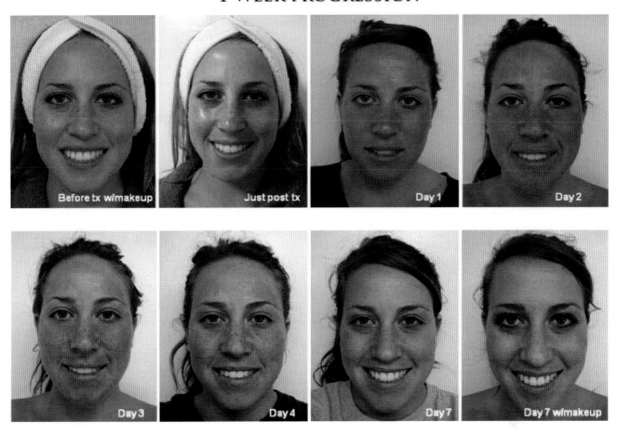

Fig. 14.5 One-week progression following treatment of acne with aminolevulinic acid-photodynamic therapy (ALA-PDT). (Courtesy Dr. Goldman.)

noninflammatory lesions. The reported efficacy of IPL on acne lesions ranged from 34% to 88% with an average improvement of 40%–60%. The number of IPL sessions in those studies ranged from four to eight.

LASER LIGHT THERAPY

Pulsed-Dye Laser

Pulsed-dye laser (PDL) is a nonablative 595-nm laser, typically used to treat vascular lesions. PDL has been reported to be effective in treatment of inflammatory acne lesions (Fig. 14.8). A study by Seaton et al revealed

a mechanism of action by which PDL improve inflammatory acne lesions through the upregulation of TGF-β, a pivotal immunosuppressive cytokine which promotes inflammation resolution. There were no direct effect on *Propionibacterium acnes* or sebaceous glands detected by this study. In a placebo-controlled trial, 41 adults with mild-to-moderate facial inflammatory acne were randomly assigned to a one PDL or sham treatment session. Those treated with PDL demonstrated 49% reduction in inflammatory lesion count. In a study by Leheta et al, 45 patients with mild to moderate acne were randomly divided into three groups: a group receiving treatment with PDL every 2 weeks for, a group receiving topical

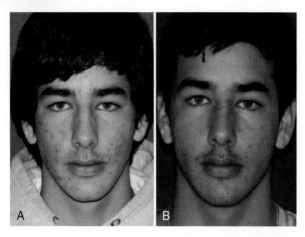

Fig. 14.6 17-year-old status post two photodynamic therapy treatments 1 year apart with 1 year follow-up after the second treatment. Patient was treated with 1 hour incubation of aminolevulinic acid, followed by pulsed-dye laser and simultaneous red and blue light. (Courtesy Dr. Goldman.)

treatments, and a group subjected to chemical peeling using trichloroacetic acid 25%. At 12 weeks, there was no statistical difference between the treatment protocols, however remission in the follow-up period was significantly higher in the PDL group.

Sami et al. treated 45 patients with moderate to severe acne with one of three treatments, PDL, IPL, or blue-red combination LED. Treatment was continued until at least 90% of the lesions was achieved. Patients treated with PDL achieved the end point of at least 90% clearance after a mean of 4 sessions, patients treated with IPL required a mean of 6 sessions, patients treated with blue-red light combination required a mean of 10 sessions.

Pulsed Green Laser

Potassium titanyl phosphate laser (KTP) is a 532 nm wavelength laser traditionally used for the treatment of rosacea and telangiectasias. There have been few studies investigating its use in treatment of ace vulgaris. Although the exact mechanism of action is unclear, selective photo-thermolysis of blood vessels or a photodynamic effect of the laser on *C. acnes* and/or sebaceous glands have all been postulated.

A split face study by Baugh et al investigated the use of KTP on one-half of the face. Each subject was treated with four laser sessions in 2 weeks. Primary outcome

analysis in the Michaëlsson acne severity score demonstrated a mean 34.9% and 20.7% reduction at the 1-week and 4-week post final treatments, respectively. No significant adverse events were reported. One side of the face of 38 patients was treated with either once weekly and twice weekly with KTP. Improvement of Michaëlsson acne severity grading score was reported in both groups, however no statistical difference was detected with once versus twice weekly treatments.

1064-nm Nd:YAG Laser

The 1064-nm neodymium-doped yttrium aluminum garnet (Nd:YAG) laser is most commonly used for tattoo and hair removal, pigmented lesions, facial rejuvenation, and acne scarring, but there is growing evidence to support its use for the treatment of acne vulgaris.

The main chromophores of the 1064-nm wavelength are water, hemoglobin, and melanin. Laser pulses penetrate deeply into the dermis and cause diffuse heating of dermal tissues, including overactive sebaceous glands. Treatment of acne with the 1064-nm Nd:YAG laser results in decreased cellular inflammation and expression of the inflammatory cytokines interleukin-8 (IL-8, associated with epidermal hyperplasia), matrix metalloproteinase-9 (MMP-9), toll-like receptor-2 (TLR-2, activated by *C. acnes*), nuclear factor-kappa B (NF-κB), and TNF-α, as well as upregulation of TGF-β, which decreases inflammation, promotes wound healing and neocollagenesis, and inhibits keratinocyte proliferation.

Several publications detail the effective use of the 1064-nm Nd:YAG laser in the treatment of acne vulgaris in patients with Fitzpatrick skin types I–VI. Laser settings vary between studies, using spot sizes of 6–15 mm, fluences of 1.1–50 J/cm^2, and pulse durations of 5 ns to 60 ms. Lower laser fluences were used for patients with darker skin types. The immediate posttreatment endpoint is an even, mild erythema over the entire treated area. Cooling of the skin, such as with cold air cooling, dynamic cooling device (DCD) spray, or a chilled sapphire tip plus cold ultrasound gel, helps to protect the epidermis while using this device. Reported side effects include edema, dryness, crusting, burning, and postinflammatory hyper- and hypopigmentation.

The 1064-nm Nd:YAG laser has been shown to reduce the number of inflammatory acne lesions in some patients by 50%–100%, while others obtain more modest results. Noninflammatory acne lesion counts

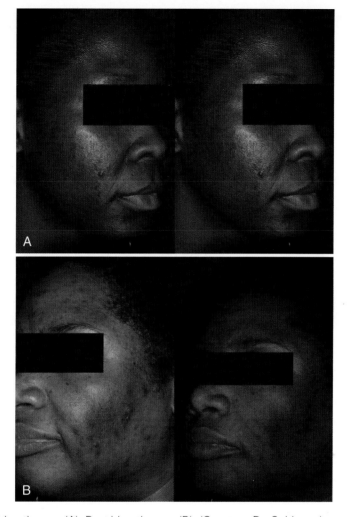

Fig. 14.7 Pre blue therapy (A). Post blue therapy (B). (Courtesy Dr. Goldman.)

also decrease, albeit to a lesser degree than inflammatory lesions (20%–75%). Maximum improvement is typically seen only after multiple treatments have been performed, but the response is sustained for several weeks to years after treatment. The device also appears to improve overall skin texture (e.g., pore size, postinflammatory erythema, sebum production, acne scarring, and skin tone).

The 1064-nm Nd:YAG laser has been compared to PDL devices used to treat acne. A split-face study found no significant difference in the reduction of inflammatory acne lesions between a combination 585/1064-nm laser and a 585-nm laser, but the former was significantly better at treating noninflammatory lesions. In another split-face study comparing 1064- and 595-nm laser treatments, both were equally effective in reducing inflammatory acne lesions and erythema, but subjects preferred the 1064-nm laser due to less discomfort during the procedure and fewer adverse effects.

1320-nm Nd:YAG Laser

Studies using 1320-nm wavelength to treat acne have been discordant. The 1320-nm wavelength has a calculated penetration depth of 1.5 mm, making it a theoretical option for targeting sebaceous glands located at a similar depth in the dermis. However, this wavelength

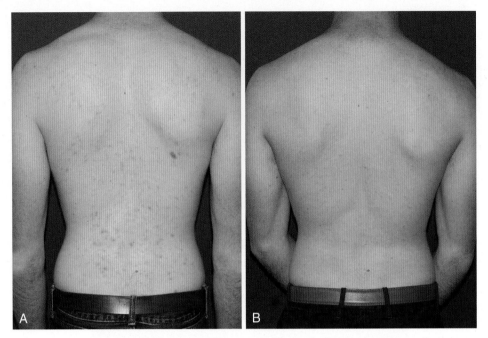

Fig. 14.8 Patient with inflammatory acne on the back successfully treated with three PDL treatments. (Courtesy Dr. Goldman.)

has a relatively low absorption coefficient for fat and significant scattering loss, requiring higher energies and heating a larger volume of tissue to cause clinically significant damage to sebaceous glands compared to longer-wavelength infrared lasers.

One 1320-nm system is based on a Q-switched Nd:YAG laser that incorporates a cryogen delivery system and real-time temperature monitoring to avoid epidermal damage. In one study using this device, three treatments were performed at 3-week intervals using a 10-mm spot size and fluences that varied to maintain peak epidermal temperatures between 40°C and 45°C. There was a modest (27%) reduction in comedones on the laser-treated sides versus untreated sides 1 week after the final treatment, but this improvement was transient and no longer appreciated after 8 weeks. There were no significant differences regarding inflammatory lesion counts, blinded evaluator scores, or sebum production between the two sides. Patients perceived at least mild improvement and less oily skin on the treated side. Adverse effects included few instances of transient dyspigmentation and blistering. Patients experienced moderate-to-extreme discomfort despite

the use of topical anesthesia, although many still indicated a preference for laser therapy over standard acne treatments, mainly citing issues of convenience.

A fractional 1320-nm Nd:YAG laser, which allows for a higher fluence and shorter treatment interval than the traditional 1320-nm laser, showed more promising results in a study of 35 patients with Fitzpatrick skin types I–IV. Six treatments performed at 2-week intervals led to a reduction in inflammatory and noninflammatory lesions of 57% and 35%, respectively, and reduced the skin sebum level by 30%. Improvement continued for up to 12 weeks after the final procedure.

1540- and 1550-nm Erbium:Glass Lasers

The use of 1540- and 1550-nm erbium:glass lasers to treat acne has shown promising results with minimal procedure-related discomfort. The 1540- and 1550-nm wavelengths are absorbed primarily by water in the dermis and sebaceous glands at a depth of approximately 400 μm. These lasers are considered safe in dark-skinned patients given their low affinity for epidermal melanin.

Two studies of patients with active acne employed a flashlamp-pumped 1540-nm erbium:glass laser that could emit a single pulse or train of pulses. Patients received four treatments at 2- to 4-week intervals. A dramatic improvement was noted shortly after the first treatment and continued until a greater than 70% reduction in acne lesions was achieved and was sustained for 24 months after treatment. Nearly all subjects reported decreased skin oiliness, and histological studies demonstrated progressive rarefaction and miniaturization of sebaceous glands and pilosebaceous follicles without appreciable epidermal damage. Treatments were well tolerated with only minimal-to-bearable pain that did not require anesthesia, attributed to the use of a 4-mm spot size along with the device's contact cooling mechanism. Discomfort is greatest when treating directly over inflamed lesions and can be reduced by allowing adequate cooling time prior to each pulse.

The 1540- and 1550-nm erbium:glass nonablative fractional lasers, which are known to improve acne scarring, have also been shown to effectively treat active acne. When four treatments (each consisting of three pan-facial passes using a 10-mm spot size with a density of 100 microbeams/cm^2, energy of 50–60 mJ/microbeam, and a 10-ms pulse duration) with a 1540-nm device were performed at 4-week intervals, most patients reported a 50%–100% improvement in their acne. The treating dermatologist and a blinded observer reported similar results. Sebum secretion, pore size, and scarring also improved significantly. Studies using a 1550-nm erbium:glass fractional laser demonstrated approximately 75% reductions in acne lesions up to 2 years after treatment, with associated biopsy-proven shrinkage of sebaceous glands.

PARTICLE-ASSISTED LASER TREATMENT

The selective delivery of an exogenous chromophore into the pilosebaceous unit may enhance the effectiveness with which lasers treat acne. A topical suspension of gold-coated silica microparticles with strong optical absorption at 800 nm has also been used for this purpose. Studies involving these microparticles demonstrate up to 61% reductions in acne lesion counts by 28 weeks after treatment. The gold microparticles, which are small enough to penetrate the follicular infundibulum but large enough to prevent nonselective diffusion through the stratum corneum, are delivered by massage, vibration, or ultrasound. The skin is then exposed

to 800-nm diode laser pulses for three treatments at 1- to 2-week intervals. Microscopic evaluation demonstrates preferential thermal injury to sebaceous glands and the follicular infundibulum at an average depth of 470 μm (maximum 1430 μm), while the adjacent dermis and epidermis are preserved. The procedure is well tolerated with low reported pain scores. Adverse effects include transient erythema and edema, but no blisters, burns, scarring, tattooing, or systemic effects have been observed. Cutaneous and internal organ gold concentrations remain below the established safety threshold and return to baseline shortly after treatment.

A 2019 review reported that two trials of a topical silver photoparticle compound used in conjunction with 810- and 1064-nm lasers achieved similar efficacy to the gold microparticles but failed to achieve primary efficacy endpoints. Both companies that developed the gold and silver nanoparticles have closed at this time. We believe that while the early experience was positive, enhancing therapeutic results by increasing penetration of the particles into the follicles is necessary. These studies are stopped at the present time.

1726-nm Lasers

While the infrared wavelengths discussed previously target water and cause nonspecific dermal damage, lasers that specifically target sebaceous glands are now being investigated. Sebum lipids have a relative absorption peak at approximately 1720 nm. At this wavelength, laser-induced heating of sebum is up to twice that of water, and the absorption coefficient for fat is at least ten times greater than that for the 1320-, 1450-, and 1540-nm devices. Lasers functioning near 1720 nm may selectively target lipid-rich sebaceous glands located up to 2 mm below the skin surface.

One of the devices in development is a 1726-nm fiber laser that uses a multiple-pulse strategy that allows for gradual heating of the sebaceous gland (Accure Laser, Boulder, CO). An air-cooling system and real-time temperature monitoring using thermal imaging prevent dangerous epidermal temperatures from being reached. Delayed red papules in the treatment zone at 24–72 hours posttreatment seem to indicate a successful clinical endpoint correlating to sebaceous gland destruction. These papules resolve without visible sequelae within 1 week.

Early studies using these lasers have shown histological evidence of total sebaceous gland necrosis with preservation of the surrounding dermis, epidermis, and other follicular structures. This selective damage appears to correlate with significant reductions in acne lesion counts, as well as high patient satisfaction with only moderate discomfort. Published results of these initial studies are forthcoming at the time of this writing.

CONCLUSION

Lasers and lights have shown to be a safe and effective option for the treatment of acne vulgaris in numerous studies. Unfortunately, none of these procedures are approved for reimbursement by medical government or private insurance companies so patients are left with the burden of bearing the cost of laser or light treatments for acne. However, with less systemic side effects, decreased risk of antibiotic resistance, faster and longer term resolution of acne in addition to simultaneous improvement in scarring we recommend the use of lasers and lights with photosensitizing agents for patients who are refractory to standard acne therapy or wish to achieve enhanced results quickly.

FURTHER READING

Alexiades-Armenakas M. Long-pulsed dye laser-mediated photodynamic therapy combined with topical therapy for mild to severe comedonal, inflammatory, or cystic acne. *J Drugs Dermatol.* 2006;5(1):45–55.

Ali MM, Porter RM, Gonzalez ML. Intense pulsed light enhances transforming growth factor beta1/S mad3 signaling in acne-prone skin. *J Cosmetic Dermatology.* 2013;12(3):195–203.

Angel S, Boineau D, Dahan S, Mordon S. Treatment of active acne with an Er:glass (1.54 μm) laser: A 2-year follow-up study. *J Cosmetic Laser Ther.* 2006;8(4):171–176.

Ashkenazi H, Malik Z, Harth Y, Nitzan Y. Eradication of *Propionibacterium acnes* by its endogenous porphyrins after illumination with high intensity blue light. *FEMS Immunology & Med Microbiology.* 2003;35(1):17–24.

Bakus AD, Yaghmai D, Massa MC, Garden BC, Garden JM. Sustained benefit after treatment of acne vulgaris using only a novel combination of long-pulsed and Q-switched 1064-nm Nd:YAG lasers. *Dermatologic Surg.* 2018;44(11):1402–1410.

Barakat MT, Moftah NH, El Khayyat MA, Abdelhakim ZA. Significant reduction of inflammation and sebaceous glands size in acne vulgaris lesions after intense pulsed light treatment. *Dermatologic Ther.* 2017;30(1):e12418.

Baugh WP, Kucaba WD. Nonablative phototherapy for acne vulgaris using the KTP 532 nm laser. *Dermatologic Surg.* 2005;31(10):1290–1296.

Bogle MA, Dover JS, Arndt KA, Mordon S. Evaluation of the 1,540-nm erbium:glass laser in the treatment of inflammatory facial acne. *Dermatologic Surg.* 2007;33(7):810–817.

Bolton JZ-LL, Goldman MP. *Atrophic Scar Management. The scar book: formation, mitigation, rehabilitation, and prevention.* Philadelphia: Wolters Kluwer; 2017:388.

Chalermsuwiwattanakan N, Rojhirunsakool S, Kamanamool N, Kanokrungsee S, Udompataikul M. The comparative study of efficacy between 1064-nm long-pulsed Nd:YAG laser and 595-nm pulsed dye laser for the treatment of acne vulgaris. *J Cosmetic Dermatology.* 2021;20(7):2108–2115.

Chang SE, Ahn SJ, Rhee DY, et al. Treatment of facial acne papules and pustules in Korean patients using an intense pulsed light device equipped with a 530-to 750-nm filter. *Dermatologic Surg.* 2007;33(6):676–679.

Choi Y, Suh H, Yoon M, Min S, Lee D, Suh D. Intense pulsed light vs. pulsed-dye laser in the treatment of facial acne: a randomized split-face trial. *J Eur Acad Dermatology Venereology.* 2010;24(7):773–780.

Dahan S, Lagarde JM, Turlier V, Courrech L, Mordon S. Treatment of neck lines and forehead rhytids with a nonablative 1540-nm Er:glass laser: a controlled clinical study combined with the measurement of the thickness and the mechanical properties of the skin. *Dermatologic Surg.* 2004;30(6):872–880.

De Leeuw J, Van Der Beek N, Bjerring P, Martino Neumann H. Photodynamic therapy of acne vulgaris using 5-aminolevulinic acid 0.5% liposomal spray and intense pulsed light in combination with topical keratolytic agents. *J Eur Acad Dermatology Venereology.* 2010;24(4):460–469.

Deng H, Yuan D-F, Yan C-L, Ding X-A. Fractional 1320 nm Nd: YAG laser in the treatment of acne vulgaris: a pilot study. *Photodermatology, Photoimmunology & Photomed.* 2009;25(5):278–279.

Friedmann DP, Goldman MP, Fabi SG, Guiha I. A retrospective study of multiple sequential light and laser sources to activate aminolevulinic acid in the treatment of acne vulgaris. *Skinmed.* 2017;15(2):105–111.

Ganceviciene R, Meskauskas R, Berzanskyte A. Treatment of acne vulgaris with 1064 nm Nd: YAG laser. *J Laser Health Acad.* 2015;15:2–5.

Gold M. The utilization of ALA-PDT and a new photoclearing device for the treatment of severe inflammatory acne vulgaris—results of an initial clinical trial. *J Lasers Surg Med.* 2003;15(suppl):46.

Gold MH. Therapeutic and aesthetic uses of photodynamic therapy part two of a five-part series: lasers and light treatments for acne vulgaris promising therapies. *J Clin Aesthet Dermatol.* 2008;1(3):28–34.

Gold MH, Andriessen A, Biron J, Andriessen H. Clinical efficacy of self-applied blue light therapy for mild-to-moderate facial acne. *J Clin Aesthetic Dermatology.* 2009;2(3):44.

Gold MH, Bradshaw VL, Boring MM, Bridges TM, Biron JA, Carter LN. The use of a novel intense pulsed light and heat source and ALA-PDT in the treatment of moderate to severe inflammatory acne vulgaris. *J Drugs Dermatol.* 2004;3(6 suppl):S15–S19.

Gold MH, Rao J, Goldman MP, et al. A multicenter clinical evaluation of the treatment of mild to moderate inflammatory acne vulgaris of the face with visible blue light in comparison to topical 1% clindamycin antibiotic solution. *J Drugs Dermatology: JDD.* 2005;4(1):64–70.

Goldman MP, Boyce SM. A single-center study of aminolevulinic acid and 417 NM photodynamic therapy in the treatment of moderate to severe acne vulgaris. *J Drugs Dermatol.* 2003;2(4):393–396.

Hong JS, Jung JY, Yoon JY, Suh DH. Acne treatment by methyl aminolevulinate photodynamic therapy with red light vs. intense pulsed light. *Int J Dermatology.* 2013;52(5):614–619.

https://www.aad.org/media/stats-numbers. Accessed March 15, 2021.

https://www.accessdata.fda.gov/drugsatfda_docs/label/2016/208081s000lbl.pdf. Accessed February 14, 2021.

https://www.levulanhcp.com/assets/pdf/levulan-prescribing-information.pdf. Accessed February 14, 2021.

https://www.levulanhcp.com. Accessed February 7, 2021.

https://www.myvibraderm.com/light-microscopy/. Accessed February 20, 2021.

Hongcharu W, Taylor CR, Chang Y, Aghassi D, Suthamjariya K, Anderson RR. Topical ALA-photodynamic therapy for the treatment of acne vulgaris. *J Invest Dermatol.* 2000;115(2):183–192.

Isarría MJ, Cornejo P, Muñoz E, Royo de la Torre J, Moraga JM. Evaluation of clinical improvement in acne scars and active acne in patients treated with the 1540-nm non-ablative fractional laser. *J Drugs Dermatol.* 2011;10(8):907–912.

Jung JY, Choi YS, Yoon MY, Min SU, Suh DH. Comparison of a pulsed dye laser and a combined 585/1,064-nm laser in the treatment of acne vulgaris. *Dermatologic Surg.* 2009;35(8):1181–1187.

Jung JY, Hong JS, Ahn CH, Yoon JY, Kwon HH, Suh DH. Prospective randomized controlled clinical and histopathological study of acne vulgaris treated with dual mode of quasi-long pulse and Q-switched 1064-nm Nd:YAG laser assisted with a topically applied carbon suspension. *J Am Acad Dermatology.* 2012;66(4):626–633.

Kalisiak MS, Rao J. Photodynamic therapy for actinic keratoses. *Dermatol Clin.* 2007;25(1):15–23.

Kawada A, Aragane Y, Kameyama H, Sangen Y, Tezuka T. Acne phototherapy with a high-intensity, enhanced, narrow-band, blue light source: an open study and in vitro investigation. *J dermatological Sci.* 2002;30(2):129–135.

Kawana S, Tachihara R, Kato T, Omi T. Effect of smooth pulsed light at 400 to 700 and 870 to 1,200 nm for acne vulgaris in Asian skin. *Dermatologic Surg.* 2010;36(1):52–57.

Kennedy JC, Pottier RH. Endogenous protoporphyrin IX, a clinically useful photosensitizer for photodynamic therapy. *J Photochem Photobiol B.* 1992;14(4):275–292.

Lee G-S. Inflammatory acne in the Asian skin type III treated with a square pulse, time resolved spectral distribution IPL system: a preliminary study. *Laser Ther.* 2012;21(2):105–111.

Lee WJ, Jung HJ, Kim JY, Lee SJ, Kim DW. Effect of photodynamic therapy on inflammatory acne using 3% liposomal 5-aminolevulinic acid emulsion and intense-pulsed light: a pilot study. *J Dermatology.* 2012;39(8):728.

Lee WR, Tsai RY, Fang CL, Liu CJ, Hu CH, Fang JY. Microdermabrasion as a novel tool to enhance drug delivery via the skin: an animal study. *Dermatol Surg.* 2006;32(8):1013–1022.

Leheta TM. Role of the 585-nm pulsed dye laser in the treatment of acne in comparison with other topical therapeutic modalities. *J Cosmetic Laser Ther.* 2009;11(2):118–124.

Liu Y, Zeng W, Hu D, et al. The long-term effect of 1550 nm erbium:glass fractional laser in acne vulgaris. *Lasers Med Sci.* 2016;31(3):453–457.

Mei X, Shi W, Piao Y. Effectiveness of photodynamic therapy with topical 5-aminolevulinic acid and intense pulsed light in Chinese acne vulgaris patients. *Photodermatol Photoimmunol Photomed.* 2013;29(2):90–96.

Mikolajewska P, Donnelly RF, Garland MJ, et al. Microneedle pre-treatment of human skin improves 5-aminolevulininc acid (ALA)- and 5-aminolevulinic acid methyl ester (MAL)-induced PpIX production for topical photodynamic therapy without increase in pain or erythema. *Pharm Res.* 2010;27(10):2213–2220.

Mohanan S, Parveen B, Annie Malathy P, Gomathi N. Use of intense pulse light for acne vulgaris in Indian skin—a case series. *Int J dermatology.* 2012;51(4):473–476.

Moneib H, Tawfik AA, Youssef SS, Fawzy MM. Randomized split-face controlled study to evaluate 1550-nm fractionated erbium glass laser for treatment of acne vulgaris—an image analysis evaluation. *Dermatologic Surg.* 2014;40(11):1191–1200.

Na JI, Suh DH. Red light phototherapy alone is effective for acne vulgaris: randomized, single-blinded clinical trial. *Dermatologic Surg.* 2007;33(10):1228–1233.

Nestor MS, Swenson N, Macri A, Manway M, Paparone P. Efficacy and tolerability of a combined 445nm and 630nm over-the-counter light therapy mask with and without topical salicylic acid versus topical benzoyl peroxide for the treatment of mild-to-moderate acne vulgaris. *J Clin Aesthetic Dermatology.* 2016;9(3):25.

Nestor MS, Swenson N, Macri A. Physical modalities (devices) in the management of acne. *Dermatologic Clin.* 2016;34(2):215–223.

Oh SH, Ryu DJ, Han EC, Lee KH, Lee JH. At comparative study of topical 5-aminolevulinic acid incubation times in photodynamic therapy with intense pulsed light for the treatment of inflammatory acne. *Dermatologic Surg.* 2009;35(12):1918–1926.

Orringer JS, Kang S, Maier L, et al. A randomized, controlled, split-face clinical trial of 1320-nm Nd:YAG laser therapy in the treatment of acne vulgaris. *J Am Acad Dermatology.* 2007;56(3):432–438.

Ozog DM, Rkein AM, Fabi SG, et al. Photodynamic therapy: a clinical consensus guide. *Dermatol Surg.* 2016;42(7):804–827.

Palm MD, Goldman MP. Safety and efficacy comparison of blue versus red light sources for photodynamic therapy using methyl aminolevulinate in photodamaged skin. *J Drugs Dermatol.* 2011;10(1):53–60.

Papageorgiou P, Katsambas A, Chu A. Phototherapy with blue (415 nm) and red (660 nm) light in the treatment of acne vulgaris. *Br J Dermatology.* 2000;142(5):973–978.

Peikert JM, Krywonis NA, Rest EB, Zachary CB. The efficacy of various degreasing agents used in trichloroacetic acid peels. *J Dermatol Surg Oncol.* 1994;20(11):724–728.

Rojanamatin J, Choawawanich P. Treatment of inflammatory facial acne vulgaris with intense pulsed light and short contact of topical 5-aminolevulinic acid: a pilot study. *Dermatologic Surg.* 2006;32(8):991–997.

Ross EV. Optical treatments for acne. *Dermatologic Ther.* 2005;18(3):253–266.

Sakamoto FH, Tannous Z, Doukas AG, et al. Porphyrin distribution after topical aminolevulinic acid in a novel porcine model of sebaceous skin. *Lasers Surg Med.* 2009;41(2):154–160.

Sami NA, Attia AT, Badawi AM. Phototherapy in the treatment of acne vulgaris. *J drugs dermatology: JDD.* 2008;7(7):627–632.

Seaton E, Charakida A, Mouser P, Grace I, Clement R, Chu A. Pulsed-dye laser treatment for inflammatory acne vulgaris: randomised controlled trial. *Lancet.* 2003;362(9393):1347–1352.

Seaton E, Mouser P, Charakida A, Alam S, Seldon P, Chu A. Investigation of the mechanism of action of nonablative pulsed-dye laser therapy in photorejuvenation and inflammatory acne vulgaris. *Br J Dermatology.* 2006;155(4):748–755.

Shaaban D, Abdel-Samad Z, El-Khalawany M. Photodynamic therapy with intralesional 5-aminolevulinic acid and intense pulsed light versus intense pulsed light alone in the treatment of acne vulgaris: a comparative study. *Dermatologic Ther.* 2012;25(1):86–91.

Shalita AR, Harth Y, Elman M, et al. Acne phototherapy using UV-free high-intensity narrow-band blue light: a three-center clinical study. Paper presented at: Lasers in Surgery: Advanced Characterization, Therapeutics, and Systems XI2001.

Shnitkind E, Yaping E, Geen S, Shalita AR, Lee W-L. Anti-inflammatory properties of narrow-band blue light. *J Drugs Dermatology: JDD.* 2006;5(7):605–610.

Taub AF. A comparison of intense pulsed light, combination radiofrequency and intense pulsed light, and blue light in photodynamic therapy for acne vulgaris. *J Drugs Dermatology.* 2007;6(10):1010.

Taub AF. Photodynamic therapy in dermatology: history and horizons. *J Drugs Dermatol.* 2004;3(1 suppl):S8–S25.

Taylor M, Porter R, Gonzalez M. Intense pulsed light may improve inflammatory acne through TNF-α down-regulation. *J Cosmetic Laser Ther.* 2014;16(2):96–103.

Wang SQ, Counters JT, Flor ME, Zelickson BD. Treatment of inflammatory facial acne with the 1,450 nm diode laser alone versus microdermabrasion plus the 1,450 nm laser: a randomized, split-face trial: TREATMENT OF INFLAMMATORY FACIAL ACNE. *Dermatologic Surg.* 2006;32(2):249–255.

Wanitphakdeedecha R, Tanzi EL, Alster TS. Photopneumatic therapy for the treatment of acne. *J drugs dermatology: JDD.* 2009;8(3):239.

Yeung CK, Shek SY, Bjerring P, Yu CS, Kono T, Chan HH. A comparative study of intense pulsed light alone and its combination with photodynamic therapy for the treatment of facial acne in Asian skin. *Lasers Surg Med: Off J Am Soc Laser Medicine Surg.* 2007;39(1):1–6.

Yeung CK, Shek SY, Yu CS, Kono T, Chan HH. Liposome-encapsulated 0.5% 5-aminolevulinic acid with intense pulsed light for the treatment of inflammatory facial acne: a pilot study. *Dermatologic Surg.* 2011;37(4):450–459.

Yilmaz O, Senturk N, Yuksel EP, et al. Evaluation of 532-nm KTP laser treatment efficacy on acne vulgaris with once and twice weekly applications. *J Cosmetic Laser Ther.* 2011;13(6):303–307.

Zhou Y, Banga AK. Enhanced delivery of cosmeceuticals by microdermabrasion. *J Cosmet Dermatol.* 2011;10(3):179–184.

Complications and Legal Considerations of Laser, Light, and Energy-Based Treatments

Saleh Rachidi and David J. Goldberg

SUMMARY AND KEY FEATURES

- Various energy-based devices in dermatology, their complications, and means to prevent them.
- Legal and professional considerations including what constitutes an informed consent and the value of such consent when legal action is taken.
- Data on medical professional liability against dermatologists.
- Act of negligence and the legal consequences arising from that.

INTRODUCTION

The applications of energy-based devices have been expanding at steadily increasing rates, with a widening spectrum of indications and patient population. Such devices include lasers which target a wide array of chromophores in the skin depending on the wavelength, radiofrequency (RF) and light-emitting devices, as well as body contouring modalities including cryolipolysis and electromagnetic energy for muscle stimulation. Over the past 3 decades, our knowledge of potential complications related to these devices has also developed, leading to safer technologies with safeguard measures that limit side effects and complications. Unfortunately, adverse events are a reality of the medical profession despite our best efforts. Here, we discuss some complications associated with energy-based devices and outline the legal framework of malpractice claims and lawsuits.

INFORMED CONSENT

We start with the informed consent because this lays the groundwork for expectations of efficacy and potential adverse effects associated with any treatment. Our intent is to always avoid adverse events and when those do occur, they would be better received by patients when education is provided a priori, yielding higher patient satisfaction, especially when such adverse effects are reversible. Discussing potential complications before a procedure not only preserves the physician–patient relationship in the event a complication occurs, but also provides context to the patient on the rationale to treat with certain settings or in a given time interval. For example, a patient might be more inclined to treat a lesion in a fewer number of sessions and using higher energy settings. Explaining potential drawbacks of such practice like scarring or pigment alteration would increase their satisfaction regardless whether a side effect develops or not.

The informed consent should meet certain minimum standards. A patient must be deemed competent by the physician obtaining the consent, and they must understand the facts, implications, and future consequences of the intervention.

The American Medical Association (AMA) outlines the following requirements in a consent: diagnosis, nature and purpose of an intervention, risks, and benefits of a proposed intervention, alternatives, risks and benefits of the alternative, and risks and benefits of not receiving or undergoing a treatment or procedure. Different states have their own version of what constitutes informed consent spelled out in statutes and case laws.

Informed consent can be verbal or written. While written consent may not be required in some states, careful documentation can provide an invaluable defense, considering that a malpractice case can be lost if a plaintiff proves that informed consent was not obtained. Importantly, patients often are overwhelmed or distracted in the period just before a procedure. Reading a written consent form provides an opportunity to take time to process the information and make a more certain decision.

PREVENTION

Initial evaluation includes accurately identifying the patient's chief cosmetic concern which could differ from that perceived by the physician. Assigning Fitzpatrick skin type based on the patient's reported history of predisposition to sun burn and tans in addition to their reported genetic heritage is more accurate than a visual estimation of their skin color. It is also important to understand the patient's expectations in term of outcomes, timeline, and downtime. Evaluation of underlying medical conditions is prudent, especially those which influence bruising, infection, and healing, as well as allergies. Other considerations include implantable devices and metals which could be affected by RF and electromagnetic energy devices. Tobacco, alcohol, or other substance use should be inquired about, as well as occupation and daily activities which could affect sun exposure and feasibility of postoperative care.

History of prior procedures is of paramount importance as it can provide insight into potential outcomes intrinsic to the procedure, allergies to anesthesia, vasovagal reactions, and postoperative care. Prior surgeries could also alter a patient's anatomy, thus affecting a treatment plan.

COMPLICATIONS

Complications from energy-based devices include those related to anesthesia, antiseptics, bruising, infection, scarring, nerve injury, pigment alteration, and interference with implantable devices.

Nearly all procedures performed by dermatologists are done under local anesthesia, with sedation in rare cases. Allergies to anesthesia include type I hypersensitivity reactions (urticaria, angioedema, anaphylaxis) or type IV (delayed hypersensitivity such as contact dermatitis). Allergy to lidocaine, an amide anesthetic, is rare and in most instances can be deciphered from history of prior procedures which the patient can recall. Most lidocaine allergies are in fact allergies to other constituents in the vial such as preservatives. Allergic reactions are more common with ester anesthetics. Some patients react to epinephrine in the local anesthetic which manifests as palpitations, tachycardia, and tremors, especially with higher doses or with inadvertent vascular injection, which can lead the patient to think they are "allergic" to lidocaine. Diluting epinephrine to 1:200,000 may minimize symptoms. No specific treatment is usually required.

Contact dermatitis manifests between 1 and 7 days after exposure to latex, skin cleansers, adhesives, or topical antibiotics. Latex allergy can present as a delayed hypersensitivity reaction or as an immediate reaction. Antiseptics are used preceding minimally invasive procedures such as RF-assisted lipoplasty or skin tightening. Chlorhexidine and povidone-iodine rarely cause allergic contact dermatitis; 0.5% for chlorhexidine and 0.4% for povidine-iodine. Postoperative topical antibiotics such as neomycin and bacitracin are probably the most common culprits. Incidence of neomycin allergy ranges from 2.5% to 11.6% and bacitracin from 7.9% to 8.7%.

Bruising is often seen with vascular lasers. While this side effect resolves inconsequentially in the vast majority of cases, deposition of hemosiderin can lead to undesirable outcomes. Starting with conservative parameters and treating test spots in the beginning can mitigate such consequences. Patients on over the counter supplements predisposing to bruising like vitamin E, fish oils, garlic and others should stop them before such procedures.

While oral arnica reduces ecchymosis postoperatively in patients undergoing rhytidectomy, topical arnica after laser treatment offered no protection.

Significant breaches in the epidermal barrier seen with ablative laser procedures predispose for potential infection, which typically shows 4–7 days after a procedure. This risk can be mitigated by counseling the patient on meticulous wound care and cleaning, and inquiring about history of herpes breakouts or any current infections such as respiratory or urinary tract infections. Prophylactic antivirals are recommended for patients with a history of herpes labialis when the face is treated.

Electrosurgery could induce firing of a defibrillator if the electric signal is falsely perceived as the heart is in asystole. Electrocautery is the safest option compared to electrodessication and electrofulguration. A survey-based study of 166 Mohs surgeons showed that 71% used short bursts and 61% used minimal power with a complication rate of 0.8 cases/100 years of surgical practice.

Energy-based devices can lead to temporary or permanent nerve damage, although the latter is extremely rare. Care should be taken to avoid the marginal mandibular nerve when treating the submental area or the face with RF or ultrasound devices. Patients can have a short-term deficit due to anesthesia in the hours following a procedure, or stunning of the nerve for the following weeks to months due to thermal and inflammatory injury.

Scarring is a dreaded consequence as it is irreversible. Hypertrophic scars and keloids can develop after aggressive ablative lasers or thermal burns from RF devices. History of keloids on the face and careful examination can guide risk management. Keloids are more prevalent in darker skin types, ranging between 4.5% and 16% in African Americans and Hispanic populations, respectively. Anatomic sites like the chest, shoulders, upper arms, jawline, and ear lobes are at a greater risk.

Pigment alteration is most often temporary but can be permanent. Care should be taken in darker skin types (Fitzpatrick types III–VI) when using melanin-targeted, vascular, and ablative lasers and intense pulsed light. Topical steroids and diligent sun protection can mitigate postinflammatory pigment alteration. Counseling patients about such a risk is extremely important as it will likely increase their adherence to sun protection. (Figs. 15.1–15.8)

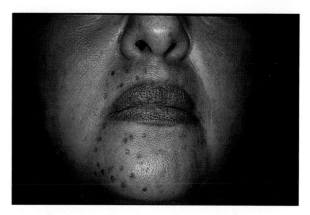

Fig. 15.1 Atrophy and hyperpigmentation.

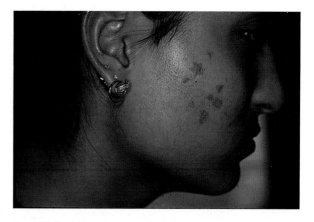

Fig. 15.2 Hyperpigmentation following use of 532 nm laser on darker skin.

RF devices including RF microneedling and subcutaneous RF used for lipoplasty and skin tightening can interfere with cardiac pacemakers and result in lethal outcomes. High intensity focused electromagnetic (HIFEM) devices used to stimulate muscle contraction and hypertrophy should also be avoided in any areas with implantable devices. Treatment overlying metal implants can also lead to internal organ damage.

Cryolipolysis implements freezing temperatures to induce adipocyte apoptosis, which yields moderate improvement in well-defined fatty areas. However, paradoxical fat hypertrophy has been reported and patients should be counseled about that before procedures. Liposuction is the treatment of choice in such instances.

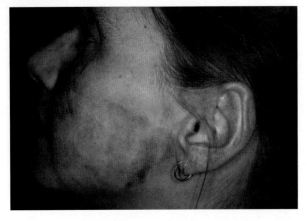

Fig. 15.3 Scar and atrophy.

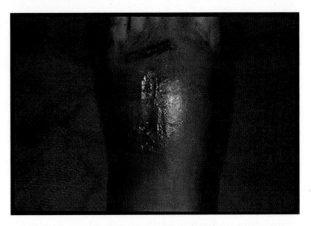

Fig. 15.6 IPL-induced burn.

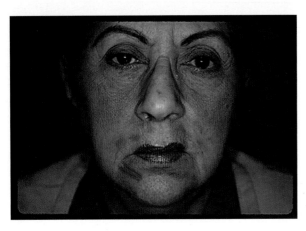

Fig. 15.4 IPL-induced scar.

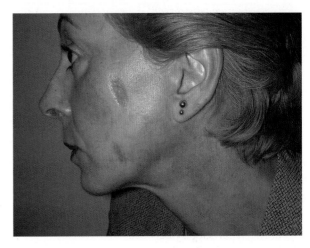

Fig. 15.7 Permanent IPL-induced scar.

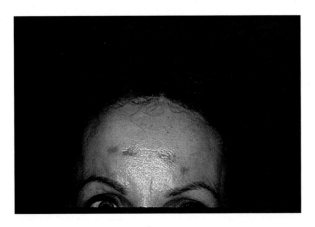

Fig. 15.5 Atrophy, erythema, and hyperpigmentation.

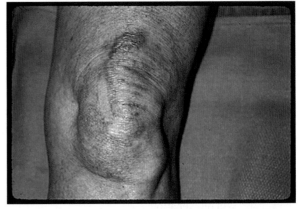

Fig. 15.8 Permanent Nd:YAG laser-induced scar.

MEDICAL PROFESSIONAL LIABILITY AGAINST DERMATOLOGISTS

In a study of the Physician Insurers Association of America registry, 2704 (1.1%) of 239,756 closed claims involved dermatologists. Of those, 28.7% resulted in an average indemnity payment of around $137,538. Improper procedure performance was the most common allegation, followed by error in diagnosis. Another study of 90,743 claims from the same database for the period 1991–2015 showed 1.2% to be against dermatologists. Full-time practitioners and those in solo practice were more likely to be sued than those in institutions and group practices, but the study did not adjust for number of patients seen within each group. The majority of claims against dermatologists (67.8%) were withdrawn, dismissed, or abandoned. Trial verdicts favoring defendants were seven times those favoring plaintiffs between 2006 and 2015. Procedure-related errors were the most common reason for claims (n = 305), of which 102 were paid. Skin operations in the broad definition was the most common reason for claims, and dyschromia was the most associated adverse outcome.

In another study of 40,916 physicians and 233,738 physician-years of coverage, dermatology was among the least likely to be sued (ahead of pediatrics, psychiatry and family medicine), and the mean indemnity payment was lowest for dermatology at $117,832.

A national database study of legal actions related to cutaneous laser surgery between 1985 and 2012 identified 174 cases due to injury secondary to laser surgery. The incidence of litigation reports increased over time, peaking in 2010. Laser hair removal was the most common litigated procedure. Importantly, non-physician operators constituted a significant proportion, and their physician supervisors were named as defendants. Failure to obtain an informed consent was the most common preventable cause of action. Half of the cases resulted in decisions in favor of the plaintiff, and the mean indemnity payment was $380,719.

A retrospective analysis of a legal database encompassing publicly available federal and state court records identified cases involving laser procedures in the head and neck. Nineteen of thirty-four cases (56%) resulted in a defendant verdict, with a median indemnity of $150,000. Skin rejuvenation, acne scarring, hair removal, and vascular lesions were the most common indications.

Analysis of ablative laser malpractice cases in the LexisNexus database in the period 1991–2015 revealed 42 claims. Alleged injuries were scarring (55%), dyschromia (14%), and infection (9.5%). Of the cases yielding verdicts favoring the plaintiff, failure to obtain informed consent was the most common type of negligence.

Dermatologists are less likely to face claims than other specialties. While dermatologists constitute 1.4% of physicians, 0.7% of claims are against dermatologists. Furthermore, around 2% of truly negligent acts lead to malpractice claims, but 17% of all malpractice claims result from true negligence. In a survey of Mohs surgeons, lawsuits were due to wrong site (n=6), functional outcome (n=6), postprocedure outcome (n=5), cosmetic outcome (n=5), recurrent tumor (n=5), improper consent (n=3), delayed diagnosis (n=2), misdiagnosis (n=1), and other (n=7).

In a 2006 study which surveyed dermatologists in 2004, there was substantial variation in medical liability premiums across states. States declared as "crisis states" by the AMA had significantly higher premiums than those "currently OK". Premiums were higher in states without $250,000 caps for noneconomic damages. Dermatologists spending more than 10% of their time in cosmetic practice or >30% non-cosmetic surgery had higher premiums. While premiums were well below those in higher risks specialties, rate of premium growth was comparable to other specialties.

LEGAL CONSEQUENCES

Complications may or may not lead to legal action. Four elements are required for a cause of action in negligence: duty, breach of duty, causation, and damage. A successful claim requires satisfaction of all four elements. A dermatologist's duty is to perform a procedure in accordance with the standard of care. The standard of care is not a well-defined practice, but is delineated by an expert in the field and what the jury ultimately believes. In a case against a dermatologist, the latter should have the knowledge and skills ordinarily possessed by a specialist in the field, and should have used these skills in the care of a patient in a similar locality under similar circumstances. Liability ensues if the jury is convinced that the dermatologist mismanaged the case and this led to damage to the patient. Conversely, if the jury is convinced by the testimony of the expert testifying for the defendant, the standard of care is met. Therefore the standard of care is often based on the testimony of an expert physician. The dermatologist is expected to perform the procedure in a reasonable manner by an objective standard, not necessarily in the best possible way. For example, if two treatments are accepted as reasonable approaches for a skin lesion, with one being superior in efficacy and side effects, the dermatologist does not fall below the standard of care for choosing the inferior method, as long as it is deemed reasonable by experts in the field. Finally, in many jurisdictions, an unfavorable outcome due to an "error in judgment" by itself is not a violation of the standard of care if the dermatologist acted appropriately prior to exercising this professional judgment.

Evidence for the standard of care in a specific case is derived from laws, regulations, medical guidelines, peer-reviewed publications, and textbooks related to a topic. The standard of care is generally recognized as a national standard, although variation among states could exist in some instances. The standard of care is the practice followed by the majority of physicians in a similar medical community and the expert is expected to reflect this reality. If the expert practices in a manner different than the majority, then they will face a difficulty providing an explanation for such deviation.

The standard of care is typically articulated by an expert witness whose basis is grounded in the following:
1. The witness' personal practice; and/or
2. The practice of others observed in their experience; and/or
3. Medical literature; and/or
4. Statutes and/or legislative rules; and/or
5. Courses discussing the subject in a well-defined manner.

Therefore the standard of care is typically an ephemeral concept resulting from differences among the medical profession, the legal system, and the public. At the extreme, the standard of care for a specific skin complaint is clearly outlined and well-defined in national guidelines or peer-reviewed publications, but even in such instances, these guidelines are general recommendations and the physician could (and often should) individualize care based on their best judgement.

Substantial efforts have been made by specialty societies such as the American Academy of Dermatology and the American Society for Dermatologic Surgery to put standard guidelines specifying treatment approaches to various conditions. Such guidelines can offer an authoritative statement of what the standard of care is, and a court would have several options when such guidelines are offered as evidence. A dermatologist acting in accordance with the guidelines would be shielded from liability to the same extent as one who can establish that she or he followed professional customs. Using guidelines as evidence of professional custom, however, is problematic if they are not necessarily consistent with prevailing medical practice. A widely accepted clinical standard may be presumptive evidence of due care, but expert testimony will still be required to introduce the standard and establish its sources and relevance.

Disclaimers are often attached to guidelines, thereby undercutting their defensive use in litigation. The AMA suggests that guidelines should not be intended to replace physician discretion. Hence, such guidelines could not be treated as conclusive.

Plaintiffs usually use their own expert, as opposed to the physician's expert, to define the standard of care. Although such a plaintiff's expert may also refer to clinical practice guidelines, the physician's negligence can be established in other manners. This includes (1) examination of the physician defendant's expert witness, (2) an admission by the defendant that he or she was negligent, (3) testimony by the plaintiff, in a rare case where they are a medical expert qualified to evaluate the physician's conduct, and (4) common knowledge in situations where a layperson could understand the negligence without the assistance of an expert.

It is often difficult to predict the outcome in any given malpractice cause of action against a dermatologist. However, a clear understanding of the aforementioned principles will decrease the chance of a physician losing any negligence cause of action brought against them.

FURTHER READING

Alonso D, Lazarus MC, Baumann L. Effects of topical arnica gel on post-laser treatment bruises. *Dermatol Surg.* 2002;28(8):686–688.

Aremu SK, Alabi BS, Segun-Busari S. The role of informed consent in risks recall in otorhinolaryngology surgeries: verbal (nonintervention) vs written (intervention) summaries of risks. *Am J Otolaryngol.* 2011;32(6):485–489.

Bendewald MJ, Farmer SA, Davis MD. Patch testing with natural rubber latex: the Mayo Clinic experience. *Dermatitis.* 2010;21(6):311–316.

Berman B, Flores F. The treatment of hypertrophic scars and keloids. *Eur J Dermatol.* 1998;8(8):591–595.

Bolognia J, Jorizzo JL, Rapini RP, et al, eds. *Dermatology.* 2nd ed. London: Mosby Elsevier; 2008.

El-Gamal HM, Dufresne RG, Saddler K. Electrosurgery, pacemakers and ICDs: a survey of precautions and complications experienced by cutaneous surgeons. *Dermatol Surg.* 2011;27(4):385–390.

Engel E, Livingston EH. Solving the medical malpractice crisis: use a clear and convincing evidence standard. *Arch Surg.* 2010;145(3):296–300.

Jalian HR, Jalian CA, Avram MM. Common causes of injury and legal action in laser surgery. *JAMA Dermatol.* 149(2): 188–193.

Jena AB, Seabury S, Lakdawalla D, Chandra A. Malpractice risk according to physician specialty. *N Engl J Med.* 2011; 365:629–636.

Juckett G, Hartman-Adams H. Management of keloids and hypertrophic scars. *Am Fam Physician.* 2009;80(3): 253–260. 2009.

Kornmehl H, Singh S, Adler BL, Wolf AE, Bochner DA, Armstrong AW. Characteristics of medical liability claims against dermatologists from 1991 through 2015. *JAMA Dermatol.* 2018;154(2):160–166.

Lachapelle JM. Allergic contact dermatitis from povidone-iodine: a re-evaluation study. *Contact Dermatitis.* 2005; 52(1):9–10.

Liippo J, Kousa P, Lammintausta K. The relevance of chlorhexidine contact allergy. *Contact Dermatitis.* 2011;64(4):229–234.

Lim KS, Kam PC. Chlorhexidine—pharmacology and clinical applications. *Anaesth Intensive Care.* 2008;36(4):502–512.

Moshell AN, Parikh PD, Oetgen WJ. Characteristics of medical professional liability claims against dermatologists: data from 2704 closed claims in a voluntary registry. *J Am Acad Dermatol.* 2012;66(1):78–85.

Perlis CS, Campbell RM, Perlis RH, Malik M, Dufresne RG Jr. Incidence of and risk factors for medical malpractice lawsuits among Mohs surgeons. *Dermatol Surg.* 2006; 32(1):79–83.

Pierce RR, Martell DW. Ablative lasers: 24 years of medical malpractice cases in the United States. *Dermatol Surg.* 2018;44(5):730–731.

Resneck JS Jr. Trends in malpractice premiums for dermatologists: results of a national survey. *Arch Dermatol.* 2006;142(3):337–340.

Seeley BM, Denton AB, Ahn MS, Maas CS. Effect of homeopathic Arnica montana on bruising in face-lifts: results of a randomized, double-blind, placebo-controlled clinical trial. *Arch Facial Plast Surg.* 2006;8(1):54–59.

Sheth VM, Weitzul S. Postoperative topical antimicrobial use. *Dermatitis.* 2008;19(4):181–189.

Svider PF, Carron MA, Zuliani GF, Eloy JA, Setzen M, Folbe AJ. Lasers and losers in the eyes of the law: liability for head and neck procedures. *JAMA Facial Plast Surg.* 2014;16(4):277–283.

Yerra L, Reddy PC. Effects of electromagnetic interference on implanted cardiac devices and their management. *Cardiol Rev.* 2007;15(6):304–309.

INDEX

Page numbers followed by "*f*" indicate figures, "*t*" indicate tables, and "*b*" indicate boxes.

A

5-Aminolevulinic acid (ALA), 129, 132
  incubation variation, 133
Ablative fractionated lasers, 195, 195*b*
Ablative laser malpractice, 225
Ablative laser skin resurfacing. *See*
  Laser skin resurfacing
Ablative lasers, 7
Ablative resurfacing, 28
Ablative systems, types of, 141*t*
Accent device, 117
AccuTite device, 115
Acne, treatment of, 206–220
  application of PDT, 133–134, 134*f*
  laser light therapy for, 213–217
  photodynamic therapy for, 206–210,
    208*f*, 212*t*
    posttreatment, 210, 213*f*, 214*f*
    pretreatment, 207
    treatment, 208–210, 209*f*, 211*f*
    introduction to, 206, 207*t*
  visible light phototherapy for,
    210–213
Acne flare, 61–63
Acne outbreaks, due to nonablative
  fractional photothermolysis, 100
Acne scars, radiofrequency micro-
  needling for, 183, 184*f*, 185*f*
Acne vulgaris, radiofrequency
  microneedling for, 183, 185*f*
Actinic cheilitis, 133
Actinic keratoses (AK), 128
  ALA, 128
  MAL, 128
Active infection
  laser resurfacing and, 146
  radiofrequency microneedling and,
    187
AK. *See* Actinic keratoses (AK)
Aktilite, 130–131
  adverse reactions, 131

Alacare, 129
Alexandrite laser, 15
  755 nm, 198, 198*b*
Aluma device, 117
Amalgam tattoos, 42
Ameluz, 129–131
  adverse reactions, 131
  incubation variation, 133
Ameluz/Metvixia and daylight, 131
Amiodarone, 41–42
Anagen, 55
Anderson, Rox, 54
Angiokeratomas, 22
Angioma
  cherry, 21–22, 22*f*
  infantile hemangioma, 12*t*, 16–19
Appendageal abnormality, laser skin
  resurfacing and, 146
Argyria, 42
Axillary hyperhidrosis, radiofrequency
  microneedling for, 183–186,
  186*f*

B

Bacterial infection, after laser skin
  resurfacing, 148
Basal cell carcinoma (BCC), 128, 132
  application of PDT, 133
  ALA, 128
  MAL, 128
BCC. *See* Basal cell carcinoma (BCC)
Beam type, 4
Becker nevus, 36
Benign pigmented lesions, 32–42
BF-RhodoLED lamp, 130–131
Bipolar electrode devices, 107, 107*b*
Bipolar radiofrequency devices, in skin
  tightening
  hybrid monopolar and, 117–118,
    118*b*, 118*f*, 119*b*
Black tattoos, 42–43, 42*f*

Blister formation, 61–63
Blue light alone, in treatment of acne,
  210–211, 215*f*
Blue nevi, 41, 42*f*
Blu-U, 129–130
BMI. *See* Body mass index (BMI)
BodyFX, 159–160
Body mass index (BMI), 153–155, 155*b*
BodyTite device, 115
Bowen's Disease (SCCis), 133
Bruising, 61–63, 160*b*
  in laser, light and energy-based
    treatment, 222–223
β-Blockers, 19*b*

C

Café au lait macules (CALMs), 35–36
Carbon dioxide full field laser, 141–142
Carbon dioxide laser, 137
Cardiac defibrillator, radiofrequency
  microneedling and, 187
Cardiac pacemaker, radiofrequency
  microneedling and, 187
Catagen, 55
Cellfina, 158
Cellfina Registry Under Investigation
  for Safety and Efficacy
  (CRUISE) study, 158
Cellulite, 153–155, 153*b*
  classification of, 155*t*
  herbal treatments for, 157*t*
Cherry angiomas, 21–22, 22*f*
Chromophore, 4–5, 6*f*
Civatte, poikiloderma of, 21, 80
Clinical endpoints, 8
Cold sores/herpes simplex 1
  laser skin resurfacing and, 146–147
Collagen fibers, 105
Collagen remodeling, in radiofrequency
  microneedling device, 177–179,
  179*f*

Combination therapy, in skin tightening, 120b
Combined electrical and optical energy devices, in skin tightening, 116–117, 116b
Congenital dermal melanocytosis, 41
Congenital nevi, 37
Cooling, 9, 9f
  epidermal, 12
  for nonablative fractional photothermolysis, 99
CoolSculpting, 163, 164f, 165b
CoolTone device, 168
Cosmetic tattoo, 44
Cryolipolysis
  in laser, light and energy-based treatment, 223
  for nonsurgical body contouring, 163–165, 163b

D

Dark blue tattoos, 42–43, 42f
Deep chemical peel/deep dermabrasion, laser skin resurfacing and, 146
Deep laser resurfacing
  previous, 146
  in radiofrequency microneedling, 188
Depilatory creams, 61
Dermal papilla, 55
Dermatitis, after laser skin resurfacing, 148
Dermatologic diseases that exhibit Koebner phenomenon, 189
Dermatosis papulosa nigra, 36
Dermoepidermal lesions, 36–40
Diffractive lens array (DLA), 27
Diode combined with RF, for hair removal, 57t–60t
Diode laser, 57t–60t
DLA. See Diffractive lens array (DLA)
Drug-induced hyperpigmentation, 41–42

E

Eckhouse, Shimon, 72–73
Ectropion, after laser skin resurfacing, 149

Eflornithine, 54
Electrodes, configuration of, 107
Electrolysis, 54
Electromagnetic muscle stimulation (EMMS), 168–169
Electromagnetic radiation, measurement of, 3–4
Electromagnetic spectrum, 1, 2f
EMMS. See Electromagnetic muscle stimulation (EMMS)
EmSculpt device, 168
Endermologie, 157–158
Epidermal lesions, 32–36
Epidermal protection to radiofrequency microneedling device, 179, 179f
Erbium:yttrium-aluminum-garnet (Er:YAG) lasers, 138, 142, 142f, 143f
  1540-nm and 1550-nm, 216–217
Er:YAG lasers. See Erbium:yttrium-aluminumgarnet (Er:YAG) lasers
Erythema, after laser skin resurfacing, 148
Erythroplasia of Querat, 133
ESWT. See Extracorporeal shock wave therapy (ESWT)
Eumelanin, 55
Excimer laser, 46
Extracorporeal shock wave therapy (ESWT), 158

F

FaceTite device, 115
Faraday, Michael, 168
Fat, 153–155, 153b
Fat-specific laser, 162–163
Flash-lamps, for IPL device, 73
Fluence, 3–4, 64, 64b, 64f
Fluorescent pulsed light, 57t–60t
Flushing, 79–80, 80f
Folliculitis, 61–63
FP. See Fractional photothermolysis (FP)
Fractional ablative technology, 143–144, 144f, 145f
Fractional laser resurfacing, 139b
Fractional microneedle radio-frequency, 101

Fractional microplasma radio-frequency devices, in laser treatment, 202, 203f
Fractional minimally invasive bipolar radiofrequency devices, in skin tightening, 112–115, 113f, 114f
Fractional photothermolysis (FP), 27–28, 34
  nonablative
    advances in technology for, 101–102
    applications of, 88–95
    complications of, 100–101
    contraindications to, 96b
    cooling for, 99
    epidemiology of, 86
    equipment for, 86–88
    experienced practitioners and, treatment tips for, 102
    fractional microneedle radiofrequency, 101
    general technique for, 98–99, 99t
    pathophysiology of, 85–86, 86f
    patient selection for, 95–97, 95b
    posttreatment for, 99–100, 100f
    pretreatment for, 97–98, 97b, 98b
    safety of, 100–101
    scarring, 90–92, 91b, 91f, 92f
Fractionation, 7
Fractora device, 113–115
Fraxel Dual, 87
Full field laser resurfacing, 139b
Fungal infection, after laser resurfacing, 147f, 148

G

Genius device, 115
Green tattoos, 43–44

H

Hair cycle, 55
Hair follicle, 55
Hair regrowth, 55
Halo, 140
Healing, slow, after laser skin resurfacing, 149
Hemangioma, infantile, 12t, 16–19
Hemoglobin, optical absorption of, 12f

Herbal treatments, for cellulites, 157t

HIFU. *See* High-intensity focused ultrasound (HIFU)

High-intensity focused ultrasound (HIFU), 120–121

Hirsutism, 55, 56f

Home-use devices, for hair removal, 57t–60t

Hori's nevus, 40–41

Hybrid lasers, in laser and light treatment, 196–197, 197b

Hyperpigmentation
   in laser, light and energy-based treatment, 223, 223f, 224f
   nonablative fractional photothermolysis for, 92–93, 93f
   periorbital, 39–40
   postinflammatory, 39
      due to nonablative fractional photothermolysis, 99–100

Hypertrichosis, 55

Hypopigmentation
   after laser skin resurfacing, 148, 148f
   nonablative fractional photothermolysis for, 92–93, 93f

I

Infantile hemangioma, 12t
   treatment of, 17–19

Infection, 61–63
   after laser skin resurfacing, 147–148, 147b–148b, 147f

Inferior segments, 55

Infini device, 113–115

Informed consent, in laser and light treatment, 221–222

Infrared light devices, in skin tightening, 119–120, 120b

Infundibulum, 55

Injectable agents, for nonsurgical body contouring, 156–157

Injectable lipolysis, 156

Intense pulsed light (IPL), 2–3, 12
   applications, 78–82
      benign pigmented lesions, 78–79, 79f
      dry eye, 81–82
      hair reduction, 81, 81f

Intense pulsed light (IPL) (*Continued*)
      poikiloderma of Civatte, 80
      rhytids and collagen stimulation, 80–81
      telangiectasias, flushing and other vascular conditions, 79–80, 79f
   complications, 78f, 82–83
   equipment, 74–75, 74f, 75b, 83
      BroadBand light (BBL), 75
      cooling mechanisms, 75
      cut-off filters and absorption filters, 74–75
      IPL hand-piece, 75
   in laser treatment, 200–201, 201b
   patient selection, 75–76, 76b
   and photodynamic therapy, 82
   sources, 57t–60t
   terminology, 73–74, 74b
   treatment, 72–84
      history of, 72–73
      of acne, 212–213
   treatment protocol, 76–78
      posttreatment, 77–78, 78f
      pretreatment, 76–77
      treatment technique, 77–78

Intensif device, 113

Isotretinoin use, in radiofrequency microneedling, 188–189

Isthmus, 55

K

KA. *See* Keratoacanthoma (KA)

Keloid/scarring history
   laser skin resurfacing and, 146
   in radiofrequency microneedling, 188

Keratoacanthoma (KA), 133

Keratoses, actinic, nonablative fractional photothermolysis for, 94–95, 95b

Klippel-Trénaunay syndrome, port-wine stains and, 14

Koebner phenomenon, 61
   in radiofrequency microneedling, 189

KTP. *See* Potassium titanyl phosphate (KTP)

Kybella, 156

L

Labial melanotic macules, 35, 35f

Lactation, radiofrequency microneedling and, 187

LAL. *See* Laser-assisted liposuction (LAL)

Lanugo, 55

Laser, 1–2, 137
   ablative, 7
   adverse effects of, 8
   beam type, 4
   in dermatology, 6t
   light, properties of, 2, 3f
   and light treatments
      650-microsecond 1064 nm laser, 198–199, 199b
      hybrid lasers, 196–197, 197b
      picosecond lasers, 199–200, 199f, 200b
      Q-switched lasers, 200, 200b
   and light treatments, complications of, 221–228
      informed consent in, 221–222
      legal consequences, 225–226
      negligence, 225
      prevention, 222
      professional liabilities against dermatologists, 225
   nonablative, 7
   for nonsurgical body contouring, 161–163
   radiofrequency *versus*, 180
   tissue interactions, 4, 5f

Laser-assisted liposuction (LAL), 161

Laser hair removal, 54–71, 197–198, 198b, 198f
   alternative technologies for, 70
   basic hair biology, 55, 55f
   future directions, 69–70
   home-use laser and light source devices for, 70
   key factors in optimizing treatment, 61–69
      complications, 67–69, 67f, 68f, 69f
      device variables, 63–66
      informed consent, 61–63, 63b
      laser safety, 63
      long-term efficacy, 67

Laser hair removal (*Continued*)
  patient selection, 61, 61*b*, 62*b*,
    62*b*–61*b*, 62*f*
  post procedure care, 66, 66*b*
  preoperative preparation, 63
mechanism of, 55–56, 56*f*, 57*t*–60*t*
medical conditions treated with,
  66–67
Laser light therapy for acne, 213–217
  1064-nm Nd:YAG laser, 214–215
  1320-nm Nd:YAG laser, 215–216
  1540-nm and 1550-nm erbium:glass
    lasers, 216–217
  pulsed dye laser, 213–214, 216*f*
  pulsed green laser, 214
Laser safety, 30–31
Laser skin resurfacing, 137–151
  absolute contraindications in, 146,
    146*b*
  complications after, 147–150
  expected benefits and alternatives of,
    141, 141*b*
  fractional, 139*b*
  full field, 139*b*
  history of, 138–140
  introduction to, 137, 138*t*
  lasers and technical overview in,
    141–144, 141*t*
  patient assessment in, 140, 140*b*
  patient selection in, 140–141, 146*b*
  pretreatment and posttreatment
    regimens in, 147
  relative contraindications in,
    146–147, 146*b*–147*b*
  safety, 144, 144*b*
  strategy in, treatment, 144–150
  summary and key features of, 137
  traditional ablative, 138–139, 139*f*
  treatment approach in, 144–146
Laser therapy, 8
Laser treatment
  benign pigmented lesions, 32–42
  complications of, 46
  for dermal lesions, 40–42
  for dermoepidermal lesions,
    36–40
  for epidermal lesions, 32–36
  of ethnic skin, 192–200

Laser treatment (*Continued*)
  fractional microplasma radio-
    frequency devices, 202, 203*f*
  intense pulsed light, 200–201, 201*b*
  laser safety, 30–31
  lasers and lights in
    ablative fractionated lasers, 195,
      195*b*
    650-microsecond 1064 nm laser,
      198–199, 199*b*
    hybrid lasers, 196–197, 197*b*
    nonablative fractionated lasers,
      195–196, 196*b*
    picosecond lasers, 199–200, 199*f*,
      200*b*
    Q-switched lasers, 200, 200*b*
    vascular lasers, 196, 196*b*, 197*f*
  lesion selection, 29–30, 29*t*, 30*t*
  microneedling, 201, 201*b*, 202*f*
  microplasma radiofrequency device,
    201–202, 202*b*, 203*f*
  particle-assisted, 217–218
  patient evaluation and selection for,
    28–29
  patient preparation in, 30–31, 31*b*
  of pigmented lesions and tattoos,
    25–53
  pigment removal principles with,
    26–28
  postoperative care in, 45–46
  preoperative considerations, 28–31
  skin tightening devices, 202
  tattoo removal outcomes and,
    45, 45*f*
  treatment techniques in, 31–45
Laugier-Hunziker syndrome, 35
Legend Pro VoluDerm device, 115
Lesions, 12–13
  vascular, 11–24
Levulan Kerastick, 129–130
  adverse reactions, 131
  incubation variation, 133
LexisNexus database, 225
Lichen sclerosus, 134
Light
  characteristics of, 1
  intense pulsed, 2–3
  properties of laser, 2

Light sources
  in photodynamic therapy, 129–130
    blue light, 129–130
    irradiation, 129
    red light, 130
Liposonix device, 161
Long-pulsed alexandrite laser, 57*t*–60*t*,
  64
Long-pulsed diode laser, 64
Long-pulsed Nd:YAG laser, 57*t*–60*t*, 64
Long-pulsed ruby laser, 63–64
Lymphangioma circumscriptum, 20

M
650-microsecond 1064 nm laser, in
  laser and light treatment,
  198–199, 199*b*
Malformations, venous, 19–20, 20*f*
Melanin, 63
Melanocytic nevi, 36–37
Melasma, 37–39, 38*f*
  nonablative fractional photothermol-
    ysis for, 94, 94*b*
Metal implants, in radiofrequency
  microneedling, 187
Methyl aminolevulinic acid (MAL),
  127–129
Methylxanthines, for cellulites, 156
Metvixia, 129, 131
  adverse reactions, 131
Microneedling, in laser treatment, 201,
  201*b*, 202*f*
Microplasma radiofrequency, in laser
  treatment, 201–202, 202*b*, 203*f*
Minocycline, 41–42
Mongolian spots, 40–41
Monopolar electrode devices, 107, 107*b*
Monopolar radiofrequency devices, for
  skin tightening
    hybrid bipolar and, 117–118, 118*b*,
      118*f*, 119*b*
Multi-colored tattoos, 44, 44*f*
Multiple sequential pulsing and pulse
  delay, for IPL device, 73
Muscle toning and contouring, 167–175
  EMMS for, 168–169
  introduction to, 167–168, 167*b*–168*b*,
    168*b*

Muscle toning and contouring (*Continued*)
NMES for, 169–172, 169*b*, 169*b*–170*b*, 172*f*
patient evaluation and expectation management, 172–173
case study, 173*b*

N

NAFR. *See* Nonablative fractional photothermolysis (NAFR)
Narrow band ultraviolet, 46
Nd:YAG laser. *See* Neodymium:yttriumaluminum-garnet (Nd:YAG) laser
Neck dyspigmentation, nonablative fractional photothermolysis for, 95
Neocollagenesis, 105, 112–113, 117, 119
Neodymium:yttrium-aluminum-garnet (Nd:YAG) laser
1064-nm, 120
1320-nm, 215–216
Neuromuscular electrical stimulation (NMES), 169–172, 169*b*, 169*b*–170*b*, 172*f*
treatment with, 170*b*–171*b*, 171*f*, 214–215
Nevus of Ito, 40–41
Nevus of Ota, 40–41, 40*f*
Nevus spilus, 35–36
Nonablative fractional laser rejuvenation, 85–103
Nonablative fractional photothermolysis (NAFR)
advances in technology for, 101–102
applications of, 88–95
actinic keratoses, 94–95, 95*b*
contraindications to, 96*b*
general technique for, 98–99, 99*t*
hyperpigmentation, 92–93, 93*f*
hypopigmentation, 92–93, 93*f*
indications for, 88*b*
melasma, 94, 94*b*
photoaging, 88–89
poikiloderma of Civatte and neck dyspigmentation, 95

Nonablative fractional photothermolysis (NAFR) (*Continued*)
scarring, 90–92, 91*b*, 91*f*, 92*f*
striae, 95
complications of, 100–101, 101*b*
cooling for, 99
epidemiology of, 86
equipment for, 86–88
experienced practitioners and, treatment tips for, 102, 102*b*
pathophysiology of, 85–86, 86*f*
patient selection for, 95–97, 95*b*
case study for, 96*b*, 96*b*–97*b*
pretreatment for, 97–98, 97*b*, 98*b*
posttreatment for, 99–100, 100*f*
safety of, 100–101
Nonablative fractional resurfacing, 142
Nonablative fractionated lasers, in laser and light treatment, 195–196, 196*b*
Nonablative lasers, 7
Nonablative resurfacing, 34
Noninvasive monopolar radiofrequency, for skin tightening devices, 108–112, 109*b*, 110*f*, 111*f*
Nonsurgical body contouring, 152–166
cryolipolysis for, 163–165, 163*b*
ESWT in, 158
fat-specific laser for, 162–163
fat *versus* cellulite in, 153–155, 154*f*, 155*f*
injectable agents for, 156–157
lasers and light sources for, 161–163
physical manipulation in, 157–158, 158*b*
radiofrequency devices for, 158–161
therapeutic options for, 155–165
topical creams for, 156, 156*b*
ultrasound devices for, 161

O

Obesity, 152
Ocular safety, 30, 30*b*–31*b*
Ohm's law, 106–107, 106*b*
Optical energy, for hair removal, 57*t*–60*t*

Optical resonator, anatomy of, 3*f*
Orolabial herpes, history of, in radiofrequency microneedling, 188

P

Pain control, advances in, 57*t*–60*t*, 69–70
Palomar brand of Cynosure, 87
Papillae adipose, 153
Paradoxical darkening, 44
Parrish, John, 54
Particle-assisted laser treatment of acne, 217–218
726-nm lasers in, 217–218
Patient evaluation and selection, 28–29
Pelleve device, 118
Peutz-Jeghers syndrome, 35, 35*f*
Pheomelanin, 55
Photoaging
case study for, 89*b*, 89*f*, 90*f*
nonablative fractional photothermolysis for, 88–89
Photodynamic therapy (PDT), 15, 127–136
5-Aminolevulinic acid blue light, 132
incubation variations, 133
for acne, 206–210, 208*f*, 212*t*
adverse reactions, 131–132
applications of, 128
approved indications, 128
basal cell carcinoma, 132
clinical applications, 133–134
clinical clearance rate, 132
contraindications to, 128
illumination variations, 133
introduction to, 127
IPL and, 82
materials and methods, 129–131
light sources, 129–130
photosensitizers, 129
mechanism of action, 128
off-label protocol variations, 132
principles of, 127–128
sactinic keratoses, 132, 132*f*
skin-preparation variations, 133

Photodynamic therapy (PDT)
      (*Continued*)
   summary and key features, 127
   in treatment of acne, 206–210, 208*f*
   treatment protocols, 129
   US FDA-approved procedures, 130
   warnings and precautions, 128–129
      mucous membranes irritation, 129
      ophthalmic adverse reactions, 129
      photosensitivity, 128
      risk of bleeding, 128
      risk of eye injury, 128
Photons, 1
Photosensitizers, 129
Photothermolysis, 27–28, 55–56
   selective, 5–7, 6*f*, 6*t*, 7*t*, 8*f*
Physical manipulation, in nonsurgical
      body contouring, 157–158, 158*b*
Picosecond laser (PS), 26–27, 32–33
   in laser and light treatment, 199–200,
      199*f*, 200*b*
PIH. *See* Postinflammatory hyperpig-
      mentation (PIH)
Plasma resurfacing systems, 142
Poikiloderma of Civatte, 21, 80
   nonablative fractional
      photothermolysis for, 95
Port-wine birthmarks (PWB), 12*t*,
      13–16, 15*f*, 16*b*
   hypertrophic, 13*f*, 15*f*, 16*f*
   treatment of, 14–16
Postinflammatory hyperpigmentation
      (PIH)
   after laser skin resurfacing, 149,
      149*b*, 149*f*
   laser treatment of, 194
Potassium titanyl phosphate (KTP), for
      infantile hemangiomas, 12
PpIX. *See* Protoporphyrin IX (PpIX)
Pregnancy, radiofrequency
      microneedling and, 187
Prep Mode for NMES device, 168
Previous deep chemical peels, in
      radiofrequency microneedling,
      188
Prior surgery or skin grafts, in radio-
      frequency microneedling, 188
Profound device, 112

Protoporphyrin IX (PpIX), 127
PS. *See* Picosecond laser (PS)
Pulsed dye laser (PDL), 12
   for infantile hemangiomas, 17
   for port-wine birthmarks, 14
   for rosacea, 20, 21*f*
   for vascular lesions, 12, 23
Pulsed dye laser, in treatment of acne,
      213–214, 216*f*
Pulsed green laser, in treatment of acne,
      214
Pulse duration, 3–4, 64–65, 65*b*
   for IPL device, 73

Q
Q-switched lasers, 4
   in laser and light treatment, 200,
      200*b*
Quality-switched (QS) lasers, 26

R
Radiofrequency (RF) devices, 176–177,
      177*t*
   for nonsurgical body contouring,
      158–161
   in skin tightening, 106–116
      depth of energy penetration in,
         107, 107*b*
      dielectric properties for human
         tissue and, 107, 108*t*
      fractional minimally invasive
         bipolar, 112–115, 113*f*, 114*f*
      hybrid monopolar and bipolar,
         117–118, 118*b*, 118*f*, 119*b*
      microneedle, 112–113, 113*f*, 114*f*
      noninvasive monopolar, 108–112,
         109*b*, 110*f*, 111*f*
      subdermal minimally invasive,
         115
Radiofrequency microneedling,
      176–191
   absolute contraindications, 187–188
   for acne scars, 183, 184*f*, 185*f*
   for acne vulgaris, 183, 185*f*
   for axillary hyperhidrosis, 183–186,
      186*f*
   characteristics of microneedles in,
      180–182, 180*f*, 181*f*, 182*f*

Radiofrequency microneedling
      (*Continued*)
   collagen remodeling, 177–179, 179*f*
   devices, 176–177, 177*t*
   epidermal protection, 179, 179*f*
   indications for, 182, 186–187
   introduction to, 176
   patient selection, 187, 187*f*, 188*f*
   polarity of, 177, 178*f*
   posttreatment regimens, 189
   pretreatment regimens, 189
   radiofrequency *versus* lasers, 180
   relative contraindications, 188–189
   for skin rejuvenation, 182–183, 183*f*,
      184*f*
Radiometry, 3–4
Red and blue light, in treatment of acne,
      211–212
Red light alone, in treatment of acne,
      211
Red tattoos, 43, 43*f*
Regional resurfacing in darker-
      skinned individuals, laser skin
      resurfacing and, 146
Rhytids and collagen stimulation,
      80–81
"R20" method, 45
Rosacea, 20–22, 21*f*

S
Scar formation, 61–63
Scarring, 36
   after laser skin resurfacing, 149, 150*f*
   in laser, light and energy-based
      treatment, 223
   nonablative fractional photothermol-
      ysis for, 90–92, 91*b*
SCCis. *See* Squamous Cell Carcinoma
      in situ (SCCis)
Scratches, due to nonablative fractional
      photothermolysis, 100
SculpSure, 162–163
Sculpt Mode for NMES device, 168
Sebaceous hyperplasia, 134
Seborrheic keratoses, 36
Selective photothermolysis, 5–7, 6*f*, 6*t*,
      7*t*, 8*f*
   in IPL device, 73

Shaving, 61
Skin
  cooling, 65–66, 65*f*, 66*b*
  eruptions, after laser skin
    resurfacing, 148
Skin grafts, in radiofrequency
    microneedling, 188
Skin rejuvenation, by radiofrequency
    microneedling, 182–183, 183*f*,
    184*f*
Skin tightening
  devices, in laser treatment, 202
  introduction to, 104–105
  major types of, technologies, 105*t*
  nonsurgical, 104–126
  radiofrequency devices in,
    106–116
    fractional minimally invasive
      bipolar, 112–115, 113*f*, 114*f*
    hybrid monopolar and bipolar,
      117–118, 118*b*, 118*f*, 119*b*
    noninvasive monopolar, 108–112,
      109*b*
    subdermal minimally invasive,
      115
  summary and key features in,
    104
  thermal collagen remodeling in,
    105–106, 105*b*, 106*f*
  tips for maximizing patient
    satisfaction, 122–124, 124*b*
SmoothShapes device, 162
Solar lentigines, 32–35, 33*f*, 34*f*
Spectral shift, in IPL device, 73–74
Spot size, 65, 65*b*
Squamous Cell Carcinoma in situ
    (SCCis), 128, 132
Striae, nonablative fractional
    photothermolysis for, 95
Sturge-Weber syndrome, 14
  port-wine stains and, 14
Subcision, for cellulite, 158
Subdermal minimally invasive
    radiofrequency devices, in skin
    tightening, 115
Synechia, after laser skin resurfacing,
    149–150

T
Tattoo, 42–45
  colors, 29*t*
Tattoo granulomas, 43*f*
Tattoo removal, outcome, 45, 45*f*
TDT. *See* Thermal damage time (TDT)
Telangiectasias, 18*f*, 20–22, 79–80, 80*f*
Telogen, 55
Terminal hair, 55
Thermage device, 108
Thermal collagen remodeling, in skin
    tightening, 105–106, 105*b*, 106*f*
Thermal damage time (TDT), 64–65
Thermal injury, 46
Thermal relaxation time (TRT), 64–65
Thulium, 140
Timolol, 17
Tissue destruction, types of, 4–5
Tissue interactions, laser-, 4, 5*f*
Titan device, 119
Tone Mode for NMES device, 168
Topical creams, 156, 156*b*
Topical retinoids, 62
  for cellulites, 156
Topical retinol, for cellulites, 156
TriActive device, 160*f*, 161–162, 162*f*
TRT. *See* Thermal relaxation time (TRT)
TruSculpt flex, 170–171
TruSculpt ID device, 161
Tweezing, 61

U
UAL. *See* Ultrasound-assisted
    liposuction (UAL)
Ulceration, 61–63
Ulthera system, 121
Ultrashape System, 161
Ultrasound-assisted liposuction (UAL),
    161
Ultrasound devices
  for nonsurgical body contouring,
    161
  in skin tightening, 120–122, 121*f*,
    122*f*, 123*f*
Unrealistic patient expectations, in
    radiofrequency microneedling,
    188

US FDA-approved procedures
  in photodynamic therapy, 130
    Ameluz and BF-RhodoLED,
      130–131
    Ameluz/Metvixia and daylight, 131
    Levulan Kerastick and Blu-U, 130

V
Vacuum-assisted bipolar
    radiofrequency devices, in skin
    tightening, 117, 117*b*
Vascular lasers, in laser and light
    treatment, 196, 196*b*, 197*f*
Vascular lesions
  classification, 12–13
  treatment of
    adverse effects of, 23
    approach to, 22–23
    complications of, 23
    laser, 11–24, 23*b*
Vascular malformations, application of
    PDT, 134
VelaSmooth and VelaShape devices,
    159, 159*f*, 160*f*, 162
Vellus, 55
Venous lakes, 20
Venous malformations, 19–20, 20*f*
Visible light phototherapy
  for acne, 210–213
    blue light alone, 210–211, 215*f*
    intense pulsed light, 212–213
    red and blue light, 211–212
    red light alone, 211
von Tappeiner, Hermann, 127

W
Wavelength, 63–64, 63*b*, 64*b*
Waxing, 61

X
Xerosis, due to nonablative fractional
    photothermolysis, 100

Y
Yellow tattoos, 43, 43*f*
Yttrium-scandium-gallium-garnet
    (YSGG) full field laser, 142